Principles of Healthcare Reimbursement and Revenue Cycle Management

Principles of Healthcare Reimbursement and Revenue Cycle Management

Eighth Edition

Anne B. Casto, RHIA, CCS and Susan White, PhD, RHIA, CHDA

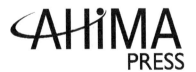

AHIMA PRESS

ISBN: 978-1-58426-915-1
eISBN: 978-1-58426-916-8
AHIMA Product No.: AB202022

AHIMA Staff:
Sarah Cybulski, MA, Assistant Editor
Jessica Ervin, MA, Senior Production Development Editor
Megan Grennan, Director, Content Production and AHIMA Press
James Pinnick, Vice President, Content and Learning Solutions
Christine Scheid, Content Development Manager
Rachel Schratz, MA, Associate Digital Content Developer

Cover image: © bestbrk, iStock

The websites listed in this book were current and valid as of the date of publication. However, webpage addresses and the information on them may change at any time. Users are encouraged to perform their own general web searches to locate any site addresses listed here that are no longer valid.

For more information, including updates, about AHIMA Press publications, visit **https://www.ahima.org/education-events/education-by-product/books/**.

American Health Information Management Association
233 North Michigan Avenue, 21st Floor
Chicago, Illinois 60601-5809
ahima.org

Contents

Detailed Contents

About the Authors

Anne B. Casto, RHIA, CCS, was the 2007 recipient of the Legacy Award, which honors significant contributions to the knowledge base in the field of health information management (HIM) through an insightful recent publication, building on the enduring tradition of the Edna K. Huffman Literary Award. Ms. Casto is president of Casto Consulting, LLC. She provides services to hospitals and other healthcare stakeholders primarily in the areas of reimbursement and coding. Additionally, Ms. Casto is associated faculty in the HIMS division at the Ohio State University School of Health and Rehabilitative Sciences. Ms. Casto teaches healthcare reimbursement and healthcare data trending and analysis. Ms. Casto is the consulting editor for the AHIMA-published *ICD-10-CM Code Book*, *ICD-10-PCS Code Book*, and *ICD-10-PCS Code Book, Professional Edition*.

Ms. Casto received her degree in health information management from the Ohio State University in 1995. She received her certified coding specialist credential in 1998 from the American Health Information Management Association (AHIMA). In 2009, Ms. Casto received the ICD-10-CM/PCS trainer certificate from AHIMA. For her commitment, creativity, and leadership to the HIM profession, Ms. Casto was honored with the 2008 OHIMA Distinguished Member Award and the 2011 Professional Achievement Award.

Susan White, PhD, RHIA, CHDA, was the 2014 recipient of the Literary Legacy Award for her text *A Practical Approach to Analyzing Healthcare Data*. Dr. White is the chief analytics officer (CAO) at the Ohio State University Wexner Medical Center. As the CAO, she has responsibility for the enterprise analytics function for the Ohio State University health system. Dr. White served on AHIMA's National Board of Directors from 2015 to 2018.

Dr. White is the author of AHIMA's *A Practical Approach to Analyzing Healthcare Data*, *Principles of Finance for Health Information and Informatics Professionals*, *Certified Health Data Analytics Exam Preparation*, *Calculating and Reporting Healthcare Statistics*, Sixth Edition, as well as numerous peer- and editor-reviewed articles.

Dr. White is a regular presenter at the state and national level on healthcare data analytics, alternative payment models, and big data. She earned her PhD in statistics from the Ohio State University. In 2016, Dr. White was honored with the Ohio Health Information Management Association (OHIMA) Professional Achievement Award and the Distinguished Member Award.

Preface

Health information management (HIM) professionals play a crucial role in the delivery of healthcare services in the US. However, to be fully effective in their roles, HIM professionals need an in-depth understanding of healthcare reimbursement systems, reimbursement methodologies, and payment processes throughout the healthcare industry.

Principles of Healthcare Reimbursement and Revenue Cycle Management makes complex topics understandable for students and professionals by clarifying the US healthcare reimbursement maze. This text integrates information about US healthcare reimbursement methodologies and processes into one authoritative source. It examines the complex financial systems within today's healthcare environment and provides an understanding of the basics of health insurance and public funding programs, managed care concepts, and how services are paid. Step-by-step details about how claims are processed, managed, and paid are provided. This gives the reader an appreciation for the complexity of the healthcare reimbursement process and an understanding of the profound effect reimbursement methodologies and policies have had on healthcare professionals and payers, consumers, public-sector policymakers, and the development of classification and information technology systems over the years.

Healthcare leaders and administrators often receive on-the-job and on-the-fly training when learning about healthcare reimbursement. While other texts feature healthcare finance and healthcare economics, they do not offer the bottom line and nitty-gritty of the healthcare payment systems themselves. This text fills the gap. This textbook can be used in the classroom for students enrolled in RHIA and RHIT programs, as well as students studying health sciences or earning the master of health administration degree. Additionally, health information professionals moving into or working in the revenue cycle arena can use this textbook to enhance their reimbursement and revenue cycle knowledge.

Part I: Foundations of Healthcare Reimbursement

A systematic approach makes the complexity of healthcare reimbursement and the revenue cycle manageable. Chapters 1 through 3 of this text discuss the structure of healthcare delivery and health insurance in the US. Next, the text dives into the complex workings of healthcare insurance. Lastly, part I ends with a discussion of the government-sponsored healthcare systems. Terms, abbreviations, and acronyms are clearly defined.

Chapter 1, "Healthcare Reimbursement and Revenue Cycle Management," introduces and explains the basic concepts and principles of healthcare reimbursement in simplified, step-by-step terms. This introduction gives the reader a solid foundation to understand the more detailed and complex discussions that follow in later chapters.

Chapter 2, "Health Insurance," explains the concepts of health insurance plans and gives you a detailed understanding of the sections of a healthcare insurance policy. Principles of managed care and the numerous types of plans that have emerged through the integration of administrative, financial, and clinical systems to both deliver and finance healthcare services are explored.

Chapter 3, "Government-Sponsored Healthcare Programs," differentiates among the various government-sponsored healthcare programs in effect today, explains their effect on the American healthcare system, and presents the history of Medicare and Medicaid programs in the US.

Part II: Reimbursement Methodologies and Payment Systems

Part II begins with providing foundational knowledge about healthcare reimbursement methodologies. The text then moves through four Medicare payment systems. The first three payment systems are designed to fit their healthcare setting (acute inpatient, skilled nursing facility, and hospital outpatient settings). The last payment system is for physicians and clinicians and spans all healthcare settings.

Chapter 4, "Healthcare Reimbursement Methodologies," differentiates among the most prevalent reimbursement methodologies in use today. The advanced concept of risk adjustment is discussed and explored through Centers for Medicare and Medicaid Services (CMS) programs.

Chapter 5, "Medicare Hospital Acute Inpatient Services Payment System," explains the model and policies of payment and defines basic language associated with reimbursement for Medicare admissions in the acute inpatient hospital setting.

Chapter 6, "Medicare Skilled Nursing Facility Services Payment System," explains the model and policies of payment for Medicare admissions and defines basic language associated with reimbursement in the skilled nursing facility setting.

Chapter 7, "Medicare Hospital Outpatient Payment System," describes the federal payment system for the outpatient hospital setting. The chapter explores the model and policies of payment and defines the basic language associated with reimbursement for Medicare admissions in the outpatient hospital setting.

Chapter 8, "Medicare Physician and Other Health Professional Payment System," explains the model and policies of payment for physicians and other health professionals, such as nurse practitioners and physical therapists. The chapter defines basic language associated with reimbursement for Medicare encounters.

Part III: Revenue Cycle Processes

Part III of this text dives into the revenue cycle processes. Each segment of the revenue cycle is discussed in detail, providing information about the tasks performed in order for a facility or practice to produce a claim for payment. By discussing the revenue cycle process after healthcare reimbursement systems, the reader is able to insert their knowledge about payment systems into the tasks and functions discussed.

Chapter 9, "Revenue Cycle Front-End Processes—Patient Engagement," explains the beginning components of the revenue cycle, which begins when the patient schedules services.

Chapter 10, "Revenue Cycle Middle Processes—Resource Tracking," provides a detailed discussion of how hospitals and physician offices track resources used to treat patients. The chapter presents baseline information about today's approved code sets and their functionality and application in the revenue cycle.

Chapter 11, "Revenue Cycle Back-End Processes—Claims Production and Revenue Collection," explores the final processes of the revenue cycle and describes in detail how claims are created, managed, and paid. This chapter defines basic language associated with claims processes and reconciliation.

Part IV: Revenue Cycle Management

Once the reader has the foundational and detailed knowledge about reimbursement systems and revenue cycle, the next topics pertain to the management of capturing data for claims and the compliance of obtaining accurate healthcare reimbursement. The functions surrounding data capture for claims production are highly regulated; therefore, sound management and compliance practices are necessary to stay in alignment with revenue integrity.

Chapter 12, "Coding and Clinical Documentation Integrity Management," explains management concepts for coding and clinical documentation integrity. These areas directly impact healthcare reimbursement and are highly regulated by federal and state laws. Therefore, sound management practices are key for success.

Chapter 13, "Revenue Compliance," explores the oversight, guidance, and management of health data used in the reimbursement process. This chapter explores compliance from both the payer and the provider perspective.

Part V: Revenue Cycle Analysis

Part V takes information from all previous sections and incorporates it into real-world examples. This allows the student to see how the pieces all fit together. Each case study is a real analysis that healthcare data analysts perform on a day-to-day basis.

Chapter 14, "Healthcare Data in Action: Real-World Analysis," uses case studies to explore common areas for analysis. The case studies allow students to see the analytics process in action and how insights can be derived from healthcare data.

Features

Throughout the chapters, key terms appear in **bold** type with a definition. An abbreviation list is provided in appendix A at the back of the textbook for students to use as a "cheat sheet" due to the high volume of acronyms and initialisms used in healthcare. A complete glossary of the healthcare reimbursement terminology used throughout the text is provided in appendix B. A detailed content index is also provided at the end of the textbook. Throughout the chapters, Check Your Understanding (CYU) question sets provide an opportunity for students and readers to self-assess their comprehension of the material presented. Appendix C provides the answers for the CYU questions.

At the end of each chapter, a Patient Connection storyline is provided. Chapter 1 introduces the main storyline characters that are followed throughout the textbook. The Patient Connection scenarios are real-world examples that show how content from the textbook is applied in the various US healthcare settings and processes.

Each chapter culminates in a review quiz to help instructors assess students' comprehension of the material presented. Instructors may use these questions as homework or as part of weekly quizzes to assess their students' grasp of concepts covered in the chapter.

Acknowledgments

AHIMA Press would like to thank **Heather Merkley, RHIA**, for her technical review of this textbook.

The authors would like to thank Sierra Welch, Calvin Herpolsheimer, and Kristina Swank for providing sample student work for the instructor materials that accompany this text.

Online Resources

For Students

A student workbook, which reinforces the topics and learning objectives from each chapter, is available online to accompany this textbook. Visit the AHIMA Learning Center at https://my.ahima.org/learningcenter and register your unique student access code that is provided behind the front cover of this text to download the files.

Medicare payment system content is provided in online chapter 15, "Other Medicare Prospective Payment Systems." This chapter covers the Medicare inpatient psychiatric facility prospective payment system, the Medicare inpatient rehabilitation facility prospective payment system, and the Medicare home health prospective payment system. Appendix G provides an overview of basic statistics to support understanding of these concepts throughout the text.

For Instructors

AHIMA provides supplementary resources to educators who use this text in their courses. In addition to the student workbook listed above, the instructor resources include the following:

- Instructor's manual. Each chapter of the instructor's manual includes lesson plans, application and data analysis exercises, discussion questions, review quizzes with answer key, and a test bank with answer key.

- Microsoft PowerPoint presentations. Provided to enhanced course lectures. These slide presentations cover the key topics presented in each chapter.

- Check Your Understanding. Each chapter of the text includes discussion questions on the chapter topics to help students recall and focus on the important points within each chapter. Answers to all Check Your Understanding questions are provided at the end of the text in appendix C.

- Course curriculum map. Each chapter of the text is mapped to the appropriate AHIMA HIM Curricula Competencies.

Instructor materials for this book are provided only to approved educators. Please visit https://www.ahima.org/education-events/education-by-product/books/ for further instruction. If you have any questions regarding the instructor materials, please contact AHIMA Customer Relations at (800) 335-5535, or submit a customer support request at https://my.ahima.org/messages.

Part I:
Foundations
of Healthcare
Reimbursement

Chapter 1
Healthcare Reimbursement and Revenue Cycle Management

Learning Objectives

- Distinguish between the social insurance, national health service, and private health insurance healthcare delivery models

- Describe the US healthcare business model

- Define health insurance

- Explain the connection between US health insurance and employment

- Define revenue integrity

- Identify the three main components of the revenue cycle

Key Terms

Beneficiary
Guarantor
Insurance
Integrated revenue cycle (IRC)
National health service (Beveridge) model
Policyholder
Premium
Private health insurance model
Reimbursement

Revenue cycle
Revenue cycle management (RCM)
Revenue integrity
Risk pool
Single-payer health system
Social insurance (Bismarck) model
Third-party payer
Universal healthcare coverage

Healthcare professionals who understand US healthcare reimbursement systems can assist their patients, their organizations, and the public with navigating the business side of healthcare encounters. This book is a guide to healthcare reimbursement and revenue cycle management (RCM). **Reimbursement** is the amount paid to a healthcare provider for services provided to a patient. **Revenue cycle** is the regular set of tasks and activities that produces reimbursement (revenue). **Revenue cycle management (RCM)** is the supervision of all administrative and clinical functions that contribute to the capture, management, and collection of patient service reimbursement. In this chapter and the chapters that follow, readers will learn about healthcare delivery systems, health insurance, government-sponsored healthcare programs, healthcare reimbursement methodologies, revenue cycle processes, RCM, revenue compliance, and revenue cycle analysis. **Insurance**, in general, is a system of reducing a person's exposure to risk of loss by having another party, an insurance company, assume the risk. Healthcare professionals must understand health insurance and the revenue cycle in the US healthcare sector because of their potential fiscal impact on people's lives.

In this chapter we discuss the national models of healthcare delivery. These models have been used to develop healthcare delivery systems throughout the world. Next, the healthcare delivery system in the US is explored. This section is an introductory view of health insurance in the US. The last section of this chapter explores the basic concepts surrounding RCM and revenue cycle integrity.

National Models of Healthcare Delivery

Three national models for delivering healthcare services exist: social insurance, national health service, and private health insurance (Kulesher and Forrestal 2014, 127). These models can be seen in various permutations in countries around the world. The models vary by sources of funding, number and types of payers involved, and levels of healthcare services. Here are descriptions of the three national models:

- **Social insurance model**, or the **Bismarck model**. Introduced in 1883 by German Chancellor Otto von Bismarck, this model is the oldest in the world. The foundation of this model is **universal healthcare coverage** for a set of benefits defined by the national government. Universal healthcare coverage is the minimum level of healthcare insurance defined by the government, which may include coverage for preventative and primary care, hospitalization, mental health benefits, and prescription drugs. In this model, every worker and employer must contribute to sickness funds, agencies that collect and redistribute money per government regulations; they are a form of social security. The amounts of the contributions are proportionate to workers' and employers' incomes. Workers can choose among competing sickness funds. With varying modifications, France, Japan, the Netherlands, and many other countries have adopted this German model. (Frogner et al. 2011, 72)

- **National health service model**, or the **Beveridge model**. In 1946, Sir William Beveridge created the national health service model for the United Kingdom (UK). In the UK, the government owns the clinics and hospitals and pays the doctors and healthcare professionals who work in these public facilities. This government-run model is a **single-payer health system**—the UK government is the only payer. In this type of system, one entity acts as an administrator of a single insurance pool. The entity collects all health fees (taxes or contributions) and pays all health costs for an entire population. The single entity can be an agency of the government or a government-run organization. In the UK, the healthcare system is financed by the country's general revenues. The general revenues come from taxes that increase in proportion to income (progressive tax). With varying modifications, Spain and the Scandinavian countries have adopted this model. (Frogner et al. 2011, 72)

- **Private health insurance model**. In this model, many private health insurance companies exist. The private health insurance companies collect premiums to create a pool of money. This pool of money is used to pay health claims. Much as with the Bismarck model, workers and employers contribute to the pool. Unlike the Bismarck system, the insurance company determines the contribution, and this contribution is not based on the employee's income. The US and Switzerland use the private health insurance model. In Switzerland, governmental regulation of health insurance is more extensive than in the US. (Frogner et al. 2011, 73)

No country's system is a pure version of these models (Kulesher and Forrestal 2014, 127). For example, a hybrid of the Bismarck and Beveridge models exists. This hybrid is used in Canada, South Korea, and other countries. Generally, however, one model dominates each country's system.

Each model has positive and negative attributes depending on the role of the observer: patient, provider, or administrator. Cram et al. (2017) discuss the pros and cons of the Canadian healthcare system. The Canadian system is primarily a national health service model. From the patient's perspective, the cons of the Canadian system are higher taxes and longer wait times for nonemergent procedures. Some of the pros include a more equitable healthcare system and no out-of-pocket treatment costs for patients (Cram et al. 2017). Although insured patients are generally able to access nonemergent care more quickly in the US system, high out-of-pocket costs and lack of insurance are barriers to care. In the Canadian system, there is little administrative burden on the physician and hospital, but the primary care physician must prioritize which patients receive high-cost tests and treatments. Chapter 4 in this text will present much of the detail around the administrative burden within the US healthcare system.

Healthcare Delivery in the US

The US healthcare sector represents a significant portion of the US economy. In 2021, the US healthcare sector accounted for $4.2 trillion, or 18.3 percent, of the nation's gross domestic product (GDP). The GDP is the value of all goods and services made within a country. National healthcare spending continues to grow each year, and it grew at a rate of 10.3 percent from 2019 to 2020 (CMS 2022) due to the COVID-19 pandemic. Growth slowed to 2.7 percent from 2020 to 2021. The trend of increased spending on healthcare has been consistent for more than a decade. Figure 1.1 demonstrates that the actual expenditures continue to increase each year. Figure 1.2, however, demonstrates that the percent increase is on a downward trend if the outlier COVID-19 year is excluded.

Figure 1.1.   Annual US national healthcare expenditures

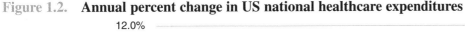

Source: Adapted from CMS 2022, Table 1.

Figure 1.2.   Annual percent change in US national healthcare expenditures

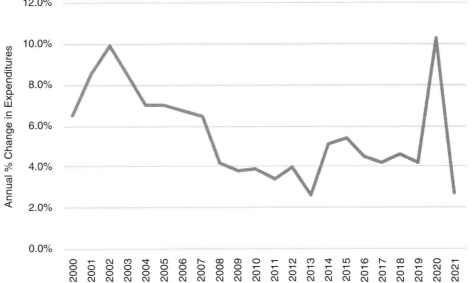

Source: Adapted from CMS 2022, Table 1.

In addition to being large, the US healthcare system is complex. Facilities and physicians typically treat patients with various types of health insurance, including commercial insurance and government-based insurance. Chapter 2, "Health Insurance," and chapter 3, "Government-Sponsored Healthcare Programs," discuss the structure of insurance in more detail. The contract between a health insurance company and facility can include a wide variety of plans, with each plan designating which reimbursement methodologies will be employed for each service. The result is the facility or physician practice managing multiple plans within its revenue cycle. Moreover, the payment rates and terms of these contracts between providers and insurance plans can be revised, updated, or renewed on different timetables, such as midyear, annually, or after multiple years. The management of the numerous insurance plans is required to ensure the financial viability of the provider and requires a significant amount of administrative burden.

Figure 1.3 depicts the relationships among the patient, the employer, the third-party payer, and the provider. The **third-party payer** is an insurance company or health agency that pays the physician, clinic, or other provider for the care or services rendered to the patient. There are transactions and communication among all four parties. Relationship (1) represents transactions between the consumer or patient and the provider. Healthcare services are provided to the patient. The patient contacts the provider to arrange services and is responsible for payment if the patient does not have insurance coverage for the service. If the patient does have coverage, then the patient pays any cost-sharing amount that may be required under the third-party payer coverage parameters. Relationship (2) represents transactions between the provider and the third-party payer. The provider submits an invoice to the third-party payer for services the patient received. The third-party payer submits payment on behalf of the patient based on any contractual relationship it may have with the provider. Relationship (3) represents the transactions between the third-party payer and the patient's employer. If the patient's healthcare coverage is a benefit of employment, then the employer may pay all or a portion of the premium to the third-party payer on behalf of the patient. The **premium** is the amount of money that a policyholder or beneficiary must periodically pay an insurance company in return for healthcare coverage. If the patient pays the third party directly, then the transactions are directly between the patient and the third-party payer; relationship (5) is a better representation of those transactions. Relationship (4) represents the transactions between the patient and the patient's employer. If the patient is responsible for a portion of the premium paid to the third-party payer, then that sum is collected via payroll processing. Another healthcare-related transaction between the patient and the patient's employer may be the selection of a plan. Many larger employers provide a menu of health plans with varying benefits and premium levels that employees may

Figure 1.3.   US healthcare business model

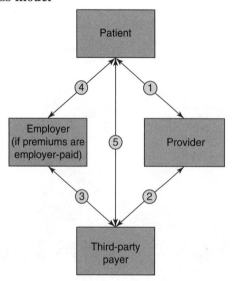

Source: White 2018.

choose from. Relationship (5) represents the issue of any precertifications that may be required by the patient's health plan prior to service as well as direct payments between the patient and the payer.

Compare this model to the traditional business-to-consumer model used in retail stores. In that model, the goods and services are received by the consumer and payment is remitted by the consumer. An example of a business model for a grocery store is depicted in figure 1.4. The incentives in the traditional model are aligned such that the consumer can withhold payment or shop elsewhere if the product is not of sufficient quality or available immediately. The provider (retailer) is free to sell the product to the consumer without approval from a third party. Compare this simple model to the one displayed in figure 1.3. Understanding the various relationships and parties that are involved in the delivery of healthcare in the US provides a valuable context for the study of healthcare finance issues.

Health Insurance

Traditionally, some portion of the payment for healthcare services is covered via health insurance. In healthcare, the risk that the health insurance company assumes is the unknown cost of healthcare for a person or group of persons.

However, the insurance company that assumes the risk reduces its exposure by distributing the risk among a larger group of persons called *insureds*. This group of individual entities, such as individuals, employers, or associations, whose healthcare costs are combined for evaluating financial history and estimating future costs is known as a **risk pool** (American Academy of Actuaries n.d.). In healthcare, the variability of health statuses across many people allows the health insurance company to make a better estimate of the average costs of healthcare. For example, a health insurance company that includes Medicare-aged people in its risk pool would likely have more expenses than one that includes only healthy people in the age group of 20 to 29. The mix of demographics such as age, gender, and disease status are all assessed when determining the amount of risk or expected health expenditures for a risk pool.

The insurance company receives a premium in return for assuming the insureds' exposure to risk of loss or expense in this case. A **policyholder** is an individual or entity that purchases health insurance coverage. A **beneficiary** is an individual who is eligible for benefits from a health plan. Both of these terms are used throughout this text. The premium payments for all the beneficiaries in the group are combined in a pool of money. Insurance companies use data about the historical healthcare expenses of beneficiaries to calculate the premiums so that the pool of money is sufficiently large enough to pay losses of the entire group. Thus, the risk is the potential that a person will get sick or require health services and will incur costs associated with treatment or services.

The concepts of risk pools and premiums are not limited to health insurance. Consider auto insurance as an example. In general, the cost of insuring young men is higher than insuring old women. The insurance company accounts for the varying risk in the pool by charging higher or lower rates to consumers based on their risk of having an accident. Health insurance companies have a similar practice, but they can spread the risk across a larger

Figure 1.4.   Grocery store business model

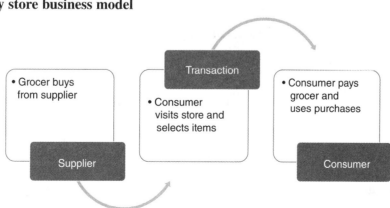

risk pool when setting rates for larger groups of insureds. In the auto insurance example, the risk is only spread across a particular driver or perhaps a family of drivers. The larger risk pool allows a health insurance company to determine a common rate for the entire risk pool.

Historical Perspectives

Health insurance in the US has been made available to help offset the expenses of the treatment of illness and injury. The first "sickness" clause was inserted in an insurance document in 1847. From then until the 1920s, the major cost associated with illness was not medical care; instead, it was the loss of wages (Thomasson 2002). Therefore, households bought into sickness funds that were like disability insurance that is offered today, and burial insurance offered by commercial insurance companies. Because Americans did not feel health insurance was necessary and instead purchased sickness funds, there was little backing for the development of compulsory, nationalized health insurance (Thomasson 2002). While many European countries had adopted forms of nationalized health insurance by 1920, proposals initiated in the US failed (Thomasson 2002). Legislation introduced in the US was opposed by physicians, pharmaceutical firms, and insurance companies.

However, health insurance was first utilized in 1929, when Blue Cross Blue Shield first covered schoolteachers in Texas. In the 1940s, during World War II, the executive and judicial branches of government issued a series of acts to address a labor shortage (Thomasson 2002). These acts became the basic structure of health insurance in the US. Moreover, these acts resulted in today's linkage of health insurance and employment. Thus, as an industry, health insurance became widespread in the US after World War II (Longest and Darr 2014, 42).

Understanding today's healthcare reimbursement environment requires examining the link between health insurance and employment, compensation for healthcare services, and the use of third-party payers.

Health Insurance and Employment

In the US, health insurance is most often provided through employers. Many larger employers, as part of a package of employment benefits, pay a portion of the health insurance premium. Medicare is also considered insurance because payroll taxes, through both employers' and employees' contributions, finance one portion of Medicare coverage. Premiums paid by eligible individuals and matched by the federal government also finance Medicare's supplemental medical insurance program.

When people lose their jobs, they often lose their health insurance. Although people can continue their health insurance by paying for it entirely by themselves, the payments are expensive. In certain circumstances, under the Consolidated Omnibus Budget Reconciliation Act of 1985 (COBRA), people can extend their health insurance for a limited period. Alternatively, under the Affordable Care Act of 2010 (ACA), they may enroll in federal marketplace health insurance.

For some employed people, adequate health insurance is an issue. Some health insurance plans require patients or their families to pay 20 percent or more of their healthcare costs. Healthcare costs can easily be in the thousands of dollars; 20 percent of $10,000 is $2,000, which is a sizable sum for many people. The median savings account value for Americans under 35 was $3,240 in 2022 (Wolfson 2022). The median value was higher for those aged 55 to 64 at $6,400. Other employees work for employers that do not offer health benefits. These individuals must purchase insurance on their own at an extremely high rate. Therefore, being able to afford adequate health insurance is a challenge for many US workers.

Third-Party Payer

Experts in healthcare finance frequently use the term *third-party payer*. Recall that a third-party payer is an insurance company or health agency that pays the physician, clinic, or other healthcare provider for the care or services provided to the patient. Discussions of the third-party payer can be confusing because often there is no mention of first parties and second parties. A party is an entity that receives, renders, or pays for health services. As shown in figure 1.5, the first party is the patient or the **guarantor**, such as a parent, responsible for the patient's health costs. Patients who are adults are often their own guarantor. Parents are the guarantor for their minor children because they guarantee payments for their children's healthcare costs.

Figure 1.5.   **Third-party payment**

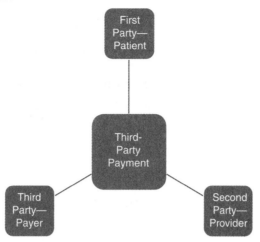

The second party is the provider, so called because they provide healthcare. The provider may be a physician, clinic, hospital, nursing home, or other healthcare entity rendering the care. The third party is the payer that provides reimbursement to the second party for healthcare provided to the first party. Often, third-party payers are referred to simply as *payers*. The payer does not provide care to the patient. Examples of payers are health insurance companies, workers' compensation, and Medicare. The terms *payer* and *third-party payer* are used interchangeably throughout this text.

Check Your Understanding 1.1

1. Which components of the Bismarck and Beveridge models does the US's private health insurance model incorporate?

2. Where and when did health insurance become established in the US?

3. What do insurance companies receive in return for assuming the insureds' exposure to risk or loss?

4. Who is the third party in healthcare situations?

   a. Patient
   b. Provider
   c. Payer

5. Insurance companies pool premium payments for all the insureds in a group. Then, they use actuarial data to calculate the group's premiums so that _____.

   a. Premium payments are lowered for insurance plan payers
   b. The pool is large enough to pay losses of the entire group
   c. Accounting for the group's plan is simplified

Revenue Cycle Management

In the US, complex payment systems have been implemented in virtually every healthcare service area. Healthcare delivery leaders understand the importance of decreasing payment delays and revenue loss through RCM. Throughout this text, a revenue cycle typical of an inpatient acute-care setting is used as an illustrative example. Though many components are similar across various healthcare settings, there may be differences in revenue cycle flow and management depending on the institution size, approach to charge capture, and availability of coding professionals.

Successful RCM programs in healthcare facilities are based on a multidisciplinary model. This approach promotes collaboration among various clinical departments by creating an RCM team composed of representatives from numerous departments in the healthcare organization. An emphasis on education encourages all team members to stay up to date on changing market forces such as payer trends, government and regulatory modifications, and organization strategy. Because each member of the team better understands other members' contributions and their importance to the revenue cycle, this modern management approach encourages the entire team to take a proactive stance regarding reimbursement issues.

Revenue Integrity

Healthcare organizations want to be reimbursed the correct amount for the services provided to patients. Thus, the concept of revenue integrity has been embraced. **Revenue integrity** is performing revenue cycle duties to obtain operational efficiency, compliance adherence, and legitimate reimbursement. Integrity is synonymous with being honest or conducting oneself with honor. Developing revenue integrity at a healthcare organization requires shared cultural attitudes and beliefs about honesty and doing what is right. In chapter 12, "Coding and Clinical Documentation Integrity Management," the text explores ethical guidelines that contribute to revenue integrity, such as the AHIMA Standards of Ethical Coding and AHIMA Ethical Standards for Clinical Documentation Improvement Professionals. Additionally, in chapter 13, "Revenue Compliance," revenue cycle compliance guidance will be discussed in detail. Oversight and guidance will be explored as well because compliant management practices are essential to ensure revenue integrity.

A key factor in establishing highly ethical behavior is a commitment to transparency. Transparency, in a business context, is honesty and openness. Openness ties directly to good communication. Stakeholders from all parts of the organization must be willing to communicate with each other and share processes and business knowledge.

The concept of "doing the right thing" is not new in the healthcare revenue cycle, but what sets revenue integrity apart is the proactive analysis and optimization of all processes within the revenue cycle. For example, organizations are shifting focus away from retrospective audits (audits done after reimbursement is received) to charge management, where monitoring and auditing activities take place while the claim is generated and up until the claim is submitted to the payer. The goal is to produce a claim that is the following:

- Clean: free of errors
- Complete: all services and supplies reflected
- Compliant: adhering to contract requirements, regulations, and laws

A claim that is clean, complete, and compliant meets the goals of revenue integrity.

Integrated Revenue Cycle

When physician practices are integrated into the revenue cycle and business practices of healthcare systems, close attention must be given to some of the nuances of the physician practice structure that can affect RCM, such as the following:

- Organization structure
- Payment methodology
- Payer classifications
- Electronic health record systems
- Metrics and monitoring systems

- Denial management

- Point-of-service patient collection opportunities

Probably the most significant difference between facility-based (hospital) and physician-based revenue cycles is the payment systems (Sorrentino and Sanderson 2011, 89). Most facility-based payment systems utilize a case-rate methodology that provides payment for each admission or encounter. Physician practices are reimbursed with a transaction-based payment system that focuses on each service rather than the encounter as a whole. Though facilities may be familiar with negotiating case rates with their payer population, physician practice contracts require more negotiation and a clear understanding of the types of services, or book of business, for the physician practice that has been acquired (Sorrentino and Sanderson 2011, 89). Incorporating the physician practice's existing expertise would provide significant benefits to healthcare organizations.

Many hospital systems are moving toward an **integrated revenue cycle (IRC)** approach. At the most basic level, an IRC coordinates revenue cycle activities under a single leadership and team structure (Colton and Davis 2015, 56). There are four areas of focus for integration. The first is a single governance structure. Second is the creation of centralized business units such as patient financial services. Third is to standardize processes. And fourth is to implement a uniform technology pattern (Bruno et al. n.d.). There are three primary benefits a system can experience from an IRC:

- Reduced cost to collect: Combine strategic and operational elements, including resources, management, overhead, vendors, IT platforms, and business intelligence.

- Performance consistency: Combine job codes and pay rates, clearly define roles and responsibilities, and strive for consistent production and quality rates through improved information sharing.

- Coordinated strategic goals: Develop a shared focus on strategic goals and promote improved coordination between financial and nonfinancial units. (Colton and Davis 2015, 57)

It will take time for a health system to move to an IRC. Not all systems move directly to a fully integrated revenue cycle. Key areas to integrate are customer engagement, business unit talent, process innovation, technology, and measurement and analytics (Bruno et al. n.d.). Some systems may face resistance from physician practices arising from a fear that low-dollar encounters will not receive the attention that high-dollar inpatient admissions receive. However, many systems will move to a form of IRC that fits the needs and environment of the individual system. For instance, a system may integrate customer engagement so that all patient-facing activities and tasks have the same look and feel. An example would be that all forms that patients sign have the same header and logos. Additionally, the system may have a centralized business unit for the medical coding function. This means physician encounters and facility admissions are all coded in the same coding department under the same coding manager. However, the system may not be under the same technology platform for all units. Physicians may continue to use the technology system they prefer rather than moving to the established facility information technology system. Therefore, this system is partially integrated.

Components of the Revenue Cycle

Each function in the revenue cycle is vital to creating efficient and compliant reimbursement processes. The basic components of the revenue cycle are similar at each facility or physician practice even though terminology used between facilities, practices, and healthcare systems varies. Size is one difference between the revenue cycles at facilities and physician practices. At a facility, numerous units and service areas, such as registration, laboratory, and coding, typically contribute to the revenue cycle. At a physician practice, one service area and one business office may complete most revenue cycle tasks and functions. Although each unit in a facility setting is responsible for its own functions and tasks, cooperation from outside departments and clinical areas is often crucial for the timely and accurate completion and submission of healthcare claims. Likewise, in a physician practice setting, each team member of the business office may be responsible for a set of tasks; however, all team members must work together to create a successful revenue cycle. The major components of the revenue cycle are displayed in figure 1.6. Notice in figure 1.6 that the revenue cycle is implemented as a linear process that spans from patient engagement to the final collection of payment for services.

Within each component of the revenue cycle are many tasks that must be completed so the provider may receive reimbursement for services provided to patients. The front-end processes, or patient engagement, include activities that occur prior to the patient receiving treatment. An example is patient registration. This component of the revenue cycle is discussed in detail in chapter 9, "Revenue Cycle Front-End Processes—Patient Engagement." The next component of the revenue cycle is the middle processes, or resource tracking. These activities take place while the patient is receiving care and shortly after discharge. An example is recording the laboratory tests ordered and completed for the patient. The tasks associated with this component of the revenue cycle are discussed in detail in chapter 10, "Revenue Cycle Middle Processes—Resource Tracking." The last component of the revenue cycle is back-end processes, or claims production and revenue collection. These tasks take place after the patient is discharged and continue until reimbursement is received for the care provided to the patient. An example is determining expected reimbursement for an admission. The details for this component of the revenue cycle are discussed in chapter 11, "Revenue Cycle Back-End Processes—Claims Production and Revenue Collection."

Figures 1.7A and 1.7B highlight the major tasks included in the revenue cycle. Figure 1.7A details the revenue cycle from the patient perspective. Figure 1.7B displays the provider perspective. Most patients are not familiar with the business operations that are required of healthcare facilities and providers, and figure 1.7B provides insight into these functions.

The healthcare revenue cycle is a strictly managed and highly monitored process by both the facility or provider and the payer community. Hospitals and physician practices closely monitor revenue cycle processes to ensure that services provided by clinicians are documented and reported to payers to ensure revenue integrity. Likewise, payers scrutinize claims and audit medical records to ensure that the reimbursement provided to the facility or provider is medically necessary and appropriate. As discussed earlier, chapters 9 through 11 of this text explore the revenue cycle in depth. Each component will be defined, and the processes will be discussed in detail.

Figure 1.6.   Components of the revenue cycle

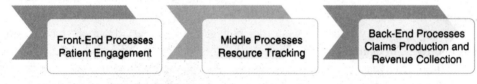

Figure 1.7A.   Detailed revenue cycle from patient perspective

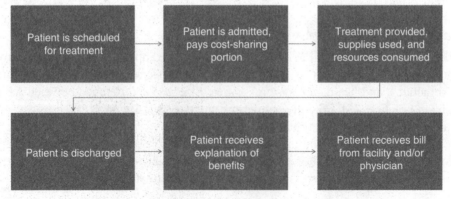

Figure 1.7B.   **Detailed revenue cycle from facility or provider perspective**

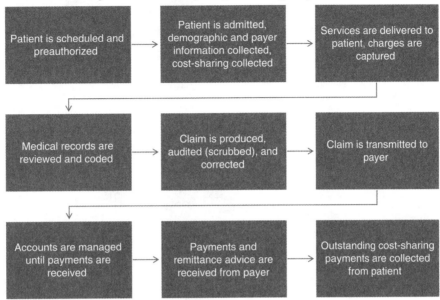

Patient Connection

At the end of each chapter, at least one topic from the chapter will be connected to example patients. In this chapter we introduce our patients. Our first patient is Malakai. Malakai is a 68-year-old male who is enrolled in Medicare. He is a retired high school math teacher who also spent 20 years coaching the boys' basketball team. Our second patient is Olivia. Olivia is a 30-year-old female who has commercial insurance for her family through her employer. The name of her insurance company is Super Payer. Olivia is a partner at a local law firm. Olivia is married, and she and her husband have one daughter, age six.

This chapter discusses the concept of third-party payment used in the US. Let's connect Malakai and Olivia to this concept. Malakai's primary care physician is Dr. Lewis. Using figure 1.5 as a model, let's apply a physician office visit for Malakai to the third-party payment concept.

(continued)

Patient Connection   *(continued)*

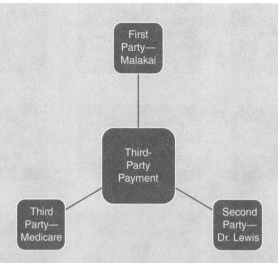

Here, Malakai is the first party. He is the patient and guarantor for his care. Malakai is responsible for cost-sharing amounts for the visit to Dr. Lewis. Dr. Lewis is the second party. He provided care to Malakai. Medicare is the third party. Medicare will reimburse Dr. Lewis for the care provided to Malakai because Malakai has enrolled in and received insurance coverage from Medicare.

Let's apply a physician office visit for Olivia's daughter to her pediatrician, Dr. King, to this concept.

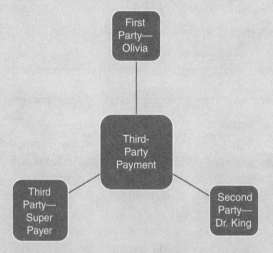

Here, Olivia and her daughter are combined as the first party. She is not the patient—rather, her daughter is the patient—but Olivia is the guarantor. Olivia is responsible for the cost-sharing amount for her daughter's visit to Dr. King. Dr. King is the second party. She provided care to Olivia's daughter. Super Payer is the third party. Olivia enrolled in and purchased healthcare coverage through her employer.

Chapter 1 Review Quiz

1. Which one of the three models of healthcare delivery is used in the US?

2. Compare the social insurance model and the national health service model. Describe their similarities and differences.

3. Describe the healthcare spending trend in the US over the past decade.

4. Provide two examples of transactions that occur between the provider and third-party payer.

5. Define *risk pool* as used in health insurance.

6. In the US, healthcare is most often connected to employment. Provide a downfall of this approach.

7. Dr. Gilbert sees a 14-year-old male with adolescent scoliosis. During today's visit, the patient was seen for mononucleosis and was started on prednisone for severe sore throat and difficulty swallowing. The patient was accompanied by his parents who have health insurance through the mother's employment at the State Department of Treasury. Who is the first party in this scenario?

8. What is a benefit of a multidisciplinary approach to RCM?

9. What are the goals of revenue integrity?

10. Describe how a healthcare organization benefits from an IRC.

References

American Academy of Actuaries. n.d. "Risk Pooling: How Health Insurance in the Individual Market Works." Accessed September 26, 2022. https://www.actuary.org/content/risk-pooling-how-health-insurance-individual -market-works-0.

Bruno, J., B. Snow, and J. Marra. n.d. "Revenue Cycle Integration." Accessed May 15, 2023. https://www2 .deloitte.com/us/en/pages/life-sciences-and-health-care/articles/revenue-cycle-integration-insights.html.

CMS (Centers for Medicare and Medicaid Services). 2022. "National Health Expenditure Data, Historical." https://www.cms.gov/research-statistics-data-and-systems/statistics-trends-and-reports/nationalhealthexpenddata /nationalhealthaccountshistorical.

Colton, B. and A. Davis. 2015. Integrating the revenue cycle for improved health system performance. *Healthcare Financial Management* 69(1):56–61.

Cram, P., I. Dhalla, and J. L. Kwan. 2017. Trade-offs: Pros and cons of being a doctor and patient in Canada. *Journal of General Internal Medicine* 32(5):563–565. https://link.springer.com/article/10.1007/s11606-016 -3874-0.

Frogner, B. K., H. R. Waters, and G. F. Anderson. 2011. "Comparative Health Systems." Chapter 4 in *Jonas and Kovner's Health Care Delivery in the United States*, 10th ed., edited by A. R. Kovner and J. R. Knickman. New York: Springer Publishing Company.

Kulesher, R. R. and E. Forrestal. 2014. International models of health systems financing. *Journal of Hospital Administration* 3(4):127–139.

Longest, B. B. and K. Darr. 2014. *Managing Health Services Organizations and Systems*, 6th ed. Baltimore: Health Professions Press.

Wolfson, A. 2022. "Here's Exactly How Much Americans Have in Savings at Every Age—And (Yikes) Here's What They Should Have. https://www.marketwatch.com/picks/heres-exactly-how-much-americans-have-in -savings-at-every-age-and-yikes-heres-what-they-should-have-01659384531.

Sorrentino, P. A. and B. Sanderson. 2011. Managing the physician revenue cycle. *Healthcare Financial Management* 65(12):88–94.

Thomasson, M. 2002. From sickness to health: The twentieth-century development of U.S. health insurance. *Explorations in Economic History* 39(3):233–253.

White, S. 2018. *Principles of Finance for Health Information and Informatics Professionals*, 2nd ed. Chicago: AHIMA.

Chapter 2
Health Insurance

Learning Objectives

❖ Discuss the major types of health insurance

❖ Differentiate individual healthcare insurance from employer-based healthcare insurance

❖ Explain the provisions of a health insurance policy

❖ Describe characteristics of managed care in terms of quality and cost-effectiveness

❖ Describe the common care management tools used in managed care

❖ Explain the cost controls used in managed care

❖ Describe the types of managed care organizations

Key Terms

Adverse selection
Appeal
Benefit
Benefit period
Certificate of insurance
Claim
Coinsurance
Community rating
Coordination of benefits (COB)
Copayment
Cost-sharing provisions
Covered condition
Covered service
Deductible
Dependent
Disease management
Eligibility
Employer-based health insurance
Enrollment
Evidence-based clinical practice guidelines
Exclusion
Family coverage
Formulary
Gatekeeper
Guaranteed issue

Health maintenance organization (HMO)
Individual health insurance
Limitation
Managed care
Maximum out of pocket
Medically necessary
Moral hazard
Open enrollment period
Other party liability (OPL)
Pharmacy benefit manager (PBM)
Point-of-service (POS) plan
Policy
Precertification
Preferred provider organization (PPO)
Primary care provider (PCP)
Primary insurer
Prior authorization
Prudent layperson standard
Qualifying life event (QLE)
Referral
Risk
Secondary insurer
Single coverage
Special enrollment period
Summary of benefits and coverage (SBC)

Supplemental insurance
Tier
Utilization management

Utilization review
Waiting period
Withhold amount

In chapter 1, "Healthcare Reimbursement and Revenue Cycle Management," insurance was defined as the reduction of a person's exposure to risk of loss by having another party assume the risk. This chapter discusses the numerous aspects of health insurance in the US. In the context of this text, **risk** is defined as the likelihood of an individual to incur a healthcare expense or the probability of the cost of healthcare exceeding the amount paid to the health insurance company for coverage.

There are three ways to obtain health insurance in the US: individual health insurance purchased from a health insurance agency, employer-based health insurance provided as part of an employment benefit package, and government-sponsored health insurance provided through a variety of programs. **Individual health insurance** is coverage that an individual or family purchases as opposed to coverage obtained through an employer. **Employer-based health insurance** is coverage that an individual or family obtains as part of an employment benefit package. Government-sponsored health insurance provides coverage when certain age, economic status, or other criteria set by the program are met. Chapter 3, "Government-Sponsored Healthcare Programs," will discuss the types of programs offered by the US government. This chapter focuses on aspects of health insurance regardless of whether it is individual, employer-based, or government-sponsored.

Types of Health Insurance

Health insurance companies sell healthcare plans to both individuals and groups of people. They allow people to purchase **single coverage**, healthcare coverage for the policyholder or employee only, or **family coverage**, which includes themselves and dependents. **Dependents** are spouses, children, and other family members. Family coverage costs more than single coverage because multiple individuals are covered under the plan.

The cost of health insurance is derived from the risk pool. Recall that a risk pool is a group of individual entities, such as individuals, employers, or associations, whose healthcare costs are combined for evaluating financial history and estimating future costs (American Academy of Actuaries n.d.). Larger risk pools or groups allow individuals with high expected healthcare costs to be combined with those with lower expected healthcare costs. Therefore, the cost of the higher-expense-generating individuals is spread across many lower-expense-generating individuals. This spreading of expenses or risk of expenses reduces the amount of expected expenses per person. Smaller pools do not provide a sufficiently wide range of diversity in terms of age, sex, and health status, so they are at risk for adverse selection. **Adverse selection** is the enrollment of an excessive proportion of persons with poor health status in a healthcare plan or healthcare organization. This results in disproportionate numbers of sick people in the risk pool. On the other hand, the diversity of the large-employer pools provides stable trends in utilization and fiscal impact. A key point is that the larger the pool, the more able it is to balance a wide variety of risks, or the probability of incurring loss from healthy individuals or individuals with chronic conditions or catastrophic illnesses. The risk is distributed across more entities.

Individual Healthcare Plans

Individuals and self-employed professionals purchase health insurance for themselves and their families. Thus, individual healthcare plans are so called because individuals purchase them. For some people, the individual healthcare plan is their only plan for self and family. Other people purchase individual healthcare plans to supplement their employer-based group insurance or their Medicare. The Affordable Care Act (ACA) established state and federal marketplaces that provide another option for individuals to purchase either single or family plans.

In general, individual health insurance plans provide **benefits** similar to employer-based group plans, but at a higher cost (see the next section). Benefits, also known as **covered services**, are healthcare services for which the insurance company will pay as outlined in the healthcare plan. Recall from chapter 1 that the individual or entity that purchases an insurance policy is known as a policyholder. A health insurance **policy** is a formal contract between the health insurance company and the individuals or groups for whom the company is assuming risk. Additional terms used for policyholder are as follows:

- Insured
- Beneficiary
- Certificate holder
- Member
- Subscriber

The terms *insured*, *policyholder*, and *beneficiary* are used interchangeably in this chapter and throughout the text.

Most policyholders of individual health insurance pay higher premiums to obtain and maintain health insurance. Premiums are the periodic payments that a policyholder must make to an insurance company in return for healthcare coverage. The level of deductibles and cost-sharing provisions may also be higher for the individual plans. A **deductible** is an annual amount of money that the policyholder must pay before the health insurance plan will assume its share of liability for the remaining charges or covered expenses. **Cost-sharing provisions** are policy points that require the beneficiary to pay for a portion of their healthcare services. Cost-sharing provisions are discussed in more detail later in this chapter.

Employer-Based Healthcare Plans

Employer-based healthcare plans are group plans for groups of employees. Often the employees enrolled in employer-based healthcare plans are referred to as members. Employer-based health insurance covers nearly 159 million people under 65 years of age in the US (KFF 2022). As the name implies, an employer-based healthcare plan is based on an individual's employment. However, occasionally, *employer-based healthcare plan* is a misnomer because this type of plan includes all plans that cover groups. Individuals may form groups through professional associations and other entities. An example is a state farm bureau. Individuals may join the state farm bureau and purchase health insurance through this larger group. Generally, though, employer-based health insurance is an employment benefit like vacation time or a retirement plan.

Employer-based healthcare plans typically have lower premiums, deductibles, and cost sharing, and greater benefits than individual healthcare plans. Moreover, the employer and employee may share the cost of the health insurance premium. Typically, the employer's share is larger than the employee's share; some employers may pay 100 percent of the premium for their employees. Thus, for beneficiaries, employer-based health insurance plans cost less than individual healthcare plans.

Analyses show that the number of employees who utilize group health insurance is declining slightly. In 1999, the percentage of workers covered by their employer's health plan was 66 percent. In 2022, just 54 percent of all employees were covered by health plans offered by their employer (KFF 2022). Although most employers offer health benefits, many workers are not eligible to enroll due to waiting periods or part-time work status. Some workers choose not to enroll because they feel the coverage costs too much or they may be covered through another source, like their spouse (KFF 2022).

Provisions and Functions of Health Insurance Plans

Health insurance companies assume the financial risk of the costs of individual and group healthcare. They assume this risk because individuals or groups purchase the insurance companies' healthcare plans. Health insurance companies issue policies to individuals or groups who purchase the healthcare plan.

The contract that describes the conditions of the insurance policy is called a **certificate of insurance**, also known as a certificate of coverage, evidence of coverage, or summary plan description.

The certificates of insurance stipulate all the covered conditions. **Covered conditions** are the health conditions, illnesses, injuries, diseases, or symptoms that the health insurance company will reimburse for treatment that attempts to maintain, control, or cure said conditions. In addition to covered conditions, the policy indicates healthcare services related to covered conditions and all other aspects of healthcare for which the healthcare plan will pay. Also, it is important to note, a certificate of insurance discloses what the policy does *not* cover, the maximum amount that will be paid for services, and the patient's responsibilities and obligations. Thus, certificates of insurance detail all procedures that patients must follow and all conditions that patients must meet to receive full benefits under their health insurance policies.

Per the ACA, health insurance companies must also provide a **summary of benefits and coverage (SBC)** to policyholders. The SBC is a document that, in plain language, concisely details information about a health insurance company's benefits and its coverage of health services. This information is presented in a simple, consistent, and uniform format across all insurance providers. The SBC's purpose is to give consumers improved information about their coverage. The SBC is only a summary; it does not replace the policy, the certificate of insurance, or other formal insurance document that governs the contractual provisions of the coverage.

Sections of a Health Insurance Policy

Health insurance policies, like all contracts, are divided into sections. Typically, these sections include definitions, eligibility and enrollment, benefits, limitations, exclusions, procedures, and appeals processes. The sections build upon one another, and one aspect of healthcare may be addressed in multiple sections. Because the sections interlock, reviewing multiple sections is often necessary to determine whether the health insurance company will cover and pay for a specific diagnostic procedure or treatment.

Definitions

Definitions are often in a dedicated section, but they may also be incorporated into the benefits section. Definitions are important because they can affect health insurance coverage and reimbursement. For example, Medicare defines **medically necessary** as "services or supplies that are proper and needed for the diagnosis or treatment of your medical condition; are provided for the diagnosis, direct care, and treatment of your medical condition; meet the standards of good medical practice in the local area; and aren't mainly for the convenience of you or your doctor" (CMS 2006). Most payers have a similar definition for medically necessary services. Terms often listed in definitions include the following:

- Accidental injury
- Medical emergency
- Medical necessity
- Prior authorization

Definitions sometimes are specific to the healthcare plan and may be more restrictive than those in everyday usage or dictionaries. For example, a dictionary definition of *emergency* is "situations or conditions requiring immediate intervention to avoid serious adverse results" (Online Medical Dictionary n.d.). The health insurance plan may define a medical emergency as a "life-threatening" event, a concept that is more extreme and less likely than one demanding immediate attention.

Differences in the definition of *medical emergency* led to legal disputes between health insurance companies and their policyholders. Health insurance companies denied coverage for services that their policyholders perceived as emergencies. For example, a man entered an emergency department for chest pain believing he was having an acute myocardial infarction (heart attack). After diagnostic tests were performed, the patient learned he had reflux esophagitis (heartburn). Sometimes, based on the principal diagnosis, health insurance companies retrospectively denied payment for this type of patient's emergency care. The patient believed they were having a heart attack when presenting to the emergency department. The conclusion of heartburn was derived only after a thorough examination in the emergency department. The patient is not a healthcare expert and could not self-diagnose. To address this situation, many states passed laws based on the **prudent layperson standard** (ACEP n.d.). In prudent layperson laws, a person possessing average knowledge about health and medicine would expect that a condition could jeopardize the patient's life or seriously impair future functioning. For example, in the Ohio Revised Code Section 3923.65, Coverage for emergency services, the following definition is provided:

> "Emergency medical condition" means a medical condition that manifests itself by such acute symptoms of sufficient severity, including severe pain, that a prudent layperson with average knowledge of health and medicine could reasonably expect the absence of immediate medication attention could result in any of the following: (a) placing the health of the individual or, with respect to a pregnant woman, the health of the woman or her unborn child, in serious jeopardy; (b) serious impairment to bodily functions; (c) serious dysfunction of any bodily organ or part." (Ohio Revised Code 2015)

This is an important standard because 90 percent of urgent and nonurgent symptoms overlap, and physicians do not know if emergency care is needed without evaluation and testing (ACEP n.d.). Further, the results of a recent poll conducted by the American College of Emergency Physicians showed that 47 percent of people are concerned that their insurance provider will refuse to cover their emergency department visit (ACEP 2021). The necessity for states' legal intervention highlights the importance of definitions for both health insurance companies and insureds.

Eligibility and Enrollment

The **eligibility** section of a health insurance policy specifies the individuals who are eligible to apply for the health insurance. The **enrollment** section specifies the procedures for obtaining health insurance.

Eligibility is a set of stipulations that qualify a person to apply for health insurance. For employer-based health insurance, these stipulations often involve the percentage of the appointment or position. A common provision is that individuals must be employed at least 50 percent of the time, or half-time (0.5 full-time equivalent). People who are eligible include the employees themselves and their dependents, if applicable. Eligible dependents include the following:

- Legally married spouses

- Children and young adults until they reach age 26. The definition of *children* includes natural children, legally adopted children, stepchildren, and children who are dependent during the waiting period before adoption. Effective September 23, 2010, per the ACA (Title I, Part A, Subpart II, Sec. 2714), children and young adults were eligible *regardless* of any, or a combination of any, of the following factors: financial dependency, residency with parent, student status, employment, and marital status. The regulation applies to all individual (private) and employer-based (group) health insurance plans created after the date of enactment of the ACA (March 23, 2010). For employer-based plans that were in existence before the date of enactment, young adults can qualify for dependent coverage only if they are ineligible for an employment-based health insurance plan.

- Dependents with disabilities. The age limit of 26 does not apply to dependents who are (1) incapable of self-sustaining employment due to a physically or mentally disabling injury, disease, or condition *and* (2) chiefly dependent on the policyholder for support and maintenance.

The ACA does *not* require the spouse of a dependent or the dependent of a dependent (grandchild) be eligible for coverage. Reimbursement analysts should carefully review the definition of *eligible dependent* in their own state. Some states extend coverage more broadly than the ACA; for example, New Jersey extends the dependent age to 30 (New Jersey State Health Benefits Program 2022, 1). The ACA does not supersede these states' expanded definitions of eligibility. The ACA does supersede states' narrower scopes of eligibility. In other words, states must include ACA-defined dependents at a minimum.

Under the **guaranteed issue** provision of the ACA, health insurance companies are required to accept every qualified individual who applies for healthcare coverage regardless of their health, age, sex, or other factors that might predict use of health services. However, some types of supplemental insurance coverage, such as short-term health insurance, do not have to follow guaranteed issue. Group healthcare plans may require a general **waiting period**. Waiting periods do not apply to individual health insurance plans. A waiting period is "the time period between when a patient signs up with an insurance company and when the coverage starts" (CMS 2006). The waiting period cannot exceed 90 days, and all calendar days are counted, including weekends and holidays.

Enrollment is the initial process by which new individuals apply for and are accepted as members of health insurance plans. Medicare uses the term *election* for enrollment. During enrollment periods, members specify whether the coverage will be single coverage or nonsingle coverage, which includes employee-plus-one coverage and family coverage.

Open enrollment periods are specific periods when applications are received and processed, usually without evidence of insurability or waiting periods. Typical open enrollment periods are as follows:

* Within 30 days of hire for initial coverage

* During defined periods that occur annually

During open enrollment, individuals may elect to enroll in, modify coverage under, or transfer between health insurance plans. The selections that individuals make during open enrollment are in effect for the upcoming coverage period, which is typically 12 months. The selections do not expire until the end of the coverage period.

Special enrollment periods are limited to certain circumstances and occur without regard to the health insurance company's regularly scheduled, annual open enrollment period. The timing of a special enrollment period is driven by specific events in individuals' lives and not employers or health insurance companies. These specific events are called **qualifying life events (QLEs)**. As in open enrollment periods, individuals may elect to enroll in, modify, or transfer between health insurance plans during special enrollment periods due to QLEs. Examples of QLEs that make an individual eligible for special enrollment follow:

* Loss of other healthcare coverage (self, spouse, or dependent)

* Marriage

* Divorce

* Birth

* Adoption

* A student moving to or from the place they attend school

* Becoming a U.S. citizen (Healthcare.gov n.d.)

Typically, individuals have 30 days after the event to request the special enrollment for the upcoming **benefit period**. The benefit period is the length of time for which the policy will pay benefits for the policyholder and family and dependents, if applicable. Often, in employer-based health insurance, the benefit period is the entire next calendar year and until the next open enrollment period. This one-year period often occurs because each year, employers renegotiate the benefits and costs of health insurance.

Self-insured people may purchase health insurance annually on their own. They may also vary their benefits depending on costs. However, some individual health insurance policies have three-year benefit periods, five-year benefit periods, and lifetime (unlimited) benefit periods. In each case, the policy will provide coverage for the period for as long as the policyholder is qualified to receive the benefits.

Benefits

Benefits are the healthcare services for which the health insurance company will cover or reimburse. Benefits may include the following services:

- Healthcare services provided by physicians, allied health practitioners, and visiting nurses
- Free care for preventive services and immunizations recommended by the US Preventive Services Task Force (USPSTF) (A or B grade), routine immunizations, childhood preventive services, and women's preventive care services including well-woman visits; mammograms; screenings for cervical cancer, osteoporosis, colorectal cancer, and domestic violence; and other preventive healthcare services
- Confinement in an acute-care hospital, long-term care hospital, partial day center, specialty hospital, or nursing home, including necessary services, supplies, and medications
- Inpatient and outpatient surgeries and associated anesthesia services
- Emergency department, physician office visits, and home healthcare
- Mental and behavioral health services and substance abuse treatment
- Vision and dental care
- Laboratory tests, x-rays, and other radiological procedures and treatments
- Rental or purchase of durable medical equipment (DME), prosthetic and orthotic appliances, prescriptions, and medical supplies
- Prescription drugs
- Rehabilitative services
- Emergency transport services

In addition to healthcare services, plans provide other types of benefits, such as a **maximum out of pocket**. The maximum out of pocket is a specific amount, in a certain time frame, such as one year, beyond which all covered healthcare services for that policyholder or dependent are paid at 100 percent by the healthcare insurance plan. The policyholder is not liable for any cost sharing beyond the maximum out-of-pocket amount. For example, if the maximum out of pocket for the policy is $4,000, once the policyholder spends $4,000, then all covered healthcare services for that policyholder or dependent after the $4,000 are paid at 100 percent by the health insurance plan. Deductibles and other cost-sharing amounts that the policyholder is responsible to pay out of pocket are included in the total. Cost-sharing provisions are discussed in detail in the section that follows. Note that premiums are not included in the maximum out-of-pocket cost. The maximum out-of-pocket cost is based on the actual insurance coverage and represents the maximum amount of money that the insured will need to pay to receive healthcare services. Benefits can be categorized into two broad classifications: essential benefits for general healthcare services and special limited benefits for specific situations. The essential benefits are the types of benefits available in employer-based health insurance and in individual health insurance. There are 10 categories of essential benefits that are required by the ACA:

- Ambulatory patient services, also referred to as outpatient care
- Prescription drugs
- Emergency care
- Behavioral health services
- Hospitalization

- Rehabilitative and habilitative services

- Preventive and wellness services

- Laboratory services

- Pediatric care

- Maternity and newborn care

Policy benefits are available at different levels, which vary widely in the range of services they cover. Premiums, deductibles, and cost-sharing provisions range accordingly. The deductible must be met before the health insurance company will pay for any covered expenses. Cost-sharing provisions, such as coinsurance and copayments, for all covered expenses must be paid until the policyholder reaches the maximum out-of-pocket cost. **Coinsurance** is a preestablished percentage of eligible expenses after the deductible has been met. The percentage may vary by type or site of service. **Copayment** is a cost-sharing measure in which the beneficiary pays a fixed dollar amount per service, supply, or procedure that is owed to the healthcare facility by the patient. The fixed amount may vary by type of service, such as a visit or a prescription. Additional covered expenses are paid in full by the health plan.

Special limited benefits include the following:

- Hospital and surgical policies cover major expenses in the hospital and expenses related to surgeries, including outpatient surgery. Health insurance payments may be percentages or specific dollar amounts. Hospitalization policies typically have high deductibles and high coverage limits.

- Major medical or catastrophic policies are designed to reduce risk associated with catastrophic illness or injury. A fixed amount is available during the lifetime of the policyholder or dependent. Major medical policies typically have high deductibles and high coverage limits.

- Hospital confinement indemnity policies pay a per diem for each day in the hospital. This policy is typically in addition to comprehensive policies, hospital and surgical policies, and major medical policies.

- Long-term care policies provide benefits for nursing home care and services.

- Disability income protection policies provide weekly or monthly payments during a lengthy illness or recovery from an injury. Disability income protection policies begin to pay only after a period established in the contract, such as 30 days or six months. Contracts usually contain maximum payment limits based on a percentage of the policyholder's salary, such as 60 percent.

- Accidental death and dismemberment policies cover expenses arising from an accident that causes a loss such as death, amputation of a limb, or blindness. Benefits vary greatly depending on the specific policy.

- Specific condition, disease, or accident policies provide coverage for diseases or accidents listed in the policy. Common examples are vision care policies, dental policies, and cancer policies.

- Medicare supplemental health insurance policies are designed to coordinate their payments with payments from Medicare. These policies "wrap around" the benefits of Medicare, filling in "gaps" in Medicare coverage, such as deductibles and coinsurance. Benefits vary by policy.

- Other **supplemental insurance** policies fill in, or supplement, the coverage in other policies. The policies "wrap around" the benefits in comprehensive policies, essential health benefits policies, hospital and surgical policies, and catastrophic policies, filling in their gaps. Gaps include high deductibles and cost-sharing amounts. The previously listed long-term policies, disability income protection policies, accidental death and dismemberment policies, and specific disease or accident policies are common examples of supplemental insurance plans. Another example is a short-term health insurance policy purchased for the duration of a vacation or trip. Supplemental policies provide cash benefits; cover deductibles, coinsurances, and copayments; or provide other forms of payment. Patients and guarantors often use the additional funds to pay incidental costs associated with healthcare, such as travel, lodging, meals, and day care.

Members purchase special limited policies based on their health status and financial standing. For example, a Medicare beneficiary with several chronic conditions who expects to have numerous healthcare visits may purchase Medicare supplementation insurance to provide coverage of their cost-sharing amounts associated with high utilization of services.

Limitations

Limitations are qualifications or other specifications that limit the extent of the benefits. Limitations can be placed on total dollar amount, time frame, duration, and number. For example, purchases of DME exceeding $500 require prior authorization. **Prior authorization**, also known as precertification or preauthorization, is the process of obtaining approval from a health insurance company before receiving healthcare services. Cost sharing, or the dollar amount the beneficiary is responsible for paying, is a common limitation. In the following section, several types of cost-sharing provisions are discussed.

Cost-Sharing Provisions

Cost-sharing provisions are a common limitation found in health insurance policies. The extent and number of cost-sharing provisions have risen as the costs of healthcare have increased. Cost-sharing provisions require beneficiaries to bear some of the costs of healthcare that they consume. Making beneficiaries bear some of the financial burden of healthcare is a mechanism to control healthcare costs. Therefore, cost sharing is a strategy to decrease the effect of moral hazard. **Moral hazard** is when "policyholders as patients have an incentive to use more services than those on which their insurance premiums are based" (Light 2021). This modern meaning of moral hazard has roots in morality, which is the principles of right and wrong behavior. Insurance companies use moral hazard as the foundation of implementing cost sharing for policyholders. The concept is, if a patient must pay for a portion of the healthcare service, then they will not abuse their benefits. In other words, the patient will think carefully before going to the emergency department for a sinus infection because they have a $150 cost-sharing amount. Instead, the patient may wait to visit an urgent care facility, where their cost-sharing amount is $35. Likewise, if the insurance company has established a cost-sharing amount of 30 percent for all radiology services, the patient will consider if they really need the MRI before registering and agreeing to pay the 30 percent cost-sharing amount. However, as a counterpoint, implementing cost-sharing provisions can have a negative effect on a patient's health. Cost sharing can deter patients, especially low-income patients, from getting necessary services if they are unable to pay the cost-sharing amounts (Chandra et al. 2021). A study by the Kaiser Family Foundation (KFF) found that even small levels of cost sharing, such as five dollars, are associated with reduced care (Artiga et al. 2017). Further, the study finds that there are additional consequences, such as increased emergency department use, reduced treatment for children with asthma, and increased rates of uncontrolled hypertension and hypercholesterolemia (Artiga et al. 2017). While insurance companies continue to increase the use of cost sharing and increase the amount of cost-sharing measures, the KFF research shows that the potential gains from cost sharing are offset by increased disenrollment, increased use of more expensive services, like emergency department services, and increased administrative expenses (Artiga et al. 2017).

The cost-sharing provisions of a policy are included in the SBC section. The SBC is included in the policy and often the policyholder has web access to this information. Figure 2.1 provides an excerpt from the cost-sharing provision section of a sample SBC.

This sample illustrates that there are two main types of cost sharing: coinsurance and copayment. Recall that coinsurance is a preestablished percentage of eligible expenses after the deductible has been met. The percentage may vary by type or site of service. An example of coinsurance is the cost-sharing amount for surgeon fees for outpatient surgery. Figure 2.1 indicates that the beneficiary will pay a 20 percent coinsurance amount for outpatient surgery surgeon fees. For example, the total reimbursement owed to the surgeon is $2,000. The beneficiary is responsible for 20 percent of this amount and the payer is responsible for 80 percent of this

Figure 2.1.   Cost-sharing provision section of a sample summary of benefits and coverage

Common Medical Event	Services You May Need	What You Will Pay	
		Network Provider (You will pay the least)	Out-of-Network Provider (You will pay the most)
If you visit a health care provider's office or clinic	Primary care visit to treat an injury or illness	$35 copay/office visit and 20% coinsurance for other outpatient services; deductible does not apply	40% coinsurance
	Specialist visit	$50 copay/visit	40% coinsurance
	Preventive care/ screening/ immunization	No charge	40% coinsurance
If you have a test	Diagnostic test (x-ray, blood work)	$10 copay/test	40% coinsurance
	Imaging (CT/PET scans, MRIs)	$50 copay/test	40% coinsurance
If you need drugs to treat your illness or condition	Generic drugs (Tier 1)	$10 copay/prescription (retail & mail order)	40% coinsurance
	Preferred brand drugs (Tier 2)	$30 copay/prescription (retail & mail order)	40% coinsurance
	Non-preferred brand drugs (Tier 3)	40% coinsurance	60% coinsurance
	Specialty drugs (Tier 4)	50% coinsurance	70% coinsurance
If you have outpatient surgery	Facility fee (e.g., ambulatory surgery center)	$100/day copay	40% coinsurance
	Physician/surgeon fees	20% coinsurance	40% coinsurance
		50% coinsurance for anesthesia	

Source: CMS 2020, 2.

amount. The coinsurance calculation is shown in figure 2.2. The beneficiary is responsible for the coinsurance amount, which is $400.

Figure 2.1 indicates that the copayment amount for a primary care office visit is $35. The copayment amount increases to $50 for a specialist office visit. Further, there is no cost sharing for a preventive care visit, such as a beneficiary's annual visit. Some health plans have tiers of benefits. A **tier** is a level of coverage. Specifically, in health insurance, tiers act as *limits*. Health insurance companies impose these limits to increase the certainty of their costs. The tiers limit their members' freedom of choice of providers, the amount of services allowed, and

Figure 2.2. **Coinsurance calculation**

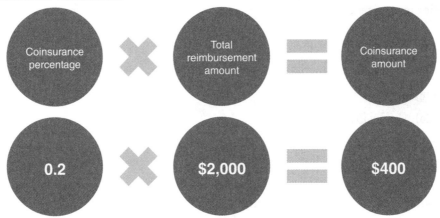

the types of drugs or other services. The number and types of tiers vary by the benefit being limited and by the health insurance company. Figure 2.1 provides an example of tiers in the prescription drugs section. This example shows that there are four prescription drug tiers. In tier 1, generic drugs, the beneficiary has the lowest copayment amount, $10. In contrast, in tier 4, specialty drugs, the beneficiary must pay a 50 percent coinsurance amount. In this scenario, the payer is using higher copayment and coinsurance amounts in tiers 2 through 4 to encourage the beneficiary to use a tier-1 generic drug when possible.

Exclusions

Exclusions are situations, instances, conditions, injuries, or treatments that the healthcare plan states will not be covered and for which the healthcare plan will not pay benefits. Specific and unique definitions may serve as exclusions. Typical exclusions include the following:

- Experimental or investigational diagnostic and therapeutic procedures

- Medically unnecessary diagnostic or therapeutic procedures

- Cosmetic procedures, except when related to accidents, disease, or congenital defects, and source-of-injury treatments, such as for war-related injuries and injuries sustained during risky recreational activities

For example, a healthcare plan may deny coverage for a prescription to remove wrinkles because the purpose is cosmetic. Coverage for experimental or investigational services is also often denied. Examples of experimental or investigational procedures or therapies include face transplants, medications used to treat conditions for which the FDA has not issued approval, and active cold therapy units using mechanical pumps and portable refrigerators.

Procedures

Procedures explain how policyholders obtain the healthcare benefit or qualify to receive the healthcare benefit. Healthcare plans may deny benefits because procedures are not followed. Moreover, the procedures can function as limitations and exclusions, even though they may be stated in the positive. For example, "All behavioral health and substance use services must be rendered by an eligible provider." Therefore, if services were provided by an ineligible provider, they would not be covered. Common procedures included in health insurance include prior authorization, coordination of benefits (COB), and other party liability (OPL).

A common procedure is obtaining prior authorization. **Prior authorization**, as defined earlier in this chapter, also known as **precertification**, is the process of obtaining approval from a health insurance company before receiving healthcare services. During this approval process, the healthcare plan determines whether the condition to be treated is a covered condition and whether the planned treatment is medically necessary. The types of services that often require prior authorization include the following:

- Outpatient surgeries

- Diagnostic, interventional, and therapeutic outpatient procedures

- Physical, occupational, and speech therapies

- Behavioral health and substance use care

- Inpatient care, including surgery, home health, private nurses, and nursing homes

- Organ transplants

Therefore, if a policy requires prior authorization for physical therapy services and the beneficiary does not obtain the prior authorization, the expenses related to the physical therapy services may be denied.

Coordination of Benefits and Other Party Liability

Other common procedures are **coordination of benefits (COB)** and determination of **other party liability (OPL)**. These procedures are used when multiple insurance companies are involved. The responsible insurance party must be determined through clauses of the policies and the circumstances of the case.

COB becomes necessary when people have multiple health insurance carriers that are providing coverage, which can occur in instances when both spouses or parents work and both employers provide health insurance. The **primary insurer** is the health insurance company responsible for the greatest proportion or majority of the healthcare expenses. The **secondary insurer** is responsible for the remainder of the healthcare expenses. The two health insurance companies are sharing the responsibility for the healthcare expenses. This integration of payments is known as COB and ensures that the payments of multiple plans do not exceed 100 percent of the amount owed by the patient.

Determining the primary or secondary insurer can be complicated. There are several common rules to follow:

- A patient's health insurance company is primary over a spouse's health insurance company.

- A dependent child's primary insurer is the insurance company of the parent whose birthday comes first in the calendar year. This is called the "birthday rule." A legal decree, such as a divorce agreement, dictates determination.

OPL is similar but differs in that the other party is totally responsible for paying the costs. The other insurance is typically not health insurance. For example, should a person incur healthcare expenses related to an injury suffered in a motor vehicle crash, the health insurance company may deny coverage because the other party, the automobile insurance, is liable (responsible) for the expenses. The two common examples of OPL are when an automobile insurance company or workers' compensation is paying for the treatment of injuries incurred during a motor vehicle crash or during work-related activities, respectively.

Appeals Processes

An **appeal** is a request for reconsideration of denial of coverage for healthcare services or rejection of a claim. A **claim** is a bill for healthcare services submitted by a hospital, physician's office, or other healthcare provider or facility. The beneficiary or the provider submits claims to the health insurance company for reimbursement. The appeals section of a policy describes the steps the beneficiary must take to appeal a decision about coverage or payment of a claim. Typically, the appeal must be in writing and within a specific time frame of the health insurance company's decision concerning the issue.

Managed Care

The purpose of **managed care** is to provide affordable, high-quality healthcare. Managed care systematically merges clinical, financial, and administrative processes to manage access, cost, and quality of healthcare. In the US between 1966 and the early 1970s, the costs of healthcare escalated quickly (Foster 2000). To control costs and provide affordable quality healthcare, federal legislation encouraged the growth of **health maintenance organizations (HMOs)**. HMOs are health entities that combine the provision of health insurance and the delivery of healthcare services using the principles of managed care. The Health Maintenance Organization Act of 1973 (HMO Act) provided federal grants and loans for new HMOs. Even though the title of the HMO Act specifies HMOs, this act initiated the proliferation of several types of managed care plans.

Since the passage of the HMO Act, managed care has increased its share of the market, in part because of economic pressures. Managed care evolved into numerous types of organizations and plans in addition to HMOs, such as preferred provider organizations (PPOs) and point-of-service (POS) plans. These multiple types of managed care plans emerged to meet the needs of consumers for freedom of choice and access to specialists and the need of employers to reduce their healthcare costs. Most health insurance companies offer managed care plans. In this section of chapter 2, we will explore the concepts of managed care.

Managed care plans are healthcare plans that attempt to manage care by integrating the financing and delivery of specified healthcare services. In the Balanced Budget Act of 1997, the Centers for Medicare and Medicaid Services (CMS) termed these plans *coordinated care plans*. Managed care plans implement provisions to manage both the costs and the outcomes of healthcare. In the following sections, the benefits and characteristics of managed care are discussed. The three main characteristics of managed care are quality patient care, cost controls, and prospective reimbursement methods.

Benefits and Services of Managed Care

Managed care plans offer the following levels of benefits, depending on the cost of their premiums and cost sharing:

- Physician services (inpatient and outpatient)

- Inpatient care

- Preventive care and wellness, such as immunizations, well-child examinations, adult periodic health maintenance examinations, and preventive gynecologic services

- Prenatal care

- Emergency medical services

- Diagnostic and laboratory tests

- Certain home health services

Beneficiaries of managed care plans typically only have access to mental and behavioral health and specialty care through referral from a primary care physician. A physician that is familiar with the patient can serve as the gatekeeper, or point person, to manage access to more expensive specialty resources. The concept of a gatekeeper is explained more later in this chapter.

Characteristics of Managed Care

Managed care plans share characteristics associated with providing quality care and cost-effective care as detailed in tables 2.1 and 2.2. Some characteristics, such as the use of **primary care providers (PCPs)** as gatekeeper, impact both quality of care and cost-effective care. A PCP is typically a physician, nurse practitioner, or physician assistant that is the primary healthcare contact for an individual. A discussion in each section is provided because the characteristic can be examined from multiple viewpoints. Managed care plans coordinate and control healthcare services to improve quality and to contain expenditures.

Quality Care

Managed care focuses on providing high-quality patient care. Plans achieve this goal through four main principles: careful selection of providers, an emphasis on the health of their beneficiary population, use of care management tools, and quality assessment and improvement.

Table 2.1. **Managed care characteristics associated with quality care**

Characteristic	Description
Selection of providers	Criteria include quality, scope of services, cost, and location
	Credentialing and periodic recredentialing
	Procedural selection process at senior clinical staff level
Health of populations	Responsible for delivery of healthcare services on continuum of care (prevention, wellness, acute, and chronic)
	Population receives recommended preventive care and appropriate care for chronic conditions
	Health and wellness management
Care management tools	Coordination of care by PCP
	Disease management
	Evidence-based clinical practice guidelines
Quality assessment and improvement	Entities are accredited and engage in performance improvement

Table 2.2. Managed care characteristics associated with cost-effective care

Characteristic	Description
Service management tools	Utilization management and utilization review
	Gatekeeper role of PCP
	Prior authorization
	Second and third opinions
	Case management
	Prescription management
Prospective reimbursement	Payment rate established in advance for an episode-of-care
Financial incentives	Providers to meet fiscal targets
	Members to use providers associated with the plan

Selection of Providers

Managed care plans stress the use of criteria in their selection of providers. Senior clinicians in the upper echelons of the plan select providers using preestablished procedures and standards. These criteria are based on quality, scope of services, cost, and location. Timelines for credentialing and recredentialing are strictly followed. This emphasis on the selection of providers ensures their members have access to superior and eminent providers throughout a geographic area.

Health of Populations

Managed care plans emphasize the health of their entire beneficiary population. These plans are responsible for the delivery of healthcare services across the continuum of care in terms of settings and types. Examples of settings include physicians' offices, home health agencies, and hospitals. Examples of types of care are preventive, wellness oriented, acute, and chronic. The plan is clinically responsible for the health outcomes of its population. Beneficiaries receive appropriate testing for preventive care, such as timely mammograms and Pap smears. Moreover, beneficiaries with chronic conditions receive appropriate assessment and therapeutic procedures, as recommended by evidence-based clinical practice guidelines. **Evidence-based clinical practice guidelines**, explicit statements that guide clinical decision-making, are the foundation of beneficiaries' care for specific clinical conditions. Systematic use of guidelines is termed *evidence-based medicine*. Evidence-based clinical practice guidelines outline the following:

- Key diagnostic indicators
- Timelines
- Alternatives in interventions and treatments
- Potential outcomes

These guidelines are discussed further in the next section.

In addition, managed care plans often support their beneficiaries' participation in health and wellness management. Wellness programs are one component of health and wellness management. These programs stress the habits of healthy lifestyles, such as exercise and proper nutrition. Other aspects of health and wellness management include smoking cessation, alcohol moderation, and harm reduction.

Care Management Tools

Care management tools include coordination of care, disease management, and the application of evidence-based clinical practice guidelines. Together, these tools foster continuity and accessibility of healthcare services and reduce fragmentation and misuse of resources and facilities.

Coordination of care is achieved using a PCP. PCPs often are family practitioners, general practitioners, internists, and pediatricians. In many managed care plans, one PCP provides, supervises, or arranges for a patient or client's healthcare and makes necessary and appropriate referrals to specialists or providers within the managed care plan. A **referral** is a process in which a PCP makes a request to a managed care plan on behalf of a patient to send that patient to receive medical care from a specialist or provider outside the managed care plan.

Disease management focuses on preventing exacerbations or flare-ups of chronic diseases and promoting healthier lifestyles for patients and clients with chronic diseases. In disease management, patients are monitored to promote adherence to treatment plans and to detect early signs and symptoms of exacerbations. Disease management programs often focus on diabetes, congestive heart failure, coronary heart disease, chronic obstructive pulmonary disease (COPD), and asthma. Often the management of chronic diseases requires treatment plans and complex medication regimens involving multiple healthcare providers. Thus, disease management is closely aligned with coordination of care because the efforts of multiple providers must be synchronized. Disease management programs have been overwhelmingly implemented across the US healthcare sector. Despite the widespread implementation of disease management programs, healthcare administrators should inspect the programs' designs and features and should closely monitor the programs' achievement of their goals and objectives.

Disease management is based on evidence-based guidelines that have been systematically developed from scientific evidence and clinical expertise to answer clinical questions. Other terms for these guidelines are *clinical practice guidelines*, *clinical guidelines*, *clinical pathways*, *clinical criteria*, and *medical protocols*. Sources of these guidelines are the USPSTF, the Agency for Healthcare Research and Quality (AHRQ), the Centers for Disease Control and Prevention, and specialty organizations such as the American College of Cardiology, the American Academy of Family Physicians, the American Academy of Ophthalmology, and the American College of Obstetricians and Gynecologists. These guidelines are benchmarks of best practices in the medical care and treatment of patients and clients.

These guidelines are used to manage the wellness of beneficiaries and to direct the care of acute illnesses and chronic conditions. The guidelines typically address the following:

- The entire plan of care across multiple delivery sites

- The appropriate diagnostic and therapeutic procedures for a disease or condition

- Reasons for referrals to specialists

- Clinical decision factors and decision points

Thus, evidence-based clinical practice guidelines serve to standardize optimal care for all patients and to deliver comprehensive, coordinated care across multiple providers.

Quality Assessment and Improvement

Managed care plans participate in rigorous accreditation processes and in performance improvement initiatives. Organizations with accreditation standards for managed care include the following:

- National Committee for Quality Assurance (NCQA)

- URAC (formerly the Utilization Review Accreditation Commission)

- Accreditation Association for Ambulatory Health Care (AAAHC, also known as the Accreditation Association)

Plans also participate in performance improvement initiatives. Two common sets of measures to assess and improve quality follow:

- AHRQ's Consumer Assessment of Healthcare Providers and Systems (CAHPS)
- NCQA's Healthcare Effectiveness Data and Information Set (HEDIS)

Often as a part of these improvement initiatives, managed care plans survey their beneficiaries to obtain feedback on such issues as the following:

- Satisfaction with administrative, clinical, and customer services
- Perceptions of the plan's strengths and weaknesses
- Suggestions for improvements
- Intentions regarding reenrollment

In addition to surveying beneficiaries, plans conduct satisfaction surveys of patients, physicians, providers, customers, employers, and disenrolled members. Commitment to accreditation and performance improvement demonstrates the managed care plan's dedication to its beneficiaries and to the delivery of quality healthcare.

Cost-Effective Care

Managed care plans strive to provide cost-effective care. To achieve this goal, managed care organizations (MCOs) implement various forms of cost controls, as shown in table 2.2. These controls include the following:

- Service management tools, which include medical necessity and utilization management, the gatekeeper role of the PCP, prior authorization, second and third opinions, case management, and prescription management
- Prospective reimbursement
- Financial incentives, which include providers meeting fiscal targets and members using providers affiliated with the plan

Managed care plans utilize a combination of these cost-control mechanisms. Combining strategies from all three categories allows managed care plans to provide cost-effective care for their beneficiaries. Although initially influenced by managed care, some strategies, such as medical necessity and utilization management, have become commonplace in the healthcare industry due to their success in controlling cost. The following sections describe strategies from the three categories of cost control: service management tools, prospective reimbursement, and financial incentives.

Service Management Tools

A primary cost-control tool is **utilization management**. Utilization management is a program that evaluates the healthcare facility's overall efficiency in providing necessary care to patients in the most effective manner. A key component of utilization management is **utilization review**. Utilization review is a process that determines the medical necessity of a procedure and the appropriateness of the setting for the healthcare service in the continuum of care. Determining the most appropriate setting is sometimes referred to as *site of service review*. Both components of utilization review are often performed concurrently. If the criteria for medical necessity are not met, then the payer will not approve or reimburse the service or treatment. Utilization review factors in patients' severity of illness and other medical conditions and illnesses. For example, utilization review assesses whether, considering the patient's severity of illness, the services could be provided more efficiently and economically in an ambulatory setting rather than in an inpatient hospital.

Managed care plans and other insurance companies use a three-step process for utilization review, which is presented in table 2.3. Step 1 is the initial clinical review. In this step the reviewer is a licensed health professional who reviews the medical case against established criteria. In step 2 a peer clinical review takes place. During this review, a peer clinician performs a clinical review of the case. In this step a qualified, expert clinician in the same specialty as the medical case provides their clinical opinion. For each step, if the result is a positive decision, meaning the service is medically necessary and a site of service is determined, then the process stops. However, if the result of the step is a negative decision, then the process moves to the next step until all steps are exhausted.

Medical necessity and site of service are reviewed using objective, clinical criteria. There are many proprietary and public domain sets of criteria for utilization review. Utilization review is often used for the following services:

- Confinement in acute-care hospital, long-term acute-care facility, long-term care facility, psychiatric hospital, or partial-day hospital, or receiving hospice or rehabilitation services

- Surgical procedures

- Emergency department services

- Emergent care received from out-of-network (out-of-plan) providers

- High-cost or high-risk diagnostic, interventional, or therapeutic outpatient procedures

- Physical, occupational, speech, and other rehabilitative therapies

- Behavioral health and substance use care

- Home health services, private duty nurses, and referrals to medical specialists

- DME, prosthetic and orthotic appliances, medical supplies, blood transfusions and administration, and medical transport

Generally, utilization review saves money through its prevention of overutilization. Overutilization is the unnecessary consumption of healthcare services or the consumption of unnecessarily expensive or sophisticated healthcare services.

Another service management tool used in managed care is a **gatekeeper**. The PCP's role as gatekeeper is to control costs. As the coordinator of all the healthcare services that a beneficiary may access, the PCP determines whether referrals are warranted. These referrals may be to (1) medical specialists, (2) other healthcare sites for diagnostic or therapeutic procedures, or (3) hospitals or other healthcare facilities. Gatekeepers determine the appropriateness of the healthcare service, the level of healthcare personnel, and the setting in the continuum of care.

Table 2.3.   Utilization review process

Step	Responsible Party	Activity or Resource
1. Clinical review	Licensed health professional	Review against established criteria
2. Peer clinical review	Peer clinician	Clinician qualified to render clinical opinion performs clinical review
3. Appeals consideration/decision	Qualified, expert clinician in same specialty	Clinician not involved in initial decision but qualified to render clinical opinion performs clinical review

Prior authorization is also a cost-control measure. Prior authorization is the formal administrative process of obtaining prior authorization for healthcare services. Inpatient admissions, surgeries, visits to medical specialists, elective procedures, and expensive or sophisticated diagnostic tests are all types of services that require prior authorization. Occasionally, for healthcare services such as mental or behavioral health, providers must submit entire treatment plans for prior authorization. Managed care plans may deny coverage or payment for healthcare services for which required prior authorization was not obtained. The beneficiary's insurance policy identifies the healthcare services for which prior authorization must be obtained.

Second and third opinions are cost-containment measures to prevent unnecessary tests, treatments, medical devices, or surgical procedures. Second or third opinions are obtained from medical experts within the healthcare plan. They are particularly sought when a service is high risk or high cost, diagnostic evidence is contradictory, or experts' opinions are mixed about efficacy.

Another service management tool is case management. Case management coordinates an individual's care, especially in complex and high-cost cases. Individuals are assigned case managers who are typically nurses or physicians. With the beneficiary and their family, case managers coordinate the efforts of multiple healthcare providers at multiple sites over time. Consultants, specialists, PCPs, ancillary services, ambulatory care, inpatient services, and long-term care may all be involved. Case managers often are assigned to beneficiaries with catastrophic illnesses or injuries, such as a severe head injury. Workers' compensation cases may involve a case manager. Goals of case management include continuity of care, cost-effectiveness, quality, and appropriate utilization.

Prescription management is also a cost-control measure. Prescription management expands the use of a formulary to a comprehensive approach to medications and medication administration. A **formulary** is a list of prescription drugs that a health insurance plan will cover or allow to be reimbursed. This approach includes patient education; electronic screening, alert, and decision-support tools; expert and referent systems, especially related to drug-drug interactions, food-drug interactions, and cross-sensitivities; and criteria for drug utilization. Some electronic prescription management systems include POS order entry, electronic transmission of the prescription to the pharmacy, and patient-specific medication profiles. As discussed earlier in the cost-sharing section, generic, less expensive drugs are preferred to brand-name, expensive drugs. However, the comprehensive approach also enhances the quality of patient care. Considering the cost of medications, prescription management is a powerful tool of cost containment.

Specialty management organizations exist to provide the comprehensive service of pharmacy benefit management. These organizations are called **pharmacy benefit managers (PBMs)**. PBMs administer health insurance companies' and self-insured employers' prescription drug benefits.

Prospective Reimbursement

Managed care plans use prospective reimbursement methodologies to reimburse providers in their network. The purpose of the prospective reimbursement method is to reduce the inflation of costs. Through prospective reimbursement, plans and providers share the risks of beneficiaries' care costs. In this method, providers receive one predetermined amount for all the care a beneficiary may receive during an episode-of-care. The managed care plan does not increase payments for the complexity or extent of healthcare services, so the incentive to provide higher volumes of services to generate higher reimbursements is eliminated.

Prospective reimbursement rates are based on the typical patient. On average, most beneficiaries will rarely or never use healthcare services within a period. These low users or nonusers offset the acutely or chronically ill members. In the aggregate, low users or nonusers balance out heavy users. Various types of prospective reimbursement methodologies are discussed in detail in chapter 4, "Healthcare Reimbursement Methodologies."

Financial Incentives

Managed care plans are fiscally accountable for the health outcomes of their populations. Thus, financial incentives exist for both providers and beneficiaries. These incentives save financial resources by preventing excessive or unnecessarily expensive healthcare services.

Incentives can be both positive and negative. As a positive incentive, providers may receive bonuses for meeting cost-containment targets. Conversely, a penalty may be assessed as a negative incentive. An example of a penalty includes a percentage reduction of the PCP's salary if the provider does not meet the benchmark target. A commonly used term for the reduction of a PCP's salary is *withhold amount*. A **withhold amount** is a part of the provider's prospective payment that the managed care plan deducts and holds to pay for excessive expenditures for expensive healthcare services, such as referrals to specialists. The use of withhold amounts transfers risk to the providers. For a group practice, the withhold amounts from individual providers are combined to form a withhold pool. At the end of the period, surplus withheld funds are dispersed for meeting efficiency or performance targets. Providers who do not meet targets do not receive withhold amounts at the end of the period.

As financial incentives to beneficiaries, managed care plans set varying rates of cost sharing. For example, managed care plans require higher cost-sharing payments when members use out-of-network providers than when they use network providers, as shown previously in figure 2.1. Other managed care plans offer beneficiaries levels of prescription drug benefits. The drug benefit with the most restrictive formulary is the least expensive, whereas the beneficiary's cost sharing increases as the formulary becomes less confining. Incentives are intended to influence beneficiaries' behavior without eliminating freedom of choice.

Although MCOs share many characteristics as discussed, there are several distinct types of MCOs. The variation in types of managed care often revolves around control of beneficiaries' choices. In the following sections three types of managed care plans will be explored.

Types of Managed Care Plans

As managed care has evolved, lines have blurred among the types of managed care plans. Thus, a continuum is a better conceptualization of managed care than individual, separate categories. The distinct types of managed care plans can be placed on a continuum of control. The continuum of control reflects the amount of control the managed care plan allows the beneficiary to have regarding healthcare provider choice. On this continuum, the HMOs represent the most controlled, and the PPOs represent the least controlled, as shown in figure 2.3. This section discusses several managed care plans across the continuum of control, including HMO, PPO, and POS plans.

Health Maintenance Organization

HMOs combine the provision of health insurance and the delivery of healthcare services. The HMO Act of 1973 was an initiative to control healthcare costs. Subsequent amendments were enacted in 1976, 1978, and 1981 to implement regulations (CFR 42, Part 417). Included in the act were conditions for becoming a federally qualified HMO. The conditions were a minimum benefits package, open enrollment, and **community rating**. In community rating, the rates for healthcare premiums are determined by geographic area (community) rather than by age, health status, or company size. This method increases the size of the risk pool. Costs are increased to younger, healthier individuals who are, in effect, subsidizing older or less healthy individuals.

Figure 2.3. Managed care plan continuum of control

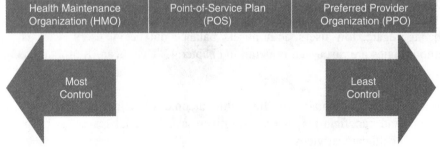

HMOs emphasize preventive care in the belief that in the long term, preventive care saves money by preventing acute illness and chronic conditions. HMOs are the most restrictive form of managed care because they allow patients and clients the least freedom in choosing a provider. This loss of freedom is offset by reduced cost-sharing payments and a wide range of benefits.

Preferred Provider Organization

A **preferred provider organization (PPO)** is an entity that contracts with employers and insurance companies to render healthcare services to a group of members. Its common characteristics are as follows:

- Virtual rather than physical entity
- Decentralized
- Flexibility of choice for members
- Negotiated fees, which may include discounts
- Financial incentives to induce members to choose preferred option
- No prepaid reimbursement per member
- Not subject to regulatory requirements of HMOs
- Limited financial risk for providers

The PPO also contracts with providers for healthcare services at fixed or discounted rates. The providers are a network of physicians, hospitals, and other healthcare providers. Members can choose to use the healthcare services of any physician, hospital, or other healthcare provider. However, the PPO influences beneficiaries to use the healthcare services of network providers. Beneficiaries' cost-sharing payments are lower if they use network providers; members' cost-sharing payments are higher if they use the services of out-of-network providers. PPOs offer greater freedom of choice for beneficiaries than HMOs.

Point-of-Service Plan

A **point-of-service (POS) plan** is one in which members choose how to receive services at the time they need them. For example, members can choose "at the point of service" whether they want an HMO, a PPO, or a fee schedule plan. They do not need to make this decision during an open enrollment period. These health insurance plans are also known as open-ended HMOs. Beneficiaries' cost-sharing payments are increased if they receive services outside of the established referral network.

Check Your Understanding 2.2

1. List three benefits or services offered by managed care plans.

2. Managed care plans focus on providing high-quality care. One principle MCOs use to ensure high quality is the use of care management tools. Describe the disease management tool.

3. Managed care plans strive to provide cost-effective care. One principle MCOs use to ensure cost-effective care is the use of financial incentives. Describe how financial incentives support cost-effective care.

4. Define utilization review.

5. Describe community rating.

Patient Connection

In chapter 1, "Healthcare Reimbursement and Revenue Cycle Management," the Patient Connection section introduced Olivia. Olivia is a 30-year-old female who has health insurance for her family through her employer. Olivia's insurance company is Super Payer. Olivia's health insurance premium is $2,000 per month. Olivia's portion of the premium is 30 percent, which totals $600 per month. Her plan has a $500 deductible for the family. Her husband, Tony, had the flu in January and sought treatment, which totaled $430. Olivia paid this amount since they had not met their deductible of $500. Therefore, Olivia still owes $70 ($500 minus $430) of the deductible before Super Payer will assume liability of paying healthcare expenses.

Additionally, Olivia's plan includes cost-sharing limitations. Following is the cost-sharing section from her SBC.

Common Medical Event	Services You May Need	What You Will Pay	
		Network Provider (You will pay the least)	Out-of-Network Provider (You will pay the most)
If you visit a health care provider's office or clinic	Primary care visit to treat an injury or illness	$35 copay/office visit 20% coinsurance for other outpatient services provided during the office visit; deductible does not apply	35% coinsurance
	Specialist visit	$50 copay/visit	50% coinsurance
	Preventive care/screening/ immunization	No charge	35% coinsurance
If you have a test	Diagnostic test (x-ray, blood work)	$15 copay/test	35% coinsurance
	Imaging (CT/PET scans, MRIs)	$60 copay/test	35% coinsurance
If you need drugs to treat your illness or condition	Generic drugs (Tier 1)	$10 copay/prescription (retail & mail order)	50% coinsurance
	Preferred brand drugs (Tier 2)	$30 copay/prescription (retail & mail order)	50% coinsurance
	Non-preferred brand drugs (Tier 3)	40% coinsurance	60% coinsurance
	Specialty drugs (Tier 4)	50% coinsurance	70% coinsurance
If you have inpatient admission or outpatient surgery encounter	Facility fee (e.g., inpatient admission, ambulatory surgery center)	$100/day copay	40% coinsurance
	Physician/surgeon fees	20% coinsurance 50% coinsurance for anesthesia	40% coinsurance

(continued)

Olivia is five months pregnant. She and Tony are reviewing healthcare costs prior to their new baby's arrival. Following is a summary of Olivia's healthcare costs for the past three months.

Date	Visit Type	Expense Type	Amount
March 15	OB	Deductible	$70.00
		Copayment	$50.00
March	N/A	Premium	$600.00
April 15	OB	Copayment	$50.00
April 25	Primary Care	Copayment	$35.00
	Prescription	Copayment	$10.00
April	N/A	Premium	$600.00
May 15	OB	Copayment	$50.00
May	N/A	Premium	$600.00
Total Healthcare Expense March–May			**$2,065.00**

On March 15, Olivia had her first prenatal visit. She paid the remaining $70 of her deductible, plus the copayment of $50 for her visit, which her plan considers a specialty service. She visits her OB each month for a prenatal visit; therefore, she also paid the $50 copayment on April 15 and May 15. On April 25, Olivia saw her PCP for seasonal allergies, and her PCP prescribed eye drops. Therefore, Olivia paid the $35 copayment for a primary care visit and the $10 copayment for generic drugs. Lastly, each month Olivia pays her portion of her family's health insurance premium, $600, through her paycheck. Olivia's total healthcare expenses from March to May totaled $2,065.

Chapter 2 Review Quiz

1. Define the term *risk pool*.
2. What is the relationship between covered conditions and covered services in health insurance plans?
3. List three synonyms for policyholder.
4. Define deductible.
5. Describe the concept of moral hazard as it relates to health insurance.
6. What is the purpose of the summary of benefits and coverage (SBC)?
7. From where do evidence-based clinical guidelines originate?
8. Name the three steps in utilization review.
9. Why is prescription management an important cost control?
10. Describe three mechanisms used by MCOs to ensure cost-effective care.

References

ACEP (American College of Emergency Physicians). 2021 (August). "Public Opinion on the Value of Emergency Physicians." https://www.emergencyphysicians.org/globalassets/emphysicians/all-pdfs/value-and-sop-august -2021-poll-final.pdf.

ACEP (American College of Emergency Physicians). n.d. "Prudent Layperson Standard." Accessed February 9, 2023. https://www.emergencyphysicians.org/article/access/prudent-layperson-standard#:~:text=The%20 Prudent%20Layperson%20Standard%20requires,symptoms%2C%20not%20the%20final%20diagnosis.

American Academy of Actuaries. n.d. "Risk Pooling: How Health Insurance in the Individual Market Works." Accessed September 26, 2022. https://www.actuary.org/content/risk-pooling-how-health-insurance-individual -market-works-0.

Artiga, S., P. Ubri, and J. Zur. 2017. "The Effects of Premiums and Cost Sharing on Low-Income Populations: Updated Review of Research Findings." https://www.kff.org/medicaid/issue-brief/the-effects-of-premiums-and -cost-sharing-on-low-income-populations-updated-review-of-research-findings/.

CFR 42 417: Health maintenance organizations, competitive medical plans, and health care prepayment plans. 2005 (Oct. 1).

Chandra, A., E. Flack, and Z. Obermeyer. 2021 (February). "The Health Costs of Cost-Sharing." NBER Working Paper Series. Cambridge, MA: National Bureau of Economic Research. https://www.nber.org/system/files /working_papers/w28439/w28439.pdf.

CMS (Centers for Medicare and Medicaid Services). 2020. Summary of Benefits and Coverage. https://www .cms.gov/CCIIO/Resources/Forms-Reports-and-Other-Resources/Downloads/Sample-Completed-SBC-Accessible -Format-01-2020.pdf.

CMS (Centers for Medicare and Medicaid Services). 2006. "Glossary." https://www.cms.gov/apps/glossary /default.asp?Letter=ALL&Language=English.

Foster, R. S. 2000. Trends in Medicare expenditures and financial status, 1966–2000. *Health Care Financing Review* 22(1):35–49.

Healthcare.gov. n.d. "Qualifying Life Event (QLE)." Accessed February 9, 2023. https://www.healthcare.gov /glossary/qualifying-life-event/.

KFF (Kaiser Family Foundation). 2022. "2022 Employer Health Benefits Survey." https://www.kff.org/health -costs/report/2022-employer-health-benefits-survey/.

Light, D. W. 2021. "The Three Moral Hazards of Health Insurance." https://www.ias.edu/ideas/three-moral -hazards-health-insurance.

New Jersey State Health Benefits Program. 2022. Health Benefit Coverage of Children Until Age 31 Under Chapter 375. Fact Sheet #74. https://www.state.nj.us/treasury/pensions/documents/factsheets/fact74.pdf.

Ohio Revised Code. 2015. Section 3923.65 Coverage for emergency services. Accessed May 13, 2023. https://codes.ohio.gov/ohio-revised-code/section-3923.65.

Online Medical Dictionary. n.d. "Emergency." Accessed February 9, 2023. https://www.online-medical-dictionary .org/definitions-e/emergencies.html.

Chapter 3
Government-Sponsored Healthcare Programs

Learning Objectives

❖ Identify the different government-sponsored healthcare programs

❖ Recall the history of the Medicare and Medicaid programs in the US

❖ Determine cost-sharing responsibility for Medicare beneficiaries

❖ Describe the effect that government-sponsored healthcare programs have on the US healthcare system

Key Terms

Children's Health Insurance Program (CHIP)
Chronic condition special needs plan (C-SNP)
Civilian Health and Medical Program of the
    Department of Veterans Affairs (CHAMPVA)
Coverage gap
Dual eligible special needs plan (D-SNP)
Federal Employees' Compensation Act of 1916
    (FECA)
Indian Health Service (IHS)
Institutional special needs plan (I-SNP)
Medicaid
Medicare

Medicare Advantage (MA)
Medicare Part A
Medicare Part B
Medicare Part C
Medicare Part D
Programs of All-Inclusive Care for the Elderly
    (PACE)
Social Security Act
TRICARE
Veterans Health Administration (VA)
Workers' compensation

State and federal government agencies administer health plans for different populations as mandated by federal and state laws and regulations. Perhaps the most well-known is Medicare, which serves individuals who qualify for Social Security benefits and who are 65 years old or older. This chapter discusses Medicare and several other federal and state-sponsored programs.

Medicare

The **Social Security Act**, established in 1935 to provide old-age benefits for workers, unemployment insurance, and aid to dependents and children with physical handicaps, was amended by Public Law 89-97 on July 30, 1965, to create the Medicare program (Title XVIII). On July 1, 1966, Medicare's coverage took effect. **Medicare** is a national health insurance program that provides health services to older adults and other qualifying individuals. Medicare benefits are available for the following:

- Individuals 65 years old or older who are eligible for Social Security or railroad retirement benefits
- Individuals entitled to Social Security or railroad retirement disability benefits for at least 24 months
- Government employees with Medicare coverage who have been disabled for more than 29 months
- Insured workers (and their spouses) who have end-stage renal disease
- Children who have end-stage renal disease

In 2010, two major laws passed that significantly affected the Medicare system. The Patient Protection and Affordable Care Act (Public Law 111-48) was enacted on March 23, 2010. In addition, the Health Care and Education Reconciliation Act of 2010 (Public Law 111-52) was passed on March 30, 2010. Together these two laws are known as the Affordable Care Act of 2010 (ACA). The ACA contains many provisions designed to do the following:

- Improve the quality of Medicare services
- Support innovation and establish new payment models
- Better align Medicare payments with provider costs
- Strengthen program integrity within Medicare
- Position Medicare on a solid financial footing (CMS 2011, 67803)

Prior to the ACA, the Medicare Prescription Drug, Improvement, and Modernization Act of 2003 (MMA) called for significant changes to the Medicare system. MMA created an outpatient prescription drug benefit, provided beneficiaries with expanded coverage choices, and improved benefits.

Medicare is divided into four parts: Part A, Part B, Part C, and Part D. Recipients of Medicare may also purchase Medigap supplemental insurance to assist with paying cost-sharing provisions. The parts of Medicare and supplemental insurance are discussed in the sections that follow.

Medicare Part A

Medicare Part A is the portion of Medicare that provides benefits for hospital inpatient services. Individuals become eligible for Medicare Part A when they or their spouse has worked and paid Medicare taxes for at least 10 years. When this criterion is met, then Part A coverage is provided with no premiums. Most services covered under this benefit require that the beneficiary pay a cost-sharing amount. Services included in this benefit are as follows:

- Inpatient hospitalization
- Long-term care hospitalization
- Skilled nursing facility services
- Home health services
- Hospice care

Each site of service has specific limitations governing cost-sharing provisions per benefit period (table 3.1).

Even though most beneficiaries do not pay a monthly premium for Part A services, cost-sharing amounts play a critical role in Medicare beneficiary healthcare costs and facility reimbursement. Example 3.1 illustrates how to calculate the cost-sharing amount for an inpatient hospital admission for a Medicare beneficiary.

Table 3.1.   **Part A services 2023**

Site of Service	Benefit Period	Beneficiary Responsibility
Hospital inpatient and long-term care hospital; includes mental health inpatient stay	First 60 days Days 61–90 Days 91–150 (lifetime reserve days*) Beyond 150 days (lifetime reserve days*)	$1,600 per benefit period $400 per day $800 per day All costs
Skilled nursing facility	First 20 days Days 21–100 Beyond 100 days	Nothing $200 per day All costs
Home health	No time limit—based on medical necessity criteria	Nothing for services; durable medical equipment (DME) is included in Medicare Part B, see table 3.2
Hospice	No time limit—based on physician certification	Limited costs for outpatient drugs and inpatient respite care

*Nonrenewable lifetime reserve of up to 60 additional days of inpatient hospital care.
Source: Medicare.gov n.d.a.

Example 3.1

Shanice is a 65-year-old female. This is her fourth acute-care inpatient admission for this year. Shanice satisfied her deductible during her first admission of the year. The first admission was 28 days. The second admission was 25 days, and the third admission was 10 days. The length of stay for the fourth admission was 15 days. The first three admissions total 63 days. Therefore, Shanice has exhausted her Medicare days for this benefit period that do not require a copayment amount per day. Her entire fourth admission is in the Days 61–90 category shown in table 3.1. Therefore, Shanice is responsible for a cost-sharing amount of $6,000 ($400 × 15) for the fourth admission.

Medicare Part B

Medicare Part B, the portion of Medicare that covers outpatient care services, is an optional and supplemental insurance package that beneficiaries may purchase. In 2023, the standard monthly premium is $164.90 (Medicare.gov n.d.a). However, the premium is modified for beneficiaries whose income is over $87,000 as indicated on a filed tax return from two years prior to the current year. Part B insurance covers physician services, medical services, and medical supplies not covered by Part A. Most of these services are provided on an outpatient basis. In addition to the monthly premium, beneficiaries are responsible for an annual deductible and for service copayments. Table 3.2 provides a summary of the services and cost-sharing provisions.

Similar to Medicare Part A, cost-sharing amounts can be significant for Part B services. Example 3.2 illustrates the cost-sharing amount for a beneficiary who had a colonoscopy in the hospital outpatient setting.

Table 3.2.   Part B services 2023

Site of Service	Benefit	Beneficiary Responsibility
Medical services	Physician services, medical and surgical services and supplies, durable medical equipment (DME)	$226 annual deductible, plus 20% of approved amount (excludes hospital outpatient; see below)
	Behavioral health care	20% of most care
		20% of approved amount
Clinical laboratory services	Blood tests, urinalysis, and more	Nothing
Home health	Intermittent skilled care, home health aide service, DME and supplies, and other services	Nothing for services, 20% for DME
Outpatient hospital services	Services for diagnosis and/or treatment of an illness or injury	Annual deductible applies (see above) plus established copayment amount per covered service, which is usually 20%
		In addition to the amount paid to the physician there is also a copayment for the hospital. However, there are certain preventive services that do not have a copayment. The facility copayment for a single service cannot be higher than the hospital Part A deductible. Beneficiary is responsible for 100% of the charges for noncovered services
Outpatient mental health services	Yearly depression screening	Nothing
	Physician services or other healthcare provider visits	20% of approved amount; annual deductible applies
	Services provided at hospital outpatient department	20% of approved amount for physician services plus additional copayment or coinsurance amount for the facility; annual deductible applies
	Partial hospitalization mental health services (provided in hospital outpatient setting or community mental health center)	Percentage of the Medicare approved amount for each service provided by physician or certain other qualified mental health professional plus coinsurance for each day of partial hospitalization; annual deductible applies

Source: Medicare.gov n.d.a.

Example 3.2

Mateo is seen in the hospital outpatient gastrointestinal (GI) endoscopy lab for a colonoscopy with biopsy. This is his first outpatient encounter for the year. However, Mateo has already satisfied his Part B deductible because he has seen his physician several times and received physical therapy services for lower back pain. Since Mateo is receiving care in the hospital outpatient setting, he will be responsible for cost sharing for both the physician services and facility services. The allowed charges for the physician services total $200.85. Mateo is responsible for 20 percent of the allowed charges, or $40.17. The allowed charges for the facility services total $1,004.22. Mateo is responsible for 20 percent of the allowed charges, or $200.84. The total cost-sharing amount for this encounter is $241.02.

Medicare Part C

Medicare Part C combines Medicare Parts A and B into a managed care option known as **Medicare Advantage (MA)**. MA is an optional managed care plan for Medicare beneficiaries who are entitled to Part A, are enrolled in Part B, and live in an area with a plan. Types of plans available include health maintenance organization, point-of-service plan, preferred provider organization, and provider-sponsored organization. Because older adults often present with complex medical conditions, MA plans typically incorporate managed care concepts, such as case management and disease management.

Several services are excluded from Part A and Part B Medicare coverage. By enrolling in MA, beneficiaries have an increased set of benefits. The Part A and Part B excluded services that may be provided under Part C are as follows:

- Long-term care (custodial care)
- Dental care including dentures
- Eye exams including contacts and eyeglasses
- Fitness benefits including exercise classes
- Routine hearing care including hearing aids
- Transportation services
- Meal benefits like cooking classes, nutrition education, or meal delivery

MA is a significant component of Medicare with participation growing in the past decade. More than 26 million Medicare beneficiaries are enrolled in MA plans (Freed et al. 2021). Additionally, 89 percent of MA plans include Parts A, B, and D (prescription drug coverage). The average premium for these plans was approximately $19 per month for 2021 (Freed et al. 2021).

Special needs plans (SNPs), a form of MA plan, were established by the MMA of 2003 (Gold et al. 2011, 1). SNPs are designed to serve a disproportionately high-need population. There are three types of SNPs for three diverse groups of Medicare beneficiaries. The first type is the **dual eligible SNP (D-SNP)** for people who qualify for both Medicaid and Medicare. The second type of SNP is the **institutional SNP (I-SNP)** for beneficiaries who live in an institution like a nursing home or require nursing care at home. The third type is the **chronic condition SNP (C-SNP)**, which is for Medicare beneficiaries with severe disabling chronic conditions. Examples of disabling chronic conditions include chronic heart failure, diabetes mellitus, end-stage liver disease, and dementia (CMS 2021a). The Centers for Medicare and Medicaid Services (CMS) posts quality and performance ratings for MA plans to help beneficiaries make informed decisions regarding their participation in managed care. The rating scale is presented as a one-to-five-star scale with one star representing deficient performance, three stars representing average performance, and five stars representing excellent performance (CMS 2021b). In 2022, 68 percent of MA plans earned an overall four-star rating or higher (CMS 2021b). MA plans that receive a four-star rating or higher are eligible for bonus payments based on their quality ratings.

Medicare Part D

Medicare Part D, Medicare's prescription drug benefit program, was created by the MMA of 2003. The benefit was fully implemented on January 1, 2006. The program offers outpatient drug coverage provided by private prescription drug plans and MA. Most beneficiaries pay a monthly premium that varies by plan. CMS uses the beneficiary's yearly income from two years prior to the current benefit year to determine the final monthly premium for the current year. For example, in 2023, those beneficiaries who earned between $97,000 and $123,000 in 2021 pay $12.20 in addition to their monthly premium. In addition to the premium, beneficiaries have an annual deductible and make copayments for their prescriptions. Low-income beneficiary provisions are built into the program for older adults who cannot afford the standard copayment amounts. MMA also established improved access to pharmacies, an up-to-date formulary, and emergency access for Medicare beneficiaries.

For some beneficiaries, there is a coverage gap for prescription drugs. The **coverage gap** is a period of expanded cost sharing based on prescription drug utilization and cost for Part D beneficiaries. This coverage gap is also referred to as the "donut hole." For 2023, once the beneficiary and their plan have paid $4,660, the beneficiary enters the coverage gap (Medicare.gov n.d.b). When a beneficiary is in the coverage gap, their cost-sharing responsibility increases to 25 percent of the cost of brand-name and generic drugs. To get out of the coverage gap, the beneficiary and plan must reach the level of $7,400 for 2023. Costs that count toward exiting the coverage gap include the deductible, coinsurance, copayments, discounts beneficiaries receive on brand-name drugs in the coverage gap, and what beneficiaries pay in the coverage gap (Medicare.gov n.d.b). When a beneficiary leaves the coverage gap, they enter catastrophic coverage, and their plan covers 95 percent of their prescription drug costs.

Medicare Supplemental Insurance

Medicare beneficiaries may elect to purchase private insurance policies to supplement their Medicare Part A or Part B coverage. This supplemental insurance specific to Medicare is also known as Medigap. Medigap decreases the beneficiary's cost-sharing expenses, which are shown in tables 3.1 and 3.2. Medigap policies must meet federal standards and are offered by various private insurance companies.

Medicaid

Originally known as the Medical Assistance Program, **Medicaid** (Title XIX) was added to the Social Security Act in 1965. Medicaid is a joint program between the federal and state governments to provide healthcare benefits to low-income individuals and families or those who meet other eligibility requirements. This program is designed to allow each individual state to develop and maintain a Medicaid program unique to its state. Each state determines specific eligibility requirements and services to be offered, so coverage varies greatly from state to state. A person qualifying for services in one state may not qualify in another state. Furthermore, coverage determination for services is state-specific. Federal funds allocated to each state are based on the average income per person for that state. However, for a state to qualify to receive Medicaid federal funds, the state's program must provide coverage to mandatory eligibility groups designated by Medicaid. The following groups are examples from the list of Medicaid eligibility groups:

- Poverty-related infants, children, and pregnant women and deemed newborns
- Low-income families (families whose income falls below the state's designated limit)
- Families receiving transitional medical assistance
- Children with Title IV-E adoption assistance, foster care, or guardianship care, and children aging out of foster care
- Disabled adult children

- Specified low-income Medicare beneficiaries
- Aged, blind, and disabled individuals in 209(b) states (Medicaid.gov n.d.a)

In addition, the state program must offer a designated set of services to members to receive federal matching funds (figure 3.1). Eligibility and services may be expanded by individual states based on that state's laws and regulations. For example, states may elect to provide members with optometry services and eyeglasses or dental

Figure 3.1. Medicaid mandatory and optional benefits

Mandatory Benefits	
Inpatient hospital	Tobacco cessation counseling for pregnant women
Outpatient hospital	Physician
Rural health clinic	Nurse-midwife
Federally qualified health center	Certified pediatric and family nurse practitioner
Laboratory and x-ray	Freestanding birth centers
Nursing facility (age 21 and older)	Home health
Family planning	Medical transportation
Early and periodic screening, diagnostic, and treatment	

Optional Benefits	
Prescription drugs	Case management
Clinic	Dental and dentures
Occupational therapy, physical therapy and speech, hearing, and language disorder services	Respiratory care services
Podiatry	Self-directed personal assistance services
Optometry and eyeglasses	Personal care
Prosthetic devices	Inpatient psychiatric services, ages less than 21
Chiropractor	Health homes for enrollees with chronic conditions
Other practitioner services	Other diagnostic, screening, preventative, and rehabilitative services
Private duty nursing services	Hospice
Intermediate care facilities for individuals with intellectual disabilities	Individuals age 65 or older in an institution for mental disease (IMD)
State plan home and community-based services	Community first choice option
TB related services	Other services approved by the secretary

Source: Medicaid.gov n.d.d.

services. States are also afforded the flexibility to determine cost-sharing (deductible and copayment) terms for their programs for certain services and members. For example, family planning services are exempt from cost sharing, as are services to pregnant women and children younger than 18 years.

Since its inception, federal law has allowed for expanded eligibility. For example, most recently, the ACA expanded Medicaid eligibility to all adults under age 65 who are not pregnant or disabled and have incomes up to 133 percent of the federal poverty level (FPL) (Medicaid.gov n.d.b). Congress has also established additional eligibility pathways, so states can expand coverage to other groups as warranted in their states. For example, the Katie Beckett option allows states to cover children under 19 years of age who are disabled and living at home (Medicaid.gov n.d.c). This special eligibility group covers children with designated long-term disabilities or special healthcare needs.

State programs may also offer managed care options. There are four main types of managed care delivery systems used for Medicaid:

- Managed care organizations (MCOs): MCOs cover all or most Medicaid-covered services.

- Primary care case management: Each beneficiary has a primary care provider who assumes responsibility for managing and coordinating their basic medical care.

- Prepaid inpatient health plan: Plans manage limited benefit packages for services such as inpatient mental health or substance abuse benefits.

- Prepaid ambulatory health plan: Plans manage limited benefit packages for services such as dental or transportation. (Medicaid.gov n.d.e)

When managed care became a primary focus in the mid-1990s, Medicaid encouraged families and children to enroll in managed care plans. As of 2022, 41 states and Washington, DC, enrolled Medicaid beneficiaries in a comprehensive risk-based MCO (Hinton and Raphael 2023). In most of these states, at least 75 percent of Medicaid beneficiaries were enrolled in the Medicaid comprehensive risk-based MCO (Hinton and Raphael 2023). Overall, in 2022 over two-thirds (72 percent) of all Medicaid beneficiaries were enrolled in a comprehensive managed care plan (Hinton and Raphael 2023). Data show that managed care penetration continues to grow for Medicaid.

Check Your Understanding 3.1

1. Match each Medicare part with the type of benefit it provides.

a. Part A	_____ Medicare drug benefit
b. Part B	_____ Physician services
c. Part C	_____ Inpatient hospital services
d. Part D	_____ Medicare Advantage

2. Arnav is a Medicare beneficiary who is covered under Part A and Part B. His first acute-care inpatient admission for the benefit period was 10 days long. This was his first healthcare encounter for the benefit year. The allowed charges for the admission were $7,845.50. What is Arnav's cost-sharing amount?

3. What benefits will a Medicare beneficiary gain by choosing Medicare Part C?

4. Describe the Part D coverage gap.

5. Why is Medicaid coverage not identical in New Jersey, California, and Idaho?

Other Government-Sponsored Healthcare Programs

The other major government-sponsored healthcare programs serve older adults, persons with disabilities, children from low-income families, veterans, active-duty military personnel, Native Americans, and sick or injured employees. Those government-sponsored healthcare programs include the following:

- Programs of All-Inclusive Care for the Elderly (PACE)
- Children's Health Insurance Program (CHIP)
- TRICARE
- Veterans Health Administration (VA)
- Civilian Health and Medical Program of the Department of Veterans Affairs (CHAMPVA)
- Indian Health Service (IHS)
- Workers' compensation

Each of these programs serves a specific target group and has specific eligibility requirements, plan requirements, and participant benefits. In the sections that follow, each program will be explored.

Programs of All-Inclusive Care for the Elderly

The Balanced Budget Act of 1997 (BBA) authorized the creation of **Programs of All-Inclusive Care for the Elderly (PACE)**. PACE is a joint Medicare-Medicaid venture that offers states the option of creating and administering this managed care option for the frail older adult population (Medicaid.gov n.d.f). PACE was designed to enhance the quality of life for the frail older adult population by enabling them to live in their own homes and communities and to preserve and support their family units. Individuals eligible for Medicare or Medicaid, or both, may join PACE if it is available in their community. PACE programs offer a robust benefit package, including all the care and services covered by Medicare and Medicaid. The following is a list of the benefits provided for all PACE beneficiaries:

- Hospital care
- Primary care services (includes doctor and nursing services)
- Home care
- Dentistry
- Laboratory and x-ray services
- Prescription drugs
- Nursing home care
- Emergency services
- Social work counseling
- Medical specialty services
- Adult day healthcare
- Personal care services
- Physical and occupational therapies
- Nutritional counseling

- Recreational therapy

- Transportation

- Meals

- Social services (Medicaid.gov n.d.g)

To have a PACE program, states must provide services in at least one facility in a geographic service area. The facilities must be accessible and offer adequate services to meet the needs of all participants in the programs. Additional facilities must be staffed and supply a full range of services when warranted by the growth of the PACE population in a service area. Beneficiaries may frequent the facility as determined by the multidisciplinary team and the patient's needs. Each facility must have in place an interdisciplinary provider team consisting of at least the following members:

- Primary care physician

- Nurse

- Physical therapist

- Occupational therapist

- Recreation therapist or activity coordinator

- Dietitian

- PACE center supervisor

- Home care liaison

- Personal care attendants

- Driver (Medicaid.gov n.d.g)

Beneficiaries of PACE, frail older individuals, must be a minimum of 55 years of age, reside in the PACE service area, be certified by the state to require nursing home–level care, and be able to live safely in the community with help from PACE.

Enrollment in PACE programs is not offered in all states, nor even in all service areas within states. The PACE program agreement between the state and CMS defines the service areas available to beneficiaries.

Children's Health Insurance Program

The **Children's Health Insurance Program (CHIP)** (formerly known as the State Children's Health Insurance Program [SCHIP]), or Title XXI of the Social Security Act, was created in 1997 by the BBA. CHIP is a state-federal partnership that targets the growing number of children not covered by health insurance. This program aims to provide health coverage to uninsured children in families whose income is too high for Medicaid but who are unable to pay for a private insurance policy for the family. CHIP was most recently renewed through the Helping Ensure Access for Little Ones, Toddlers, and Hopeful Youth by Keeping Insurance Delivery Stable Act of 2017 (HEALTHY KIDS Act). This act extended CHIP through 2027.

Currently, CHIP provides healthcare coverage to nearly 10 million children. Income requirements vary from state to state but range from 170 percent of the FPL to 400 percent of the FPL. This program targets children in low-income families. To qualify for the program, a child must meet the following requirements:

- Under 19 years of age

- Uninsured

- Citizen or meet immigration requirements

- Resident of the state where the child is seeking coverage

- Eligible within the state's CHIP income range, based on family income, and any other state-specified rules in the CHIP state plan (Medicaid.gov n.d.h)

CHIP varies from state to state. Each state may determine how it would like to deliver the healthcare benefit to qualifying individuals. The state may elect to expand Medicaid eligibility to children who would qualify for CHIP. The state may design a separate program to provide the benefit, or the state may combine the Medicaid expansion and separate program concepts; regardless of the individual program design, CMS must approve state plans and revisions. With several delivery options comes multiple benefit options. States with a Medicaid expansion of CHIP provide the Early and Periodic Screening, Diagnostic, and Treatment services (EPSDT) benefit. This benefit package is comprehensive and designed to provide early detection of health problems so children are diagnosed and treated as promptly as possible.

There are mandatory benefits for separate CHIP programs developed by states. They must provide well-baby care and well-child care, dental coverage, behavioral healthcare, and vaccines. Additionally, states have three options for benefit packages: benchmark coverage, benchmark-equivalent coverage, or secretary-approved coverage. Benchmark coverage includes a benefits package that is equal to the health benefits found in one of three specified plans as shown in table 3.3.

Benchmark-equivalent coverage plans have the same actuarial value as the benchmark coverage plans in table 3.3. The benchmark-equivalent benefits package must include mandatory coverage benefits and additionally include the following:

- Inpatient hospital services

- Outpatient hospital services

- Physicians' medical and surgical services

- Laboratory and radiology services (Medicaid.gov n.d.i)

In secretary-approved coverage, the "secretary" refers to the secretary of Health and Human Services. This coverage consists of the health benefits coverage that the secretary has determined to provide appropriate coverage for low-income children covered under CHIP. This coverage may be the same as the coverage provided under the state Medicaid plan, but it may also include expanded benefits.

States may elect to require cost-sharing provisions for beneficiaries enrolled in the program. Types of cost sharing include enrollment fees, premiums, deductibles, coinsurance, and copayment. States' FPL requirements

Table 3.3.   Benchmark coverage plans

Federal Employees Health Benefit Plan	Standard Blue Cross Blue Shield preferred provider option service benefit plan offered to federal employees
State Employee Plan	Health benefits plan that is offered and generally available to state employees in the state
Health Maintenance Organization (HMO) Plan	Health insurance coverage plan that is offered through an HMO, as defined in the Public Health Service Act, and has the largest insured commercial, non-Medicaid enrollment in the state

Source: Medicaid.gov n.d.i.

vary, so there are different cost-sharing maximum thresholds. For families with incomes at or below 150 percent of the FPL, premiums cannot exceed the amount permitted in Medicaid. For families with incomes above 150 percent of the FPL, cumulative state cost-sharing provisions cannot exceed 5 percent of a family's income. There are, however, cost-sharing limitations. Beneficiaries cannot be asked to cost share, in any form, for well-baby and well-child services. States may not require cost sharing of American Indian or Alaskan Native children. And states cannot establish cost sharing in any way that favors children from higher-income families over children from lower-income families (Medicaid.gov n.d.j).

TRICARE

The Department of Defense provides a healthcare program for active-duty and retired members of the eight uniformed services of the US: Air Force, Army, Coast Guard, Marine Corps, Navy, Space Force, National Oceanic and Atmospheric Administration (NOAA) Commissioned Corps, and Public Health Service Commissioned Corps. In addition, coverage is provided for such members' families and survivors. The healthcare program is now titled **TRICARE**, replacing the Civilian Health and Medical Program of the Uniformed Services (CHAMPUS), which was enacted in 1966 by amendments to the Dependents Medical Care Act of 1956. TRICARE provides comprehensive coverage for all beneficiaries:

- Outpatient visits

- Hospitalization

- Preventive services

- Maternity care

- Immunizations

- Mental and behavioral healthcare

TRICARE offers several different health plan options to provide coverage for beneficiaries around the globe. Active-duty service members (ADSMs) may enroll only in a TRICARE prime plan, but several additional plans are available for active-duty family members (ADFMs), retirees, and their family members and retirees' survivors. In the sections that follow, each TRICARE option will be discussed.

TRICARE Prime Options

TRICARE Prime and TRICARE Prime Remote are the program's managed care options. All ADSMs and activated Guard or Reserve members are automatically covered by one of these programs, although the individual must complete an enrollment form and submit it to the regional contractor. TRICARE Prime is required when ADSMs live and work within 50 miles, or less than an hour's drive, from a military treatment facility.

TRICARE Prime Remote is required when ADSMs live and work in remote areas. By using this option, a member may access primary care from an out-of-network provider if in-network providers are unavailable in the area. There are no enrollment fees, deductibles, or copayments for authorized medical services and prescriptions with either TRICARE option.

TRICARE Prime Overseas and TRICARE Prime Remote Overseas follow the same concept as Prime and Prime Remote, but the ADSMs and ADFMs, if applicable, are located overseas.

ADFMs may also enroll in TRICARE Prime, Prime Remote, Prime Overseas, and Prime Remote Overseas. This is the most economical program available for military families because there are no enrollment, deductible, or copayment fees for covered services. To participate in the managed care option, ADFMs must enroll during an open enrollment period.

The US Family Health Plan is a component of the TRICARE Prime plan that is available to all ADFMs, retirees, and retiree family members. After enrolling, beneficiaries will not access Medicare providers, military treatment facilities, or TRICARE network providers. They will instead receive care (including prescription drug coverage) from a primary care manager (PCM) for most of their care. The PCM is a military or network provider that provides care, coordinates care, and initiates referrals to specialists when necessary.

TRICARE Select and TRICARE Select Overseas

If ADFMs do not want to enroll in the managed care options, they can participate in TRICARE Select, which requires members to pay an annual outpatient deductible as well as a cost share of allowed charges. The cost-sharing provisions vary by type of service. For most services, there is a copayment amount for in-network providers and a coinsurance amount for out-of-network providers. The ADFM need not enroll in the plan. Rather, each family member is included in the Defense Enrollment Eligibility Reporting System (DEERS), which outlines eligibility dates. Service members are responsible for maintaining up-to-date information in DEERS.

The National Defense Authorization Act for federal fiscal year 2005 expanded TRICARE coverage, making it available for Reserve Component (RC) members and their dependents when the RC member is called to active duty (on orders) for more than 30 consecutive days. RC dependents become eligible for TRICARE Select on the first day of the RC member's orders if the orders are for more than 30 days. RC dependents may choose to enroll in TRICARE Select any time during the first month of the RC member's activation.

TRICARE Young Adult

This plan option is available for young adult children of ADSMs, Reserve members, and military retirees. For young adults to qualify, they must be a child of a qualified military member, 21 to 25 years old, unmarried, and not eligible to enroll in an employer-sponsored health plan based on their own employment (TRICARE 2021). TRICARE Young Adult is a premium-based plan with additional cost-sharing services. The Prime option allows for lower cost sharing per visit: free care at military treatment facilities (with a few exclusions), a small copayment for in-network outpatient providers, and a small per-day copayment for in-network inpatient providers. The Select option allows greater flexibility by allowing out-of-network providers but requires a percentage coinsurance for in-network and out-of-network visits.

TRICARE Reserve Select and TRICARE Retired Reserve

TRICARE Reserve Select is a premium-based health plan that qualified National Guard and Reserve members may purchase. Individual plans and a family plan are available. In addition to the monthly premium, there is a copayment amount for in-network providers that varies by the healthcare setting or type of provider. The Retired Reserve plan is similar but has higher premiums and higher coinsurance and copayment amounts for services. Additionally, for both plans, there are separate cost-sharing provisions for overseas care.

TRICARE for Life

TRICARE for Life (TFL) is TRICARE's secondary coverage (Medicare-wraparound coverage) for TRICARE beneficiaries who have Medicare Part A and Part B. Essentially, TRICARE becomes the secondary payer to Medicare. TFL minimizes cost-sharing amounts, such as deductibles and copayment amounts for services that are covered by both Medicare and TRICARE. ADSMs, ADFMs, and retirees are eligible for TFL. Medicare, TFL, and TRICARE Prime work together as primary and secondary insurance plans based on the ADSM's or ADFM's eligibility status.

Veterans Health Administration

The **Veterans Health Administration (VA)** is the nation's largest integrated healthcare system, with over 1,200 care sites serving over 9 million veterans each year (VA 2023). The VA encourages all veterans to apply to determine eligibility for health benefits. Basic eligibility includes veterans who served in active military service and were separated under any condition other than dishonorable, as well as current and former members of the Reserves or National Guard called to active duty by federal order and having completed the full period for which they were called or ordered to active duty. The minimum duty requirement for most who enlisted after September 7, 1980, or entered active duty after October 16, 1981, is service of 24 continuous months or the full period for which they were called to active duty. There are, however, many exceptions to the eligibility and minimum duty requirements, so all veterans are encouraged to apply. The VA program requires enrollment for participation in the program, but after enrolling, the member remains enrolled and has access to certain VA health benefits. Program members are placed into one of eight priority groups based on their individual service and circumstances. Figure 3.2 provides a sampling of the priority groups and those who qualify for each level.

The VA provides healthcare services at little or no cost to its members. There are copayments for treatment of nonservice-connected conditions. At the time of enrollment, veterans complete a financial assessment that determines their level of copayment for services. The cost-sharing amounts are matched to the priority group in which the veteran is placed. For example, in 2023, a member in priority group 7 has a copayment rate of $15 for primary care (outpatient) services. Members in priority group 8 have a copayment amount of $5 for Tier 1 medications, which include preferred generic prescription medicines (VA 2022b). Having private insurance does not affect a veteran's eligibility for VA services. Veterans can choose to use their private insurance to supplement their VA benefits. For example, many private insurance plans will cover VA copayment requirements.

Civilian Health and Medical Program of the Department of Veterans Affairs

The Department of Veterans Affairs provides covered healthcare services and supplies to eligible beneficiaries through the **Civilian Health and Medical Program of the Department of Veterans Affairs (CHAMPVA)**. This benefits program is available for the spouse or widow(er) and children of a veteran who meets or met one of the following criteria:

- Permanently and totally disabled due to a service-connected disability

- At the time of death, the veteran was permanently and totally disabled due to a VA-rated service-connected condition

- Died of a VA-rated service-connected disability

- Died on active duty, not due to misconduct (most often these family members are eligible for TRICARE instead of CHAMPVA)

Individuals eligible for TRICARE benefits cannot participate in CHAMPVA. This program covers most healthcare services and supplies that are medically and psychologically necessary. There are deductibles and

Figure 3.2. **Sample of VHA priority groups**

Priority Group 1
- Veterans with service-connected disabilities rated by the VA as 50% or more disabling
- Veterans determined by the VA as unable to work due to service-connected conditions
- Veterans who have received the Medal of Honor (MOH)

Priority Group 2
- Veterans with service-connected disabilities rated by the VA as 30% or 40% disabling

Priority Group 3
- Veterans who are former prisoners of war (POWs)
- Veterans awarded a Purple Heart medal
- Veterans whose discharge was for a disability that was incurred or got worse because of active duty
- Veterans with service-connected disabilities rated by the VA as 10% or 20% disabling
- Veterans awarded special eligibility classification under Title 38, USC Section 1151, "benefits for individuals disabled by treatment or vocational rehabilitation"

Source: Adapted from VA 2022a.

cost-sharing provisions. For example, there is an outpatient coinsurance amount of 25 percent of the allowable amount (VA 2021, 62). CHAMPVA becomes a secondary payer when another health insurance benefit is available. For example, when a beneficiary reaches age 65, Medicare is the primary payer and CHAMPVA becomes the secondary payer.

Indian Health Service

The **Indian Health Service (IHS)** was created to uphold the federal government's obligation to promote healthy American Indian and Alaskan Native people, communities, and cultures (IHS n.d.a). A government-to-government relationship between the US and American Indian nations was established in 1787 based on Article I, Section 8, of the US Constitution. From this relationship came the provision of health services for members of federally recognized nations. Principal legislation for authorizing federal funds for the IHS is the Snyder Act of 1921. The IHS is an agency within the Department of Health and Human Services.

The strategic goals of the IHS include the following:

- to ensure that comprehensive, culturally appropriate personal and public health services are available and accessible to American Indian and Alaska Native people;

- to promote excellence and quality through innovation of the Indian health system into an optimally performing organization; and

- to strengthen IHS program management and operations. (IHS n.d.b)

Healthcare services offered by the IHS include inpatient and outpatient care, immunization, and physical rehabilitation. The federal IHS healthcare delivery system consists of hospitals, health centers, health stations, and residential treatment centers.

Workers' Compensation

The **workers' compensation** benefit is provided to most employees to cover healthcare costs and the loss of income that results from a work-related injury or illness. Federal government employees are covered under the **Federal Employees' Compensation Act of 1916 (FECA)**, a benefit program that ensures civilian employees of the federal government are provided medical, death, and income benefits for work-related injuries and illnesses. Other employees are covered under state workers' compensation insurance funds if that program is established in the state in which the employees work.

The Office of Workers' Compensation Programs (OWCP), a division of the Department of Labor, administers FECA. OWCP also administered the Longshore and Harbor Workers' Compensation Act of 1927 and the Black Lung Benefits Reform Act of 1977.

State workers' compensation insurance funds are established by each state. Benefits may include burial, death, income, and medical. Rather than contracting individually with insurance companies for coverage, employers pay premiums into the nonprofit workers' compensation fund for their state. This allows the workers' compensation premiums to remain low and affordable for small-business owners.

Check Your Understanding 3.2

1. Match each TRICARE health plan on the right with its description on the left.

a.	ADFM aged 21–25 years old	_____ TRICARE for Life
b.	Traditional insurance plan for ADFMs (non-managed care)	_____ TRICARE Prime
c.	Managed care plan for ADSMs and ADFMs	_____ TRICARE Select
d.	Secondary payer for Medicare Part A and B eligible beneficiaries	_____ TRICARE Young Adult

(continued)

Check Your Understanding 3.2   *(continued)*

2.   Which population is targeted by the PACE program? Why was this population selected?

3.   How are veterans placed into different health plans?

4.   Provide two examples of how CHIP varies from state to state.

5.   How many children are enrolled in CHIP?

Patient Connection

In chapter 1, "Healthcare Reimbursement and Revenue Cycle Management," the Patient Connection section introduced Malakai. Malakai is a 68-year-old male who is enrolled in Medicare. Malakai is enrolled in traditional Medicare Part A and has purchased Parts B and D. Malakai's Part B premium is $170 per month. His Part D premium is $30 per month. As discussed earlier in this chapter, tables 3.1 and 3.2 provide cost-sharing amounts applicable for Medicare beneficiaries in 2023. We will use these figures in this Patient Connection.

Malakai's friend Zach is enrolled in a Medicare Advantage (MA) plan through Best Insurance Company. Zach told Malakai that he only pays $50 per month for his Medicare premium. Remember that MA (Medicare Part C) includes Medicare Parts A, B, and D and is a managed care option. Zach helps Malakai arrange a meeting with his Best Insurance Company representative to discuss his options for the next open election period. Malakai decides to investigate why his premium is so much higher for traditional Medicare and wants to understand the impact of switching to an MA plan prior to his meeting.

To begin, Malakai researches the costs for MA plans on the Medicare.gov website. Here he finds there are several qualifiers for how much it actually costs a beneficiary in an MA plan. This information leads Malakai to list the following questions for his meeting with a Best Insurance Company representative:

- Does the MA plan offered by Best Insurance Company have a yearly deductible?
- How much do beneficiaries pay for each visit or service (copayment or coinsurance)?
- Do you limit the physicians that I can see? Can I only see certain doctors?
- What extra benefits are offered? How much do I have to pay for these benefits?

Malakai's biggest concerns are being able to continue to see his long-term primary care physician and how much he will have to pay for each visit. During his meeting with Best Insurance Company he finds out the following:

- He has to pay more to see out-of-network providers.
- Office visits and physical therapy will have a copayment amount of $15 for the upcoming year.
- There is one annual deductible amount of $150 for all types of services (inpatient, outpatient, and pharmacy).

Malakai's physician, Dr. Lewis, is not included in the Best Insurance Company's network of providers. Instead of a $15 copayment, Malakai will have to pay a 30 percent coinsurance amount to see Dr. Lewis. Currently, Malakai only pays 20 percent coinsurance. To help him decide, Malakai compares estimates of his medical expenses from last year to MA rates offered by Best Insurance Company.

(continued)

Last Year's Services for Malakai	Traditional Medicare (estimate)	Medicare Advantage (estimate)
Outpatient visits (4) with Dr. Lewis	$226 deductible + $120 for coinsurance. [Total allowed charges were $600. $600 × 0.20 = $120]	$150 deductible + $180 for coinsurance. [Total allowed charges were $600. $600 × 0.30 = $180]
Physical therapy visits (6) in network	$180 in coinsurance. [Total allowed charges were $900. $900 × 0.20 = $180]	$90 in copayment. [6 visits × $15 = $90]
Depression screening	$0	$0
TOTAL	$526	$420

Overall, even with Dr. Lewis being out-of-network, Malakai would most likely pay less under MA. But what if he has to see the doctor more often? Currently, he is not required to take any prescription drugs. What if that changes? He has played basketball his whole life; what if his knee pain gets worse? Is the reduction in premium enough to offset the higher coinsurance amount for seeing Dr. Lewis? Malakai has four more months to decide if he wants to switch, so he decides to do more research and give his decision more thought.

Chapter 3 Review Quiz

1. Katrina is a Medicare Part A beneficiary. She has met her Part A deductible. During March and April, Katrina had a 22-day stay in a skilled nursing facility. What is her cost-sharing amount?

   a. $0—Katrina's cost-sharing obligation does not apply to skilled nursing care

   b. $352

   c. $1,408

   d. $1,760

2. Which part of Medicare is the managed care option?

3. When was Medicare Part D added to the Medicare benefit package? What services did it add?

4. List at least three eligibility requirements mandated for states to qualify for federal matching funds.

5. List three examples of services provided under PACE.

6. What is the target population of the Children's Health Insurance Program (CHIP) (Title XXI)?

7. Which TRICARE program is the most economical program for military families, and why is it less expensive than the other options?

8. What program covers healthcare costs and loss of income from work-related injuries or illness of federal government employees?

9. What services must be included in CHIP plans?

10. Which act set regulations for injured federal workers?

References

CMS (Centers for Medicare and Medicaid Services). 2021a. "Special Needs Plans." https://www.cms.gov/Medicare/Health-Plans/SpecialNeedsPlans.

CMS (Centers for Medicare and Medicaid Services). 2021b. "CMS Releases 2022 Medicare Advantage and Part D Star Ratings to Help Medicare Beneficiaries Compare Plans." https://www.cms.gov/newsroom/press-releases/cms-releases-2022-medicare-advantage-and-part-d-star-ratings-help-medicare-beneficiaries-compare.

CMS (Centers for Medicare and Medicaid Services). 2011. Medicare program: Medicare shared savings program: Accountable care organizations; Final rule. *Federal Register* 76(212):67802–67990.

Freed, M., A. Damico, and T. Newman. 2021. "Medicare Advantage Spotlight: First Look." Kaiser Family Foundation. https://www.kff.org/medicare/issue-brief/medicare-advantage-2022-spotlight-first-look/.

Gold, M., G. Jacobson, A. Damico, and T. Neuman. 2011. "Special Needs Plans: Availability and Enrollment." http://www.kff.org/medicare/upload/8229.pdf.

Hinton, E. and J. Raphael. 2023. "10 Things to Know about Medicaid Managed Care." https://www.kff.org/medicaid/issue-brief/10-things-to-know-about-medicaid-managed-care/.

IHS (Indian Health Service). n.d.a. "About IHS." Accessed February 9, 2023. https://www.ihs.gov/aboutihs/.

IHS (Indian Health Service). n.d.b. "Agency Overview." Accessed February 9, 2023. https://www.ihs.gov/aboutihs/overview/.

Medicaid.gov. n.d.a. "List of Medicaid Eligibility Groups." Accessed February 9, 2023. https://www.medicaid.gov/sites/default/files/2019-12/list-of-eligibility-groups.pdf.

Medicaid.gov. n.d.b. "Medicaid Eligibility." Accessed February 9, 2023. https://www.medicaid.gov/medicaid/eligibility/index.html.

Medicaid.gov. n.d.c. Implementation Guide: Medicaid State Plan Eligibility Children under Age 19 with a Disability. Accessed June 19, 2023. https://www.medicaid.gov/resources-for-states/downloads/macpro-ig-children-under-age-19-with-a-disability.pdf.

Medicaid.gov. n.d.d. "Mandatory & Optional Medicaid Benefits." Accessed February 9, 2023. https://www.medicaid.gov/medicaid/benefits/mandatory-optional-medicaid-benefits/index.html.

Medicaid.gov. n.d.e. "Managed Care Entities." Accessed February 9, 2023. https://www.medicaid.gov/medicaid/managed-care/managed-care-entities/index.html.

Medicaid.gov. n.d.f. "Program of All-Inclusive Care for the Elderly." Accessed February 9, 2023. https://www.medicaid.gov/medicaid/long-term-services-supports/program-all-inclusive-care-elderly/index.html.

Medicaid.gov. n.d.g. "Program of All-Inclusive Care for the Elderly Benefits." Accessed February 9, 2023. https://www.medicaid.gov/medicaid/long-term-services-supports/pace/programs-all-inclusive-care-elderly-benefits/index.html.

Medicaid.gov. n.d.h. "CHIP Eligibility." Accessed February 9, 2023. https://www.medicaid.gov/chip/eligibility/index.html.

Medicaid.gov. n.d.i. "CHIP Benefits." Accessed February 9, 2023. https://www.medicaid.gov/chip/benefits/index.html.

Medicaid.gov. n.d.j. "CHIP Cost Sharing." Accessed February 9, 2023. https://www.medicaid.gov/chip/chip-cost-sharing/index.html.

Medicare.gov. n.d.a. "Your Medicare Costs." Accessed January 27, 2023. https://www.medicare.gov/your-medicare-costs.

Medicare.gov. n.d.b. "Costs in the Coverage Gap." Accessed January 27, 2023. https://www.medicare.gov/drug-coverage-part-d/costs-for-medicare-drug-coverage/costs-in-the-coverage-gap.

TRICARE. 2021. "TRICARE Plans & Eligibility." https://www.tricare.mil/Plans.

VA (Veterans Health Administration). 2023. "Veterans Health Administration." https://www.va.gov/health/.

VA (Veterans Health Administration). 2022a. "VA Priority Groups." https://www.va.gov/health-care/eligibility/priority-groups/.

VA (Veterans Health Administration). 2022b. "VA Health Care Copay Rates." https://www.va.gov/health-care/copay-rates/.

VA (Veterans Health Administration). 2021. CHAMPVA Guide. https://www.va.gov/COMMUNITYCARE/docs/pubfiles/programguides/champva_guide.pdf.

Part II:
Reimbursement
Methodologies and
Payment Systems

Chapter 4
Healthcare Reimbursement Methodologies

Learning Objectives

- ❖ Define retrospective reimbursement
- ❖ Define prospective reimbursement
- ❖ Compare the types of healthcare reimbursement methodologies
- ❖ Differentiate retrospective reimbursement methodologies from prospective reimbursement methodologies
- ❖ Illustrate how diagnosis coding is used in risk adjustment models
- ❖ Describe how accountable care organizations combine reimbursement methodologies to create a hybrid payment system

Key Terms

Accountable care organization (ACO)
Allowable charge
Attribution
Billed charges
Bundled payment
Capitation
Case-rate methodology
CMS hierarchical condition categories (CMS-HCC) model
Fee schedule

Global payment method
One-sided risk
Payment
Per diem payment
Per member per month (PMPM)
Percent of billed charges
Prospective reimbursement
Retrospective reimbursement
Risk adjustment
Two-sided risk

Healthcare reimbursement in the US is a complex topic. Before exploring the various reimbursement methods, it is important to review some terms that are used regularly. **Billed charges**, or charges, refers to the price assigned to a unit of medical or health service, such as a visit to a physician or a day in a hospital. This is analogous to the retail price or price tag on an item one may purchase at a store. **Allowable charges**, or allowable amount, is the amount that the third-party payer or insurance company will pay for a service. This term is typically used in the physician setting. The terms **payment** and reimbursement are often used interchangeably; both refer to the amount paid to a healthcare provider for services provided to a patient. In this chapter, the terms third-party payer and payer are used interchangeably. Both terms are commonly used in practice and are interchanged in most healthcare settings. The basic concepts of the most popular reimbursement methodologies are presented in this chapter.

Types of Healthcare Reimbursement Methodologies

The fundamental concepts in healthcare reimbursement methodologies are discussed in this section. Third-party payers such as Medicare, Medicaid, and commercial payers use a variety of reimbursement methodologies to set reimbursement rates for services. The type of reimbursement methodology to be used is first introduced by the third-party payer during contract negotiations with the provider. The third-party payer and the provider negotiate the reimbursement methodology and terms to be used for the provider's fiscal year. Therefore, the type and level of reimbursement greatly varies from payer to payer and provider to provider. This results in different reimbursement levels among Medicare, Medicaid, and commercial payers. This section is organized by the two major types of payment: retrospective reimbursement and prospective reimbursement. **Retrospective reimbursement** is based on the actual resources expended to deliver the services and is finalized after the services are delivered. **Prospective reimbursement** is established prior to the healthcare delivery and does not change based on the costs of the actual services delivered to the patient. Table 4.1 lists the most common reimbursement methodologies organized by type. In the upcoming sections, retrospective reimbursement and prospective reimbursement methodologies will be discussed.

Retrospective Reimbursement

In the retrospective reimbursement methodology, the third-party payer bases reimbursement on the actual resources expended to deliver the services. Since the total amount of resources is not known until after the services are delivered, the payer reviews the services delivered and determines the reimbursement amount. Determining total reimbursement after service delivery is the foundation of retrospective reimbursement. Historically, this was the predominant method of reimbursement. Although still used today, fewer payers utilize retrospective reimbursement methodologies.

In retrospective reimbursement methodologies, the payer has established rates for each service that may be provided to the patient, but the total reimbursement for the health services is based on procedure and service mix and level of utilization. For example, it is known that the patient will receive preoperative laboratory services, but the actual laboratory services the physician orders and completes for the patient is unknown until after the visit. The number of services the patient receives could also be unknown until delivery, such as for inpatient admissions. For example, it is known that the patient will be admitted for heart surgery, but the number of days the patient stays in an acute-care setting is unknown until the patient is discharged. Examples of retrospective reimbursement methodologies are fee schedule, percent of billed charges, and per diem. Table 4.2 provides characteristics of the different retrospective reimbursement methodologies.

Fee schedule, percent of billed charges, and per diem payment methodologies and criticisms are discussed in the sections that follow.

Fee Schedule

In a retrospective reimbursement environment, third-party payers establish a **fee schedule**. A fee schedule is a predetermined list of fees that the third-party payer allows for payment for a set of healthcare services. Fee schedules are most often used for physician or clinician reimbursement or outpatient facility ancillary services, such as radiology or laboratory tests. Figure 4.1 provides an example of a physician office fee schedule. The contracting unit in this methodology is the service. The fee (third column in figure 4.1) or allowable charge represents the average or maximum amount the third-party payer will reimburse providers for the service. It may appear as if the fee schedule methodology is a blend of retrospective and prospective payments, as the fee is set in advance for a given service via the fee schedule. However, the type of services and the volume of services are unknown until the visit or encounter is completed. This results in the payer not knowing the exact services delivered until after the care has been provided. Therefore, fee schedules are considered a retrospective reimbursement methodology.

Table 4.1.   **Reimbursement methodologies examples**

Retrospective Reimbursement Methodologies	Prospective Reimbursement Methodologies
Fee schedule	Capitated payment
Percent of billed charges	Case rate
Per diem	Bundled payment
	Global payment

Table 4.2.   **Characteristics of retrospective reimbursement methodologies**

Reimbursement Methodology	Contracting Unit	Alternative Terminology
Fee schedule	Service	Fee-for-service
Percent of billed charges	Claim	Discounted fee-for-service, discounted rate
Per diem payment	Day	Daily rate, or per day rate

Figure 4.1.   **Sample fee schedule for physician office**

HCPCS Code	Service Description	Fee*
99201	Office visit, new patient, level 1	$35.00
99202	Office visit, new patient, level 2	$50.00
99203	Office visit, new patient, level 3	$95.00
99204	Office visit, new patient, level 4	$115.00
99205	Office visit, new patient, level 5	$145.00
90632	Hepatitis A vaccine, adult	$55.00
90636	Hepatitis A and hepatitis B vaccine, adult	$105.00
71045	Chest x-ray, single view	$45.50
71046	Chest x-ray, 2 views	$52.75
71047	Chest x-ray, 3 views	$61.35
71048	Chest x-ray, 4 or more views	$80.25
81000	Urinalysis, by dip stick or tablet; non-auto with microscopy	$7.00
81001	Urinalysis, by dip stick or tablet; auto with microscopy	$7.00
81002	Urinalysis, by dip stick or tablet; non-auto without microscopy	$5.00
81003	Urinalysis, by dip stick or tablet; auto without microscopy	$5.00

*Fee is fictitious and should not be used for rate setting.

Percent of Billed Charges

To control their costs, third-party payers negotiate reduced fees for their members or beneficiaries. Specifically, the payer reimburses the facility or provider a percentage of the charge amount for a service, supply, procedure, or admission. This methodology is commonly referred to as **percent of billed charges**. In this methodology, the contracting unit is the claim. Figure 4.2 illustrates one example, in which a third-party payer agrees to pay 64 percent of all covered charges. In this example, the covered charges for this admission total $11,791.08. The reimbursement is $7,546.29 or 64 percent of the total covered charges. Contracts that use the percent of billed charges methodology are now rare; however, there are still service lines, such as cancer care and children's hospitals, where its use is prevalent by commercial payers. This reimbursement methodology may be applied in both inpatient and outpatient settings.

Per Diem Payment

Per diem payment, or per day (daily) rate, is a type of retrospective payment method that is commonly used in the hospital inpatient setting. The third-party payer reimburses the provider a fixed rate for each day a beneficiary is hospitalized. Therefore, the contracting unit is an inpatient day. All services rendered within a day are reimbursed with the daily rate. Since a hospital admission may include a very expensive surgical procedure in the first days, this methodology is most commonly applied to medical or obstetric admissions. This reimbursement methodology is a blend of retrospective payment and prospective payment. The daily rate is established in advance; however, the type of care (for example, intensive care, cardiac care, general surgery) may not be known in advance. Additionally, the number of days a patient is treated in each type of care is unknown until the patient is discharged. Therefore, this is considered a retrospective reimbursement methodology since the number of days at each level of service, and any subsequent reimbursement, is unknown until after the care is provided.

Third-party payers set the per diem rates using historical data. For example, to establish an inpatient per diem, the total costs for all inpatient services for a population during a period are divided by the number of patient days in the period.

$$Traditional\ Per\ Diem\ Rate = \frac{Total\ cost\ for\ all\ inpatient\ services}{Total\ patient\ days}$$

Figure 4.2.   Sample claim reimbursement using the percent of billed charges methodology

Revenue Code	Service Description	HCPCS Code	Unit of Service	Covered Charges*	Reimbursement %	Total Reimbursement (Covered Charge × 0.64)
250	Pharmacy		7	$93.08	64%	$59.57
258	Pharmacy, IV solutions		1	$15.00	64%	$9.60
320	Diagnostic radiology	77003	1	$353.50	64%	$226.24
360	Operating room	64490	1	$11,102.75	64%	$7,105.76
370	Anesthesia, general	01992	1	$226.75	64%	$145.12
Totals				**$11,791.08**	**64%**	**$7,546.29**

*Charge is fictitious and should not be used for rate setting.

Figure 4.3.   **Illustration of per diem reimbursement methodology**

Charge Category	Charge*	Reimbursement
Day 1—ICU	$6,500	$5,000
Day 2—ICU	$6,500	$5,000
Day 3—Medical	$4,500	$2,500
Day 4—Medical	$4,500	$2,500
Day 5—Medical	$4,500	$2,500
Ventilation procedure	$6,000	$0
Ancillary	$500	$0
Pharmacy	$3,700	$0
Totals	$36,700	$17,500

*Charge is fictitious and should not be used for rate setting.

The payment is determined by multiplying the per diem rate by the number of days of hospitalization. Figure 4.3 illustrates the per diem reimbursement methodology. In this example, the payer has established that the reimbursement rate for an ICU day equals $5,000 and a Medical day equals $2,500.

Criticism of Retrospective Reimbursement

For third-party payers, the retrospective reimbursement methodology has the disadvantage of great uncertainty. The payers do not have advance notice of the exact number and type of days or services that will be delivered. This uncertainty has resulted in third-party payers moving toward prospective payment methodologies, which are discussed in the next section. Critics of retrospective reimbursement assert that the method provides few incentives to control costs. In a retrospective environment, providers are reimbursed for each service they provide. The more services a provider renders, the more reimbursement the provider receives. Moreover, critics argue that there is little incentive to order less expensive services rather than more expensive services. Therefore, some critics contend that retrospective reimbursement does not incentivize providers to control costs of healthcare because the payment method rewards providers for more services regardless of whether such services are warranted.

Prospective Reimbursement

Prospective reimbursement is a healthcare payment method in which providers receive a predetermined amount for all the services they provide during a defined time frame. There are four guiding principles of prospective payment:

1. Payment rates are to be established in advance and fixed for the fiscal period to which they apply.

2. Payment rates are not automatically determined by the hospital's past or current actual cost.

3. Prospective payment rates are payment in full.

4. The hospital retains the profit or suffers a loss resulting from the difference between the payment rate and the hospital's cost, creating an incentive for cost control. (Averill et al. 2001, 106)

In the prospective payment method, the unit of payment is the encounter, established period of time, or insured, not each individual service provided. The prospective payment methods provide incentives to providers to provide more cost-effective care due to the fixed payment rate.

Forms of prospective reimbursement are capitation, case rate, global payment, and bundled payment. Table 4.3 provides a summary of characteristics of the types of prospective reimbursement. The types of prospective reimbursement and the criticisms to these methodologies are discussed in the next section.

Capitation

The capitated payment method, or **capitation**, is a method of payment for health services in which the third-party payer reimburses providers a fixed, per capita amount for a period. "Per capita" means "per head" or "per person." A common phrase in capitated contracts is **"per member per month" (PMPM)**, which is the amount of money paid to the provider each month per individual enrolled in the health insurance plan. Alternative terminology for this method is *global capitation*. In this methodology, the contracting unit is the person or insured.

In capitation, the actual volume or intensity of services provided to each patient has no effect on the payment. More services do not increase the payment, nor do fewer services decrease the payment. In a limited capitation methodology, a provider or provider group contracts with a payer to provide a specified set of services, such as primary care, to a group of enrollees or beneficiaries for a capitated rate. The provider receives the payments for each member of the group regardless of whether all the members receive the provider's services. Example 4.1 illustrates how capitation is applied.

Example 4.1

Z Company has a health insurance plan for its workers and their families through Wellness Insurance. Wellness Insurance has contracted with Dr. T to provide health services (care) to members of the Z Company group for the capitated rate of $25 per month ($25 PMPM).

Dr. T is under contract to receive $25 per month for every member of the Z group. The members of the Z group total 100. Each month, Dr. T receives $2,500 ($25 × 100 members) from Wellness Insurance for the Z group. Dr. T receives $2,500 each month regardless of whether no members of the group see him in the clinic, or all members of the group see him in the clinic. Dr. T receives $2,500 each month whether all the members receive complex care for cancer, or all the members receive simple care for preventive flu shots.

Other PMPM contracts utilize a full-service capitation methodology. Medicare Advantage (MA) (Medicare Part C) is a good example, as illustrated in figure 4.4. The capitation contract is between the Centers for Medicare and Medicaid Services (CMS) and the MA payer. CMS contracts with the MA payer to provide all services, inpatient and outpatient, to the Medicare beneficiary for a PMPM rate. The MA payer negotiates separate contracts with providers and healthcare facilities to provide the care. These contracts may use a variety of reimbursement methodologies.

The advantages of capitated payment are that the payer has no uncertainty about the total reimbursement amount for the provider and that the provider has a guaranteed customer base. The payer knows exactly what the costs of healthcare for the group will be, and the providers know that they will have an established group of customers to manage. Since providers will be reimbursed a set amount for the group of patients, they may want to engage in activities to help control healthcare spending. Providers can somewhat control the utilization of

Table 4.3.   Characteristics of prospective reimbursement methodologies

Reimbursement Methodology	Contracting Unit	Alternative Terminology
Capitation	Person or insured	Per member per month (PMPM), global capitation
Case rate	Encounter	Case-based payment, case-rate methodology
Global payment	Episode	Global package, global payment method
Bundled payment	Episode	Episode payments, episode-of-care payment

Figure 4.4.   Medicare Advantage as example of full-service capitation

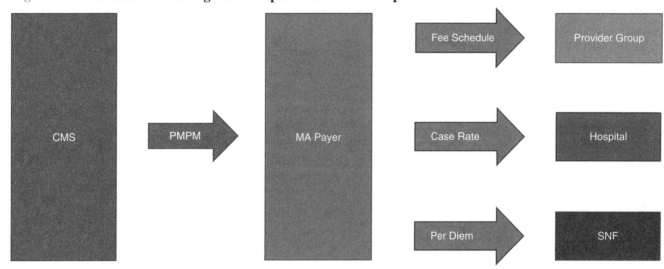

services by engaging in population health activities such as preventive care and case management for patients with chronic diseases. Providers can encourage patients to receive screenings and other preventive care services, and to participate in wellness care. By encouraging population health activities, providers hope to keep their group of patients healthier and prevent spending more on treatment and care than they receive in reimbursement from the payer. Some payers use a risk adjustment model that varies capitation rates based on a beneficiary's demographic data and health status. A section later in this chapter will discuss risk adjustment models.

Case-Rate Methodology

In the **case-rate methodology**, the third-party payer reimburses the provider one amount for the entire visit or encounter regardless of the number of services or length of the encounter. The contracting unit is the encounter (inpatient stay or outpatient visit or procedure). The case-rate methodology, sometimes known as *case-based payment*, is most often utilized for inpatient admissions but can also be applied for hospital outpatient encounters for same-day surgery. The facility will not receive an increased payment for each day the patient remains in the acute-care setting. Likewise, the facility will receive the predetermined amount even if the cost of care is less than the set reimbursement rate. Example 4.2 illustrates how the case-rate methodology is applied in the inpatient hospital setting.

Example 4.2

Two patients were hospitalized with pneumonia. One patient was hospitalized for three days, the other for 30 days. Each patient is a case. The third-party payer has established a case-rate payment of $3,500 for cases with pneumonia. The hospital would receive a payment of $3,500 for each of the two cases.

The case rate is determined by the historical resource needs of the typical patient for a given set of conditions or diseases. Case-rate payment can be one flat rate per case or can be multiple rates that represent categories of cases (sets of conditions or diseases). The case-rate payment method rewards effective and efficient delivery of health services and penalizes ineffective and inefficient delivery. Case-rate payment rates are based on the typical costs for patients within the group. Generally, costs for facilities that treat patients efficiently and effectively are beneath the average costs. The providers earn profit in this situation. On the other hand, providers that commonly exceed average costs lose money. Inefficiencies that may hinder profit include duplicate laboratory work, scheduling delays, and lost reports. Many healthcare organizations have implemented procedures to streamline the delivery of health services to offset inefficiencies.

Global Payment Method

In the **global payment method**, like case-rate payments, the third-party payer makes one combined payment to cover the services of multiple providers, typically physicians, who are treating a single episode-of-care. Thus, this payment method consolidates payments. This methodology is typical for physician services and outpatient care. The contracting unit in this methodology is the episode. In the global payment method, there is no additional payment for higher volumes of services or more expensive or complex services.

An example of global payment is the global surgical package. The global surgical package encompasses an operation, local or topical anesthesia, a preoperative clinic visit, immediate postoperative care, and usual postoperative follow-up. Figure 4.5 provides an illustration of the global payment method. In this example, the charges for the services provided in the preoperative, operative, and postoperative periods total $9,050. However, the payer has contracted with the provider to pay the global amount of $5,430.

Another example is in outpatient dialysis facilities, where bundling combines the costs of dialysis services, injectable drugs, laboratory tests, and medical equipment and supplies into a single prospective payment (MedPAC 2022, 1). Another common package is for obstetrical services that includes prenatal care, the delivery, and usual postpartum care.

Bundled Payment Methodology

A **bundled payment** is "a payment structure in which different health care providers who are treating you for the same or related conditions are paid an overall sum for taking care of your condition rather than being paid for each individual treatment, test, or procedure. In doing so, providers are rewarded for coordinating care, preventing complications and errors, and reducing unnecessary or duplicative tests and treatments" (CMS n.d.). The course of the treatment is referred to as an *episode*. This means that all treatment provided for the condition, illness, or medical event during the specified time frame is an episode. The payment methodology for the episode is bundled payment. Therefore, some alternative terms for bundled payments are *episode payments* and *episode-of-care payments*. The contracting unit for this methodology is the episode.

There is a trigger event, typically a service or onset of a condition, that initiates the episode-of-care. Once triggered, the bundle includes payment for the trigger event plus a predetermined, predefined set of services for a set time frame. The provider controls the amount of variation in care by including or excluding patients from the bundle based on predefined criteria. For example, patients with a history of an organ transplant may be excluded from a bundle since the likelihood of an infection due to the patient's immune-compromised status is greater. The set of services and treating providers requires careful consideration to ensure the bundled payment is sufficient to cover the services provided *and* is also fair for the third-party payer. For example, services that are part of a clinical trial are typically excluded from bundled payment. Additionally, there is a well-defined time frame that varies by bundle in which all services must be performed for the provider to be eligible to receive the bundled payment.

Figure 4.5.   Illustration of the global payment method

Preoperative clinic visit	Surgery (includes pre- and postoperative services)	Routine postoperative follow-up visit
Charge = $250.00	Charge = $8,500.00	Charge = $300.00

Total Reimbursement = $5,430.00

For example, it must be determined if the episode ends after a specified number of days post-surgery or when the condition or illness is resolved.

CMS supports several bundled payment methods. The Comprehensive Care for Joint Replacement (CJR) Model is a bundle that CMS first defined in 2015 (CMS 2023a. The model will be in effect through December 31, 2024. This program was voluntary in 2015 but moved to a requirement in certain geographic areas in 2018. The trigger for this bundle is an inpatient admission with a Medicare severity diagnosis-related group (MS-DRG) of 469 or 470. These are the two MS-DRGs that include the majority of total hip and knee replacements. The services related to the joint replacement that occur within 90 days of the hospital discharge for MS-DRG 469 or 470 are included in the bundled payment. The CJR model is shown in figure 4.6.

Exclusion criteria for both patients and services are a part of the CJR design. For instance, patients with a cancer diagnosis are included in the bundle, but the services received to treat the cancer are excluded. CMS supplies an extensive list of the diagnosis codes that are excluded from each of the bundles they design. An example of the design, including inclusion and exclusion criteria, may be found on the CMS website (CMS 2023a).

The CJR represents a bundle that has a well-defined trigger event and a treatment pathway that is relatively predictable. Cancer treatment is not as predictable and, therefore, bundle design in that area is not as developed. Recently, the University of Texas MD Anderson Cancer Center and UnitedHealthcare published the results of their bundled payment pilot in an article titled, "Development and Feasibility of Bundled Payments for the Multidisciplinary Treatment of Head and Neck Cancer: A Pilot Program" in the *Journal of Oncology Practice*. In this pilot program, the participants tested whether a comprehensive cancer center and a national payer could successfully pilot a comprehensive (professional and technical services), one-year prospective bundled payment methodology for head and neck cancer (Spinks et al. 2017, 2). The results of the pilot were positive, with 88 patients enrolled in the program during the three-year period. However, a major takeaway from the project was that the facility expended significant administrative effort for claims processing, systems functionality issues, and other processes (Spinks et al. 2017, 1). Extra administrative burden adds directly to the cost of providing services and, therefore, could limit the use of the bundled payment methodologies by hospitals.

Criticisms of Prospective Reimbursement

Some consumer advocates have voiced concerns about prospective reimbursement. They believe that the payment method creates incentives to substitute less expensive diagnostic and therapeutic procedures. Other concerns include

Figure 4.6.   **CMS's CJR model**

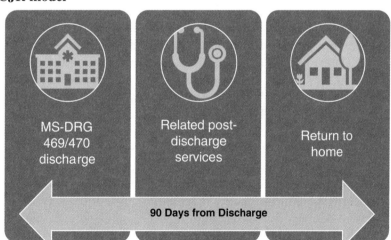

Source: Adapted from CMS 2023a.

the inappropriate elimination of laboratory and radiological tests. Further concerns include the delay or denial of procedures and treatments, such as new and innovative devices or medications. Additionally, concerns have been raised about inappropriate premature discharge in the inpatient setting. In response, Medicare and other third-party payers have included access to care provisions to ensure their beneficiaries receive new technologies. Typically, a quality component is attached to prospective reimbursement to ensure not only efficient care, but also high-quality care. For example, Medicare includes a hospital readmission reduction program to hinder inappropriate discharges (CMS 2022).

Payers often may adjust or combine reimbursement methodologies to build payment systems. The upcoming sections will discuss Medicare's risk adjustment models, which are applied to the capitation methodology and accountable care organizations (ACOs), which combine multiple methodologies to create a payment system that covers the continuum of care.

Check Your Understanding 4.1

1. Which of the following is not a type of retrospective reimbursement?

    a. Global payment
    b. Per diem
    c. Fee schedule
    d. Percent of billed charges

2. Why is the fee schedule reimbursement methodology retrospective instead of prospective?

3. Explain how bundled payment methodology differs from the case-rate methodology.

4. Create an illustration of the global payment method for outpatient dialysis. Exact dollar figures are not required.

5. List two criticisms of prospective reimbursement methodologies.

Risk Adjustment Models

Risk adjustment is a statistical process that considers the underlying health status and health spending of patients when examining their healthcare outcomes or healthcare costs (HealthCare.gov n.d.). Healthcare facilities and providers often use risk adjustment to benchmark against other entities. Risk adjustment models are used in many commercial and government-sponsored payment systems. The Department of Health and Human Services (HHS) has developed several risk adjustment models. Risk adjustment of a patient population allows external benchmarking to be more relevant, since outcome variables such as length of stay and mortality rates can be normalized to remove the impact of patient mix. Risk adjustment is also important for tracking internal improvement efforts at a healthcare facility. Using risk adjustment methods can normalize for patient mix over time within a facility.

CMS, as part of HHS, developed the **CMS hierarchical condition categories (CMS-HCC) model**. The CMS-HCC model uses patient demographic characteristics and medical conditions to predict the patient's healthcare costs. This model was implemented in 2004 and is utilized with MA. As discussed in chapter 3, "Government-Sponsored Healthcare Programs," MA is Medicare's managed care plan executed under Medicare Part C. The purpose of the CMS-HCC risk adjustment model is to provide fair and accurate payments while rewarding efficiency and high-quality care for Medicare's chronically ill population (Pope et al. 2004, 140). The basis of risk adjustment is to predict which beneficiaries will be most costly to treat during the following year and then to increase capitated payments for those individuals. This allows CMS to redirect payments from managed care payers that may target healthy populations to managed care payers that provide insurance for the most ill patients (Pope et al. 2004, 140). Table 4.4 provides a representative sample of *International Classification of Diseases, Tenth Revision, Clinical Modification* (ICD-10-CM) codes that are assigned to version 24 of the CMS-HCC model.

Table 4.4. **Representative sample of ICD-10-CM diagnosis codes and assigned HCC category**

ICD-10-CM Code and Description	HCC Category and Description 2023
C25.0, Malignant neoplasm of head of pancreas	HCC 9, Lung and Other Severe Cancers
J15.212, Pneumonia due to methicillin-resistant Staphylococcus aureus	HCC 114, Aspiration and Specified Bacterial Pneumonias
M00.272, Other streptococcal arthritis, left ankle and foot	HCC 39, Bone/Joint/Muscle Infections/Necrosis
N18.6, End-stage renal disease	HCC 136, Chronic Kidney Disease, Stage 5
T87.42, Infection of amputation stump, left upper extremity	HCC 189, Amputation Status, Lower Limb/ Amputation Complications

Source: CMS 2023b.

The following 10 principles determined which codes would be included in the HCC categories and were utilized to create the CMS-HCC model:

- Principle 1: Diagnostic categories should be clinically meaningful; the codes in a category should be related.

- Principle 2: Diagnostic categories should predict medical expenditures; the codes in a category should be homogeneous with respect to predicting cost.

- Principle 3: Diagnostic categories that will affect payments should have adequate sample sizes to permit accurate and stable estimates of expenditures; codes should have adequate sample sizes in available data sets.

- Principle 4: When creating a person's clinical profile, hierarchies should be used to characterize the person's illness level within each disease process, while the effects of unrelated disease processes accumulate; most significant manifestation is placed above less significant manifestations within a disease category.

- Principle 5: The diagnostic classification should encourage specific coding; correct coding at the highest level of specificity is encouraged.

- Principle 6: The diagnostic classification should not reward coding proliferation; the risk adjustment is not based on code volume.

- Principle 7: Providers should not be penalized for recording additional diagnoses (monotonicity); no condition category should result in a decrease in payment, and higher-ranked diagnoses within a disease category should have a higher weight than lower-ranked diseases.

- Principle 8: The classification system should be internally consistent (transitive); category A is higher ranked than category B, and so on.

- Principle 9: The diagnostic risk adjustment classification should consider all ICD codes for inclusion in the model.

- Principle 10: Discretionary diagnostic categories should be excluded from payment models; reduce the sensitivity of the model due to incorrect coding, coding proliferation, or coding variations. (Pope et al. 2004, 121–122)

Principles 7, 8, and 9 were followed absolutely in the design of the CMS-HCC model. The other principles were weighed against each other and compromises were made to create a risk adjustment system that met the needs of goals for a capitated payment system in the Medicare environment, where most beneficiaries are 65 years or older. Determining which HCCs apply to a beneficiary requires diagnosis data that are collected from five sources: principal hospital inpatient, secondary hospital inpatient, hospital outpatient, physician, and clinically trained nonphysician (Pope et al. 2004, 124).

In addition to the CMS-HCC model that is used to risk adjust capitated MA payments, CMS has developed the Medicare Prescription Drug Hierarchical Condition Categories (RxHCC) classification to predict Medicare Part D spending (see chapter 3 of this text, "Government-Sponsored Healthcare Programs," for a detailed discussion on Part D). In 2014, HHS implemented the HHS-HCC model used for health plans in the individual and small group markets inside and outside the State-based Marketplaces and the Federally-facilitated Marketplaces, as enacted by the Affordable Care Act of 2010 (CMS 2016, 1). The HHS-HCC model is based on the CMS-HCC and RxHCC systems but is designed to predict expenditures for medical and drug spending for a commercial population primarily under age 65 (CMS 2016, 17). Recently, the CMS-HCC risk adjustment model has moved beyond setting capitated payment rates and into the quality arena. CMS-HCCs are utilized in ACO systems and in CMS value-based purchasing programs such as the Hospital Readmission Reduction Program.

The CMS-HCC model is used to create a risk score for each beneficiary. The risk score indicates how costly an individual is expected to be relative to an average beneficiary (MedPAC 2023, 324). The risk score is broken into two components: demographic and health status. The demographic portion is based on the beneficiary's characteristics, such as age, sex, and Medicaid status. The health status portion is derived from ICD-10-CM diagnosis codes reported for the beneficiary in the hospital inpatient, hospital outpatient, and physician office settings. The codes are collected during the base year. The base year is the year preceding the year that the beneficiary's health status will adjust payment rates (prediction year). The ICD-10-CM codes that are included in the HCC categories have a risk score. The risk score correlates to expected cost of treating the condition. The higher the risk score, the more costly it is to provide treatment and services for the condition. Figure 4.7 provides the risk score for two patients.

Each component of the risk score, demographic and health status, is calculated for each beneficiary during the base year. The final risk score is then used to determine PMPM payments during the prediction year. For example, data collected during 2023 (base year) are used to create a final risk score that is utilized for reimbursement during 2024 (prediction year). The higher the risk score, the higher the PMPM payment will be for the beneficiary because a higher risk score signals a beneficiary is expected to be costlier than the average beneficiary, whose risk score is 1.0.

ICD-10-CM diagnosis codes are the foundation of CMS-HCC, as they directly impact the risk score calculation. Therefore, the accurate and complete reporting of diagnosis codes is crucial to the financial health of an MA organization. Good coding relies on two factors: complete and legible physician documentation and well-educated coding professionals. MA plans must educate their providers on the importance of addressing all conditions for a patient, acute and chronic, during their encounters. All conditions, including chronic conditions, must be monitored, evaluated, and assessed during the base year to be eligible as part of the final risk score. It is imperative that MA programs support a coding management program that encourages complete and accurate coding practices among coding professionals and healthcare professionals, which includes physicians and clinicians who code encounters on their own in their offices. Failure to properly support and code HCC diagnoses may result in a loss of reimbursement. Figure 4.8 is a case study that compares the impact of good and poor documentation and coding practices on the health status risk score component for an MA program. This example shows how good documentation yields more complete and specific coding for the encounter. The monitoring, evaluation, and assessment of chronic conditions results in the ability for the MA program to report HCC codes that will positively impact its PMPM amounts for the next prediction year.

As risk-adjusted payment models have spread to programs outside of MA, healthcare professionals have begun to increase awareness of HCC documentation and coding. Documentation practices for HCCs are now covered under many clinical documentation integrity (CDI) plans, and coding management is placing a greater emphasis

Figure 4.7.   Risk score determination

Patient A				
Diagnostic Data				
	ICD-10-Code	*Description*	*HCC*	*Risk Score*
	A02.1	Salmonella sepsis	2 – Septicemia, Sepsis, Systemic Inflammatory Response Syndrome/Shock	0.352
	R65.20	Severe sepsis		
	L23.4	Contact dermatitis due to dyes	N/A	---
	J44.9	COPD, unspecified	111 – Chronic Obstructive Pulmonary Disease	0.335
	I10	Essential hypertension	N/A	---
	M71.111	Infective bursitis, right shoulder	N/A	---
Health Status Score				0.687
Demographic Score*	Patient age 64			0.378
	Total Patient Risk Score			1.065

Patient B				
Diagnostic Data				
	ICD-10-Code	*Description*	*HCC*	*Risk Score*
	M80.051A	Osteoporosis with pathological fracture, right femur	170 – Hip Fracture/ Dislocation	0.35
	I12.0	Hypertensive CKD with stage 5 CKD	136 – Chronic Kidney Disease Stage 5	0.289
	N18.5	Stage 5 CKD		
	N80.02	Deep endometriosis of the uterus	N/A	---
	E11.3292	Type 2 diabetes with mild nonproliferative diabetic retinopathy, left eye	18 – Diabetes with Chronic Complications	0.302
	I48.4	Atypical atrial flutter	96 – Specified Heart Arrhythmias	0.268
	E59	Dietary selenium deficiency	N/A	---
	D63.1	Anemia in CKD	N/A	---
	F51.5	Nightmare disorder	N/A	---

(continued)

Figure 4.7.   *(continued)*

Patient B	
Health Status Score	1.209
Demographic Score* Patient age 65	0.350
Total Patient Risk Score	1.559

* Demographic score is fictitious.
Source: CMS 2023b; CMS 2023c.

on coding professionals' knowledge of HCCs. Coding and CDI management are discussed in greater detail later in chapter 12, "Coding and Clinical Documentation Integrity Management."

Accountable Care Organization

Around 2005, researchers at Dartmouth first coined the term *accountable care organization* (MacKinney et al. 2011, 132). An **accountable care organization (ACO)** is a population-based model for healthcare delivery and payment. In an ACO, a set of providers "are jointly held accountable for achieving measured quality improvements and reductions in the rate of spending growth" (McClellan et al. 2010, 982). The purpose of ACOs is to provide coordinated high-quality care to Medicare beneficiaries. ACOs bring together physicians, hospitals, and other healthcare providers to provide efficient (low cost) and effective (free of duplication and errors) care. The goal of coordinated care is to ensure that patients get the right care at the right time (CMS 2023d). An ACO is accountable for all the healthcare costs of its attributed population of Medicare beneficiaries.

Successful ACOs have the following characteristics:

1. High-value culture

    a. Physician and community practice engagement

    b. Clinical partnerships

2. Proactive population health management

    a. System for identifying high-risk patients

    b. Care management functions

    c. Specific disease management programs

3. Structure for continuous improvement

    a. Operational infrastructure for performance improvement

    b. Tying performance to compensation and network contracts

    c. Participation in shared learning opportunities (HCTTF 2018)

Local healthcare providers in a city or region are integrated in an ACO. The integrated providers may include primary care physicians, specialists, hospitals, healthcare insurance plans, suppliers of durable medical equipment or other services and items, and other stakeholders. The exact makeup of the ACO depends on its sponsoring healthcare organization. The Affordable Care Act, per Section 3022, required CMS to promote the development

Figure 4.8.   **Case study for HCC documentation coding**

Poor Documentation/Coding Scenario			Good Documentation/Coding Scenario		
Chief Complaint: 74-year-old African American male, with BPH with ongoing symptoms of frequent urination. Returning to my office for follow-up visit. PMH: Stable diabetes mellitus, arteriosclerosis BKA. HPI: Patient has been experiencing frequent and urgent need to urinate. This increased at night. His urine stream is very weak when he urinates. PSA test results show 5.0 ng/mL. PVR showed 120 m. Ultrasound confirmed enlarged prostate. Plan: Avodart for LUTS associated with BPH. Referral to oncologist to rule out prostate cancer.			Chief Complaint: 74-year-old African American male, with benign prostatic hyperplasia with lower urinary tract symptoms; returning to my office for follow-up visit. PMH: Type 2 diabetes mellitus, stable BKA, right leg, arteriosclerosis with history of AMI (3 years prior). HPI: Patient has been experiencing a frequent and urgent need to urinate due to BPH. This need to urinate is increased at night. His stream is very weak when he urinates. PSA test results show 5.0 ng/mL. Post-void residual volume test showed 120 m, which indicates incomplete bladder emptying. Ultrasound confirmed enlarged prostate. Patient states DM is stable, review of blood sugar reading from patient shows good management of DM with Glucophase 500 mg b.i.d for DM. Patient is exercising 3× per week to help with the control of DM. Right leg BKA is stable, scar is within normal limits without signs of inflammation or infection. Lipid panel with LDL/HDL Ratio: Cholesterol, Total 191 mg/dl, Triglycerides 103 mg/dL, HDL Cholesterol 45 mg/dL, VLDL Cholesterol 21 mg/dL, LDL Cholesterol Calc 125 mg/dL (high), LDL/HDL Ratio 2.8. Patient will continue with low-sugar diet to control weight, heart disease, and DM. Plan: Avodart for LUTS associated with BPH. Referral to oncologist for prostate biopsy due to high PSA.		
Condition	ICD-10-CM Code/HCC Category	Risk Score	Condition	ICD-10-CM Code/HCC Category	Risk Score
BPH with LUTS	N40.1 No HCC	0.000	BPH with LUTS	N40.1 No HCC	0.000
			Urinary frequency	R35.0 No HCC	0.000
			Nocturia	R35.1 No HCC	0.000
			Weak urinary stream	R39.12 No HCC	0.000
			Incomplete bladder emptying	R39.14 No HCC	0.000

(continued)

Figure 4.8.   *(continued)*

Poor Documentation/Coding Scenario		Good Documentation/Coding Scenario		
		Type 2 diabetes mellitus	E11.9 HCC 19	0.105
		Coronary arteriosclerosis	I25.10 No HCC	0.000
		Old myocardial infarction	I25.2 No HCC	0.000
		BKA	Z89.511 HCC 189	0.519
Total medical conditions risk score	0.000	Total medical conditions risk score		0.624

Source: CMS 2023b; CMS 2023c.

of ACOs by establishing the Medicare Shared Savings Program (MSSP). The MSSP has a triple aim: (1) better quality of care for individuals, (2) better health for populations, and (3) lower growth in healthcare costs (CMS 2011, 67803–67804). The general concept of shared savings programs is that providers are rewarded with a portion of the savings if they reduce the total healthcare spending for their patients below the level that the payer expected. The overarching result is that the payer spends less money than is expected and the provider receives more revenue than is expected.

CMS has refined and further delineated the general definition of an ACO. Per CMS, an ACO is a legal entity recognized under state law. It is composed of a group of ACO participants (providers of services and suppliers) that have established a mechanism for shared governance. Under a three-year agreement with CMS, the ACO participants coordinate the care of traditional Medicare fee-for-service beneficiaries. The ACO is accountable for the quality, cost, and overall care of all the beneficiaries assigned to it (CMS 2011, 67974). Expanding on the specific components of this definition yields the following:

- ACOs are legal entities that are recognized and authorized under applicable state, federal, or tribal law.

- ACOs are identified by a taxpayer identification number (TIN).

- ACOs are formed by one or more of the following ACO participants (providers or suppliers) or others:
  - Group practice of ACO professionals (physicians, physician assistants, nurse practitioners, clinical nurse specialists, or a combination)
  - Network of individual practices
  - Partnership or joint venture arrangements between hospitals and ACO professionals
  - Hospital employing ACO professionals
  - Critical access hospitals (CAHs) that bill outpatient services under the optional method for outpatient services with the cost based on the facility services plus a 115 percent fee schedule payment for professional services (Method II)
  - Rural health clinic
  - Federally qualified health center

- ACO participants work together to manage and coordinate care for Medicare fee-for-service beneficiaries.

- ACOs are accountable for the quality, cost, and overall care for the assigned Medicare fee-for-service beneficiaries.

- ACOs operate under a risk model.
  - One-sided model (available to ACOs only for their *initial* agreement period): ACOs share savings with the Medicare program, if they meet the requirements, but the ACOs do *not* share losses.
  - Two-sided model: ACOs share savings with the Medicare program, if they meet the requirements, and ACOs share losses with the Medicare program.

- ACOs maintain shared governance through an identifiable, authoritative governing body (at least one Medicare beneficiary and 75 percent ACO participants) with transparent processes that promote evidence-based medicine and patient engagement, that report on quality and cost measures, and that coordinate care.

- ACOs have a leadership and management structure that includes clinical and administrative systems supportive of the triple aim; the executive officer, senior-level medical director, and other ACO participants must demonstrate meaningful commitment to the ACO's mission.

- ACOs provide primary care (outpatient, home, and wellness visits) to at least 5,000 assigned Medicare beneficiaries with at least a sufficient number of primary care ACO professionals for at least three years (term of agreement).

- ACOs are explicitly required to do the following:
  - Promote evidence-based medicine
  - Promote beneficiary engagement adopting patient-centeredness
  - Report on quality and cost metrics
  - Coordinate care across providers

ACOs are present in most healthcare markets. In 2023, there were 456 ACOs with 10.9 million beneficiaries attributed to them (CMS 2023d). In this context, **attribution** is the assignment of a beneficiary to a particular organization or ACO (CMS 2019, 14). Beneficiaries may voluntarily enroll in an ACO during the Medicare open enrollment period. For all other beneficiaries, CMS attributes individuals to an ACO via a prospective method with retrospective reconciliation. At the beginning of a model year, CMS makes assignments based on claims data for each year following the flow outlined in figure 4.9.

The MSSP is divided into tracks that define the type of risk that the ACO assumes. Basic track A/B and track 1 ACOs are subject to **one-sided risk**. That means that they can share in any savings generated by the ACO, but are not subject to any cost sharing if there is no savings or if the cost of care is higher while patients are attributed to the ACO. In 2023, 33 percent of ACOs were in one of the one-sided risk tracks. All other ACO tracks include **two-sided risk**. This means that the ACO must share in the loss if the cost of care for their attributed beneficiaries is greater than the benchmark or share in any savings if the cost of care is lower than the benchmark. Most of the two-sided risk tracks are considered advanced payment models (APMs). Two-sided risk ACOs make up 67 percent of the total.

The amount of shared savings for an ACO is determined by calculating the risk adjusted expected healthcare expenditures for the set of patients attributed. Each beneficiary's expected expense is risk adjusted based on the CMS-HCC risk scores. It is then trended forward based on the historical increase in Medicare expenses year over year. This expected expense calculation yields a baseline, or benchmark, year and is based on three years of expenses for the attributed beneficiaries. The amount that Medicare reimburses any provider for fee-for-service care during the year is totaled to determine the actual expenses. The actual is compared to the benchmark expenses to determine if any savings is available to share or if any expenses must be paid to CMS in the case of a two-sided risk ACO. Example 4.3 outlines shared amounts for a two-sided risk agreement.

Figure 4.9.   CMS attribution flow diagram

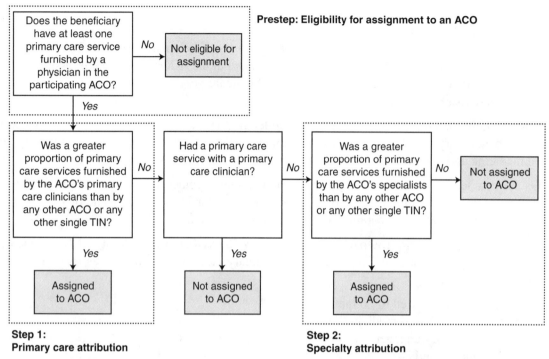

Source: MedPAC 2019, 186.

Example 4.3

Giant ACO participates in a two-sided risk agreement with CMS with a shared savings rate of 50% and a shared loss rate of 30%. Last year, 23,500 Medicare beneficiaries were attributed to Giant ACO. The target expense amount for each beneficiary was $12,500.

a. If expenditure per beneficiary during the measurement period was $15,000, then what is the shared loss amount?

Total target expenditures = 23,500 beneficiaries × $12,500 = $293,750,000

Total actual expenditures = 23,500 beneficiaries × $15,000 = $352,500,000

Total target – actual expenditures = -$58,750,000

Shared loss amount = -$58,750,000 × 0.30 = -$17,625,000

Giant ACO must repay $17,625,000 to CMS

b. What is the shared savings amount if the actual expenditure per beneficiary was $11,000 and Giant ACO achieved the quality metric benchmarks?

Total target expenditures = 23,500 beneficiaries × $12,500 = $293,750,000

Total actual expenditures = 23,500 beneficiaries × $10,000 = $235,000,000

Total target – actual expenditures = $58,750,000

Shared savings amount = $58,750,000 × 0.50 = $29,375,000

Figure 4.10.   Geographic distribution of ACO population

Medicare Shared Savings Program ACO Assigned Beneficiary Population by County

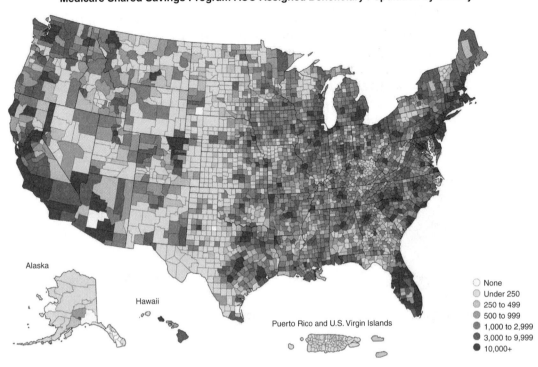

Source: CMS 2023e, 2.

In order to share in the savings derived from reducing the cost of care for an ACO's attributed beneficiaries, the organization must meet a quality performance score threshold. In 2021, the average quality score for ACOs was 91 percent, and ACOs earned $2 billion in shared savings payments (CMS 2023e). There is a significant amount of regional variation in the distribution of ACOs throughout the country. The map in figure 4.10 shows the distribution of Medicare beneficiaries assigned to ACOs by county.

Third-party payers use a variety of reimbursement methodologies to pay for healthcare services. Some payment systems, like those used for ACOs, use multiple methodologies. Risk adjustment methods are layered on top of reimbursement methodologies to enhance reimbursement rate accuracy based on individual beneficiary health status. (In the next four chapters, the text explores four Medicare payment systems.) These payment systems will illustrate case-rate, per diem, and fee schedule reimbursement methodologies.

Check Your Understanding 4.2

1. List two risk adjustment models developed by HHS.

2. Describe how diagnosis codes are utilized to determine risk scores in the CMS-HCC risk adjustment model.

3. Explain how the beneficiary's CMS-HCC risk score impacts the MA PMPM rate.

4. What is the difference between one-sided and two-sided risk in the ACO payment model?

5. How are Medicare beneficiaries attributed to ACOs?

Patient Connection

As mentioned in chapter 2's Patient Connection, Olivia is pregnant. Her insurance company, Super Payer, reimburses Olivia's OB physician group, Baby Doctors, with a global payment methodology. The global package for pregnancy includes prenatal visits, the delivery admission, and postpartum visits. Prenatal visits begin as soon as the woman is pregnant and ends at delivery. The postpartum period begins immediately after delivery and continues for six weeks. Super Payer will reimburse Baby Doctors one amount for all care provided during the global period. Figure 4.5 illustrates global payment for surgery. Let's recreate that figure for pregnancy and insert hypothetical dollar amounts for Super Payer.

Prenatal Visits	Delivery	Routine postpartum follow-up visit
Weeks 4–28; total of 7 visits Weeks 28–36; total of 4 visits Weeks 36–40; total of 4 visits	Vaginal delivery Cesarean delivery	Vaginal delivery—1 visit Cesarean delivery—2 visits
Total visits = 15	Charge vaginal delivery = $8,775	Charge vaginal visit = $175
Total charges= $2,625	Charge cesarean delivery = $12,687	Charge cesarean visit = $300

Total Reimbursement Vaginal Delivery = $6,610

Total Reimbursement Cesarean Delivery = $8,970

The reimbursement rates in this illustration represent the negotiated rates between Super Payer and Baby Doctors. Most third-party payers reimburse at varying amounts based on the type of delivery. Since cesarean deliveries require an operating room, the costs are higher for this type of delivery and, in turn, so are the reimbursement rates. However, the varying rates are predetermined. If the patient requires more prenatal visits, more reimbursement is not provided. Likewise, if the patient requires additional postpartum visits, more reimbursement is not provided. This concept of prospective reimbursement methodologies incentivizes the physicians at Baby Doctors to appropriately manage patients and provide high-quality care. Remember that this is the amount Super Payer will reimburse Baby Doctors. Olivia is responsible for the cost-sharing amounts. From the chapter 2 Patient Connection we know Olivia has a $35 copay for each office visit and a $100 per day copay for inpatient admissions.

Malakai visits Dr. Lewis, his primary care physician, about four times per year. Malakai is enrolled in traditional Medicare, so his office visits with Dr. Lewis are reimbursed via a fee schedule reimbursement methodology. A sample office visit fee schedule is provided below.

(continued)

Visit Level	Fee Schedule Reimbursement
Level 1	$23.46
Level 2	$46.19
Level 3	$76.15
Level 4	$110.43
Level 5	$148.33

The fee schedule amount is the total amount Dr. Lewis will receive. Remember that Dr. Lewis is a Medicare provider. In chapter 3, "Government-Sponsored Healthcare Programs," we examined and calculated cost-sharing amounts for Medicare beneficiaries under Medicare Parts A and B. Table 3.2 indicates that Malakai's cost-sharing amount for Part B medical services is 20 percent of the approved amount. The Medicare fee schedule amount is the approved amount. In our illustration, $46.19 is the approved amount for a level 2 visit. So, if Malakai has a level 2 clinic visit with Dr. Lewis, Malakai is responsible for $9.24 ($46.19 × 0.20) and Medicare is responsible for $36.95 ($46.19 × 0.80).

Chapter 4 Review Quiz

1. Define prospective reimbursement. How is this methodology different from retrospective reimbursement?

2. Calvin saw his primary care physician, Dr. Washington, because he had a fever and a sore throat. Dr. Washington ordered and performed a rapid strep test. Calvin's test was positive, and he was diagnosed with streptococcal pharyngitis (strep throat). Dr. Washington wrote Calvin a prescription for amoxicillin to treat the pharyngitis. Dr. Washington submitted the following charges to Calvin's insurance company, Super Payer:

   • Clinic visit, level 2—$145

   • Rapid strep test—$50

   Dr. Washington's practice has a contract with Super Payer and the reimbursement methodology is a fee schedule. The fee schedule rate for a level 2 clinic visit is $70 and the fee schedule rate for a rapid strep test is $10. What is the total reimbursement Dr. Washington will receive for Calvin's office visit?

3. Super Payer has a contract with Community Hospital to provide inpatient care for their beneficiaries. They have agreed to a per diem reimbursement methodology. ICU days are reimbursed at $5,000 per day, and medical bed days are reimbursed at $3,500 per day. Community Hospital submitted a claim for a six-day length of stay (LOS). Two of the six days were ICU days and four of the six days were medical bed days. What is the total reimbursement owed to Community Hospital for this admission?

4. Super Payer has a contract with Memorial Hospital for inpatient surgical admissions. They have agreed to a case-rate methodology for these admissions. The case rate for a coronary artery bypass graft surgical admission is $28,500. Memorial Hospital submitted claims for the following admissions:

(continued)

Chapter 4 Review Quiz   *(continued)*

Admission #	Surgery	LOS	Charges	Cost
123	Coronary artery bypass graft	5	$78,050	$27,317
124	Coronary artery bypass graft	6	$84,400	$29,540
126	Coronary artery bypass graft	5	$79,450	$27,808

What is the total reimbursement Memorial Hospital will receive for each admission?

5. Dr. O'Neil's physician practice has a PMPM contract with Super Payer to provide primary care services. Super Payer uses a risk adjustment model to determine the PMPM amounts. The beneficiary risk score breakouts are provided below:

Number of Beneficiaries	Risk Score Level	PMPM Amount
100	1 – 1.00 risk score	$200.00
135	2 – 1.25 risk score	$250.00
150	3 – 1.50 risk score	$300.00
125	4 – 1.75 risk score	$350.00
90	5 – 2.00 risk score	$400.00

How much reimbursement will Dr. O'Neil's physician practice receive each month from Super Payer to provide primary care for the 600 beneficiaries?

6. What is the main goal of the CMS-HCC risk adjustment model?

7. Describe how diagnosis coding impacts reimbursement under the CMS-HCC risk adjustment model.

8. Super-ACO had benchmark expenses of $2.5 million and performance year expenses of $2.2 million. How much total savings was achieved by Super-ACO? If the shared saving percentage is 50 percent, how much shared savings would Super-ACO receive?

9. Super-ACO is deciding whether to convert to a two-sided risk for the next year. The shared saving rate is 75 percent and the shared loss rate is 30 percent for the track that is under consideration. Estimate the gain for the two-sided risk model if the actual expenses for the next year are 10 percent below the benchmark of $2.5 million.

10. Super-ACO is deciding whether to convert to a two-sided risk for the next year. The shared saving rate is 75 percent and the shared loss rate is 30 percent for the track that is under consideration. Estimate the loss for the two-sided risk model if the actual expenses for the next year are 10 percent above the benchmark of $2.5 million.

References

Averill, R. F., N. I. Goldfield, J. Eisenhandler, J. S. Hughes, and J. Muldoon. 2001. "Clinical Risk Groups and the Future of Healthcare Reimbursement." In *Reimbursement Methodologies for Healthcare Services* [CD-ROM], edited by L. M. Jones. Chicago: AHIMA.

CMS (Centers for Medicare and Medicaid Services). 2023a. "Comprehensive Care for Joint Replacement Model." https://innovation.cms.gov/innovation-models/cjr.

CMS (Centers for Medicare and Medicaid Services). 2023b. "2023 Midyear Software Model." https://www.cms .gov/medicare/health-plans/medicareadvtgspecratestats/risk-adjustors/2023-model-software/icd-10-mappings.

CMS (Centers for Medicare and Medicaid Services). 2023c. "2023 Midyear-Final ICD-10-CM Mappings." https://www.cms.gov/medicare/health-plans/medicareadvtgspecratestats/risk-adjustors/2023-model-software /icd-10-mappings.

CMS (Centers for Medicare and Medicaid Services). 2023d. "Accountable Care Organizations (ACOs)." https://innovation.cms.gov/innovation-models/aco.

CMS (Centers for Medicare and Medicaid Services). 2023e. Shared Savings Program Fast Facts – As of January 1, 2023. https://www.cms.gov/files/document/2023-shared-savings-program-fast-facts.pdf.

CMS (Centers for Medicare and Medicaid Services). 2022. "Hospital Readmissions Reduction Program (HRRP)." https://www.cms.gov/Medicare/Quality-Initiatives-Patient-Assessment-Instruments/Value-Based -Programs/HRRP/Hospital-Readmission-Reduction-Program.

CMS (Centers for Medicare and Medicaid Services). 2019 "Shared Savings and Losses and Assignment Methodology Specifications. February 2019 Version #7." https://www.cms.gov/Medicare/Medicare-Fee-for -Service-Payment/sharedsavingsprogram/Downloads/Shared-Savings-Losses-Assignment-Spec-V7.pdf.

CMS (Centers for Medicare and Medicaid Services). 2016. HHS-Operated Risk Adjustment Methodology Meeting, Discussion Paper. https://www.cms.gov/CCIIO/Resources/Forms-Reports-and-Other-Resources/ Downloads/RA-March-31-White-Paper-032416.pdf.

CMS (Centers for Medicare and Medicaid Services). 2011. Medicare program; Medicare shared savings program: Accountable care organizations; Final rule. *Federal Register* 76(212):67802–67990.

CMS (Centers for Medicare and Medicaid Services). n.d. "Payment Bundling." HealthCare.gov Glossary. Accessed June 19, 2023. https://www.healthcare.gov/glossary/payment-bundling/.

HCTTF (Health Care Transformation Task Force). 2018. *Levers of Successful ACOs: Insights from the Health Care Transformation Task Force.* https://hcttf.org/wp-content/uploads/2018/01/LeversofSuccessfulACOs6.pdf.

HealthCare.gov. n.d. "Risk Adjustment." Glossary. Accessed January 27, 2023. https://www.healthcare.gov /glossary/risk-adjustment/.

MacKinney, A. C., K. J. Mueller, and T. D. McBride. 2011. The march to accountable care organizations—how will rural fare? *Journal of Rural Health* 27(1):131–137.

McClellan, M., A. N. McKethan, J. L. Lewis, J. Roski, and E. S. Fisher. 2010. A national strategy to put accountable care into practice. *Health Affairs* 29(5):982–990,

MedPAC (Medicare Payment Advisory Commission). 2023 (March). *March 2023 Report to Congress: Medicare Payment Policy.* https://www.medpac.gov/document/march-2023-report-to-the-congress-medicare-payment -policy/.

MedPAC (Medicare Payment Advisory Commission). 2022. Outpatient Dialysis Services Payment System. https://www.medpac.gov/wp-content/uploads/2021/11/MedPAC_Payment_Basics_22_dialysis_FINAL_SEC.pdf.

MedPAC (Medicare Payment Advisory Commission). 2019 (June). Assessing the Medicare Shared Savings Program's Effect on Medicare Spending. https://www.medpac.gov/wp-content/uploads/import_data/scrape_files/docs/default-source/reports/jun19_ch6_medpac_reporttocongress_sec.pdf.

Pope, G. C., J. Kautter, R. Ellis, A. Ash, J. Ayanian, L. Lezzoni, M. Ingber, J. Levy, and J. Robst. 2004. Risk adjustment of Medicare capitation payments using the CMS-HCC model. *Health Care Financing Review* 25(4):119–141.

Spinks, T., A. Guzman, B. Beadle, S. Lee, D. Jones, R. Walters, J. Incalcaterra, E. Hanna, A. Hessel, R. Weber, S. Denney, L. Newcomer, and T. Feeley. 2017 (December). Development and feasibility of bundled payments for the multidisciplinary treatment of head and neck cancer: A pilot program. *Journal of Oncology Practice* 14(2): https://ascopubs.org/doi/full/10.1200/jop.2017.027029.

Chapter 5
Medicare Hospital Acute Inpatient Services Payment System

Learning Objectives

❖ Describe the structure of the Medicare hospital acute inpatient services payment system

❖ Illustrate MS-DRG assignment

❖ Describe severity of illness levels of MS-DRGs

❖ Describe the Medicare hospital acute inpatient services payment system provisions

❖ Articulate Medicare value-based purchasing programs related to the hospital acute inpatient setting

Key Terms

Arithmetic mean length of stay (AMLOS)
Base payment rate
Case mix
Case-mix index (CMI)
CC/MCC exclusion lists
Comorbidity
Complication
Complication and comorbidity (CC)
Cost report
Cost-of-living adjustment (COLA)
Disproportionate share hospital (DSH)
Federal Register
Final rule
Geometric mean length of stay (GMLOS)
Grouper
Hospital-acquired condition (HAC)
Indirect medical education (IME)
Labor-related share
Major complication and comorbidity (MCC)
Major diagnostic category (MDC)
Measure
Medicare administrative contractor (MAC)

Medicare severity diagnosis-related group (MS-DRG)
MS-DRG family
New technology
Nonlabor share
Outlier
Performance achievement
Performance improvement
Post-acute-care transfer (PACT)
Present on admission (POA) indicator
Principal diagnosis
Proposed rule
Quality reporting program
Relative weight (RW)
Resource intensity
Severity of illness (SOI)
Total performance score (TPS)
Transfer
Value-based purchasing (VBP)
Wage index
Withhold

Medicare employs different payment systems for the various settings in which Medicare beneficiaries are treated. This chapter discusses the Medicare hospital acute inpatient services payment system. This payment system includes a reimbursement component and multiple quality, or **value-based purchasing (VBP)**, components. VBP includes programs that link quality to reimbursement by holding healthcare providers accountable for both the cost and the quality of the care they provide. Most payment systems have a similar structure. The Medicare Payment Advisory Commission (MedPAC) Payment Basics webpage is a good place to find more information about Medicare payment systems that are used today and may be added in the future. Before the Medicare hospital acute inpatient services payment system is explored, some basic Medicare payment system and VBP concepts are discussed. These basic concepts are applicable to all Medicare payment systems.

Basic Medicare Payment System Concepts

Every Medicare payment system follows an annual maintenance process. It is important to understand this process because as modifications are made to the payment systems, coding and revenue cycle professionals must adjust their corresponding processes. This section provides an overview of the annual maintenance process for Medicare payment systems. Additionally, it is valuable to have a basic understanding of Medicare **cost reports**. The Medicare cost report is a required form for institutional providers and must be submitted on an annual basis. The Medicare cost report is completed and filed based on all services provided by a healthcare system. There are elements of the cost report that directly impact Medicare payment systems. Therefore, a brief overview of cost reports is provided later in this section.

Annual Maintenance of Medicare Payment Systems

The federal government issues information about its payment systems in the *Federal Register*. The *Federal Register* is the official journal of the US government. Published every federal business day, the publication reports all regulations (rules); legal notices of federal administrative agencies, of departments of the executive branch, and of the president; and federally mandated standards, including Healthcare Common Procedure Coding System (HCPCS) and *International Classification of Diseases, Tenth Revision, Clinical Modification* (ICD-10-CM) codes. The stages of a prospective payment system (PPS) update are displayed in figure 5.1.

Proposed changes to federal payment systems must be publicized in advance of the effective date through a process known as notice of proposed rulemaking. Federal agencies disclose **proposed rules** in the *Federal Register*. In proposed rules, agencies publicize their intended rules and allow the public and interested organizations to comment and to provide relevant information. The update typically includes the following:

1. Changes to payment rates

2. Revisions to covered services

3. Changes to quality and other nonpayment regulations associated with the payment methodology

After the comment period for the proposed rule has concluded, the agency reviews the comments and then publishes the final rule, including its analysis of the comments and information, in the *Federal Register.* The **final**

Figure 5.1.   **Stages of annual prospective payment update**

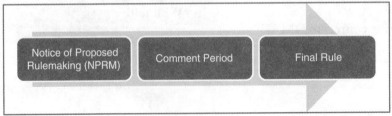

rule is a regulation issued by a regulatory body (such as the Centers for Medicare and Medicaid Services [CMS]). A regulation has the force of a law (Law.com n.d.).

Cost Reports

Medicare-certified providers are required to submit an annual cost report to their assigned **Medicare administrative contractor (MAC)** (CMS 2023a). A MAC is a contracting authority that administers Medicare Part A and Part B as required by Section 911 of the Medicare Prescription Drug, Improvement, and Modernization Act of 2003 (MMA). These companies process and manage Part A and Part B claims. The Medicare cost report is a form that collects information about institutional providers to make proper determination of amounts payable under its provisions in various PPSs. The types of institutional providers that are required to submit cost reports include the following:

- Hospital
- Skilled nursing facility
- Renal facility
- Hospice
- Home health agency (HHA)
- Health clinics, including rural health clinics
- Community mental health centers
- Federally qualified health centers

Physicians and ambulatory surgical centers are not required to submit cost reports to Medicare. However, in the 2016 Report to the Congress, MedPAC recommended that ambulatory surgical centers should be added to the list of providers required to submit cost reports (MedPAC 2016, 137).

Providers submit a variety of information including facility characteristics, utilization data, cost and charges by cost center, Medicare settlement data, and financial statement data (CMS 2023a). Cost reports are due within five months of the end of the facility's fiscal year (FY) and must be compiled using an approved software vendor. Cost report data are maintained in Medicare's Health Provider Cost Reporting Information System (HCRIS). Data are available for download from the CMS website. Cost report data can be used for research with limitations imposed by CMS (CMS 2023a). The Research Data Assistance Center (ResDAC) provides free assistance, such as workshops and seminars, to academic, government, and nonprofit researchers that want to utilize HCRIS data in their studies.

Basic Medicare Value-Based Purchasing Concepts

CMS has developed a mission and vision for healthcare quality. The quality mission is that all persons receive equitable, high-quality care. The quality vision is that as a trusted partner, CMS will shape a resilient, high-value American healthcare system to achieve high-quality, safe, equitable, and accessible care for all beneficiaries (CMS 2023b). CMS works with partners, such as the MACs, healthcare community stakeholders, private payers, and others, to support and work toward their quality goals. CMS has established eight national quality strategy goals to guide their work, which are the following:

1. Embed quality into the care journey – Incorporate quality as a foundational component to delivering value as a part of the overall care journey. Quality includes ensuring optimal care and best outcomes for individuals of all ages and backgrounds as well as across service delivery systems and settings. Quality also extends across payer types.

2. Advance health equity – Address the disparities that underlie our health system, both within and across settings, to ensure equitable access and care for all.

3. Promote safety – Prevent harm or death from health care errors.

4. Foster engagement – Increase engagement between individuals and their care teams to improve quality, establish trusting relationships, and bring the voices of people and caregivers to the forefront.

5. Strengthen resilience – Ensure resilience in the healthcare system to prepare for, and adapt to, future challenges and emergencies.

6. Embrace the digital age – Ensure timely, secure, seamless communication and care coordination between providers, plans, payers, community organizations, and individuals through interoperable, shared, and standardized digital data across the care continuum.

7. Incentivize innovation & technology – Accelerate innovation in care delivery and incorporate technology enhancements (e.g. telehealth, machine learning, advanced analytics, new care advances) to transform the quality of care and advance value.

8. Increase alignment – Develop a coordinated approach to align performance metrics, programs, policy, and payment across CMS, federal partners, and external stakeholders to improve value. Strive to create a simplified national picture of quality measurement that is comprehensible to individuals, their families, providers, and payers. (CMS 2023b)

From this mission and vision and these aims and goals, and with the support of various laws, CMS has made significant strides to link quality to reimbursement. As mentioned earlier, VBP programs link quality to reimbursement by holding healthcare providers accountable for both the cost and the quality of the care they provide. The MMA established the framework for CMS to meld together quality and reimbursement. The MMA established the pay for reporting program. The move to a VBP component in the acute inpatient setting and other medical settings was further strengthened by the Deficit Reduction Act of 2005 (DRA) when a call for a VBP program was signed into law. CMS has three broad categories of VBP programs:

- Paying for reporting
- Paying for performance
- Paying for value

In the following section, an overview of pay for reporting will be provided. Then, the pay for performance or pay for value VBP component(s) will be discussed in detail for each Medicare payment system.

Quality Reporting Programs

The development of quality measures is the first step in the establishment of a VBP program. A **measure** is quantifiable data about a function or process. In VBP, measures are used to determine an organization's performance over time. CMS has established **quality reporting programs** in several service areas; that is, CMS allows a facility to maintain the full payment for services when it successfully participates in a quality-measure reporting program. In this type of program, quality is not measured per se; rather, the action of reporting data in the proper format in the given time frame is what allows facilities to receive full payment. Each payment system's quality reporting program has its own set of measures that must be reported to CMS. The measures are site-specific and relate to quality-of-care issues relevant to the healthcare delivery in a specific service area. Each year, CMS publishes in the *Federal Register* the new, modified, and retired quality measures for each program in the respective PPS final rule. The final rule includes full discussions on the intent, structure, and use for all measures considered for adoption.

Table 5.1 lists the various Medicare quality reporting programs, the law that initiated the program, and the penalty for noncompliance.

The data facilities submit must pass the validation requirement of a minimum of 80 percent reliability. This means that the submitted data must be an accurate representation of the performance of the facility. CMS uses a two-step process, which may include a chart review, to validate the submitted quality data. Some facilities have been instructed to submit data through the QualityNet Exchange secure website. Other facilities, such as post-acute-care facilities, have been instructed to use the data submission tools specific to their respective payment systems. The data populate the Hospital Compare website, which is linked to the Medicare website.

In addition to quality measures, CMS requires survey data for the hospital inpatient and home health settings. The Hospital Quality Alliance Hospital Consumer Assessment of Healthcare Providers and Systems (HCAHPS) patient survey is the first national, standardized, publicly reported survey of patients' perspectives of hospital care. HCAHPS, also known as CAHPS Hospital Survey or Hospital CAHPS, is designed to make apples-to-apples comparisons of patients' perspectives on hospital care, including communication with doctors, communication with nurses, hospital staff responsiveness, hospital cleanliness and quietness, pain control, communication about medicines, and discharge information. The Home Health Care Consumer Assessment of Healthcare Providers

Table 5.1. **Medicare quality reporting programs**

Initiative	Law*	Penalty
Hospital Inpatient	MMA 2003 / DRA 2005 / ARRA 2009 / ACA 2010	One-quarter of the applicable annual payment rate update
Hospital Outpatient	MIEA-TRHCA 2006	2% reduction to OPPS conversion factor
Ambulatory Surgical Center Quality Reporting (ASCQR)	MIEA-TRHCA 2006	2% reduction to ASC PPS conversion factor
Long-Term Care Hospital (LTCH)	ACA 2010	2% reduction to LTCH base rate
Inpatient Rehabilitation Facility (IRF)	ACA 2010	2% reduction to standard payment conversion factor
Hospice	ACA 2010	2% reduction to standard base payment rate
Home Health	DRA 2005	2% reduction to home health market basket
Inpatient Psychiatric Facility Quality Reporting (IPFQR)	ACA 2010	2% reduction to standard federal rate
PPS-Exempt Cancer Hospital	ACA 2010	No penalty
Skilled Nursing Facility	IMPACT 2014	2% reduction to payment rate

*ACA = Affordable Care Act; ARRA = American Recovery and Reinvestment Act; DRA = Deficit Reduction Act; IMPACT = Improving Medicare Post-Acute Care Transformation Act; MIEA-TRHCA = Medicare Improvements and Extension Act under Division B of Title I of the Tax Relief and Health Care Act; MMA = Medicare Modernization Act.
Source: CMS n.d.

and Systems Survey (HHCAHPS) data are collected for home health providers. Like HCAHPS, the HHCAHPS considers patients' perspectives about the care they receive from an HHA.

Medicare Hospital Acute Inpatient Services Payment System

The Medicare hospital acute inpatient services payment system is the Medicare PPS for inpatient services provided in an acute-care setting. MedPAC and others use this name on webpages and documents. However, this payment system is also referred to as the inpatient prospective payment system (IPPS) throughout CMS webpages, CMS documents, and the *Federal Register*. In this chapter the acronym IPPS is used for this payment system. IPPS provides payment to facilities but does not include payment for professional services. Some acute-care hospitals, such as those providing primarily cancer care and pediatric hospitals, are exempt from the IPPS. IPPS is a PPS that uses a case-rate methodology for reimbursement. The rate year for IPPS is October 1 through September 30, which is the same as the federal FY. In the following sections we explore the structure of the payment system, the classification system utilized, and the provisions of the system.

Medicare Severity Diagnosis-Related Group Classification System

The IPPS uses a classification system to organize inpatient admissions into large groups for reimbursement purposes. An inpatient admission starts when the patient is formally admitted to the hospital with a physician's order. The inpatient admission ends when the physician discharges the patient. IPPS utilizes the **Medicare severity diagnosis-related group (MS-DRG)** system, which takes into consideration the role that a hospital's composition of patients plays in influencing costs (Averill et al. 2001, 83). **Resource intensity** measures the amount of resources required to treat a patient. The resource intensity of a classification group, such as an MS-DRG, is represented by the **relative weight (RW)**. An RW is an assigned weight that reflects the relative resource consumption associated with a payment group. Therefore, each MS-DRG is assigned an RW that is intended to represent the resource intensity of the clinical group. It is also used to determine the payment level for the group. **Case-mix index (CMI)** is a single number that compares the overall complexity of the healthcare organization's mix of patients with the complexity of the average of all hospitals. Typically, the CMI is for a specific period and is derived from the sum of all MS-DRG weights divided by the number of cases. An example CMI for a facility would be expressed as 1.8749. Notably, how **case mix** is defined varies by the healthcare perspective. From a clinician's or physician's perspective, case-mix complexity can be used to describe the patient population. The patient population is described by the severity of illness (SOI), risk for mortality, prognosis, treatment difficulty, or need for intervention. This viewpoint used by many clinicians and physicians uses sickness as a proxy for resource consumption.

However, from the MS-DRG perspective, the case-mix complexity is a direct measure of resource consumption and, therefore, the cost of providing care. A high case mix in the MS-DRG system means patients are consuming more resources, so the cost of care is higher. However, it is a weak measure of the SOI, risk for mortality, prognosis, treatment difficulty, or need for intervention for the patient population (Averill et al. 2001, 84). Therefore, this case-mix complexity viewpoint from the MS-DRG perspective allows MS-DRGs to be an adequate system for hospital reimbursement because it measures the resources consumed for clinically similar patients.

MS-DRGs allow the IPPS to be a fully packaged system, meaning there is one payment per admission and all treatment costs are included in that payment amount. Therefore, there is only one MS-DRG assigned per encounter, and the reimbursement rate covers all services provided during the patient's admission. Additionally, this payment system uses a case-rate reimbursement methodology, which is prospective. Facilities must accept profit or loss based on the predetermined reimbursement amount for the assigned MS-DRG. If the MS-DRG reimbursement amount is greater than the facility's costs, then the facility will keep the profit. If the MS-DRG reimbursement is less than the facility's costs, then the facility will incur a loss. The case-rate prospective payment concept drives facilities to practice cost management to mitigate financial loss. In the following sections we will discuss the structure of the MS-DRG classification system, the SOI component of MS-DRGs, and the steps for MS-DRG assignment.

Structure of the MS-DRG Classification System

The MS-DRG classification system is hierarchical in design (figure 5.2). The first level in the hierarchy is **major diagnostic categories (MDCs)**, which represent the body systems treated by medicine. There are 25 MDCs, as displayed in table 5.2.

The second level in the hierarchy divides each MDC group into surgical and medical sections. The third and final level in the hierarchy divides the surgical or medical sections of the 25 MDC groups into MS-DRGs. Table 5.3 presents a sample of MS-DRGs.

Each version of the system defines the components for each MS-DRG: title, geometric mean length of stay (GMLOS), arithmetic mean length of stay (AMLOS), RW, and the *International Classification of Diseases, Tenth Revision, Clinical Modification* (ICD-10-CM) or *International Classification of Diseases, Tenth Revision, Procedure Coding System* (ICD-10-PCS) code range that drives the MS-DRG assignment (see figure 5.3).

The **arithmetic mean length of stay (AMLOS)** is the sum of all lengths of stay (LOSs) in a set of cases divided by the number of cases. The **geometric mean length of stay (GMLOS)** is the *n*th root of a series of *n* LOSs. For example, if there are five LOS data points, multiply the LOS data points together, and then take the fifth root of the product. The GMLOS is less influenced by large **outliers**—cases in payment systems with unusually long LOSs or exceptionally high costs—than the AMLOS and, therefore, is a good measure of the center of the distribution. Example 5.1 illustrates the differences between GMLOS and AMLOS.

Example 5.1. GMLOS vs. AMLOS

Suppose there are five patients with lengths of stay of 3, 5, 6, 6, and 30 days. Calculate the AMLOS and GMLOS.

$$AMLOS = \frac{3+5+6+6+30}{5} = \frac{50}{5} = 10.0 \ days$$

$$GMLOS = \sqrt[5]{3 \times 5 \times 6 \times 6 \times 30} = \sqrt[5]{16200} = 6.9 \ days$$

Notice that the GMLOS is not as influenced by the 30-day LOS outlier as the AMLOS.

Severity of Illness Component of MS-DRG Classification System

The MS-DRG classification system includes a **severity of illness (SOI)** component. SOI refers to the extent of physiological decompensation or organ system loss of function (AHIMA 2017, 215). SOI differentiation in MS-DRGs is assigned using complication and comorbidity (CC) conditions that are reported with ICD-10-CM

Figure 5.2.   Hierarchical MS-DRG system

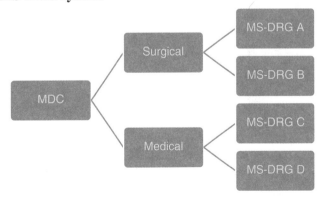

Table 5.2.   **Major diagnostic categories**

MDC	Title
01	Diseases and Disorders of the Nervous System
02	Diseases and Disorders of the Eye
03	Diseases and Disorders of the Ear, Nose, Mouth, and Throat
04	Diseases and Disorders of the Respiratory System
05	Diseases and Disorders of the Circulatory System
06	Diseases and Disorders of the Digestive System
07	Diseases and Disorders of the Hepatobiliary System and Pancreas
08	Diseases and Disorders of the Musculoskeletal System and Connective Tissue
09	Diseases and Disorders of the Skin, Subcutaneous Tissue, and Breast
10	Endocrine, Nutritional, and Metabolic Diseases and Disorders
11	Diseases and Disorders of the Kidney and Urinary Tract
12	Diseases and Disorders of the Male Reproductive System
13	Diseases and Disorders of the Female Reproductive System
14	Pregnancy, Childbirth, and the Puerperium
15	Newborns and Other Neonates with Conditions Originating in the Perinatal Period
16	Diseases and Disorders of the Blood and Blood-Forming Organs and Immunological Disorders
17	Myeloproliferative Diseases and Disorders and Poorly Differentiated Neoplasms
18	Infectious and Parasitic Diseases, Systemic and Unspecified Sites
19	Mental Diseases and Disorders
20	Alcohol/Drug Use and Alcohol/Drug-Induced Organic Mental Disorders
21	Injury, Poisoning, and Toxic Effects of Drugs
22	Burns
23	Factors Influencing Health Status and Other Contacts with Health Services
24	Multiple Significant Trauma
25	Human Immunodeficiency Virus Infections

Source: CMS 2023c.

diagnosis codes. For MS-DRG purposes, a **complication** is a medical condition that arises during the hospital stay that prolongs the LOS at least one day in approximately 75 percent of the cases. A **comorbidity** is a pre-existing condition that, because of its presence with a specific diagnosis, causes an increase in the LOS by at least one day in approximately 75 percent of the cases.

Table 5.3. **Sample of MS-DRGs**

MS-DRG	MS-DRG Title
194	Simple Pneumonia & Pleurisy with CC
291	Heart Failure & Shock with MCC
292	Heart Failure & Shock with CC
293	Heart Failure & Shock without CC/MCC
392	Esophagitis, Gastroenteritis & Misc. Digestive Disorders without MCC
470	Major Joint Replacement or Reattachment of Lower Extremity without MCC
683	Renal Failure with CC
690	Kidney & Urinary Tract Infections without MCC
871	Septicemia or Severe Sepsis without MV 96+ Hours with MCC
885	Psychoses
945	Rehabilitation with CC/MCC

Source: CMS 2023c.

The MS-DRG system groups secondary conditions into three categories: **complications and comorbidities (CCs)**, **major complications and comorbidities (MCCs)**, and conditions that are not a complication or a comorbidity (non-CC/MCCs). In general, CCs are secondary conditions that have a moderate SOI and impact on resource use. MCCs are secondary conditions that have a major or extensive SOI and impact on resource use. The remaining secondary conditions (non-CC/MCCs) are conditions that have a minor SOI and impact on resource use (HHS 2007, 47158).

SOI is applied by dividing MS-DRGs into MS-DRG families, also called MS-DRG sets. An **MS-DRG family** is a group of MS-DRGs that have the same base set of principal diagnoses with or without operating room (OR) procedures, which are divided into levels to represent SOI. There may be one, two, or three SOI levels in an MS-DRG family. MS-DRGs 291, 292, and 293 are an example of a three-SOI-level MS-DRG family that may be found in table 5.3. Figure 5.4 illustrates how MS-DRG families are divided into SOI levels.

Therefore, CC diagnosis codes, when reported as a secondary diagnosis, have the potential to impact the MS-DRG assignment by increasing the MS-DRG assignment up one severity level (see example 2 and example 3 in figure 5.4). Like CCs, MCC diagnosis codes impact MS-DRG assignment but have the potential to increase the MS-DRG assignment by one or two severity levels depending on the structure of the MS-DRG family (see example 2 and example 3 in figure 5.4). MCC secondary conditions are the highest level of severity in the MS-DRG system (HHS 2007, 47158).

Assigning MS-DRGs

Computer programs that assign patients to classification groups are generically called groupers. **Groupers** have internal logic, or an algorithm, that determines the patient groups. Although groupers are available and widely used for MS-DRG assignment, a good understanding of the assignment process is necessary to help coding and reimbursement professionals ensure proper payment for services rendered. A four-step process is used to assign MS-DRGs for hospital inpatient admissions (figure 5.5). The following sections detail this four-step process.

Figure 5.3.   **MS-DRG components**

MS-DRG 293 FY 2023		
Title: Heart Failure and Shock without Complication/Comorbidity or Major Complication/Comorbidity		
Geometric Mean Length of Stay (GMLOS):	2.1	
Arithmetic Mean Length of Stay (AMLOS):	2.5	
Relative Weight:	*0.5603*	
Principal Diagnosis		
ICD-10-CM Codes		
I09.81	I50.31	I50.813
I11.0	I50.32	I50.814
I13.0	I50.33	I50.82
I13.2	I50.40	I50.83
I50.1	I50.41	I50.84
I50.20	I50.42	I50.89
I50.21	I50.43	I50.9
I50.22	I50.810	R57.0
I50.23	I50.811	R57.9
I50.30	I50.812	

Source: CMS 2023c; HHS 2022.

Figure 5.4.   **Structure of MS-DRG families**

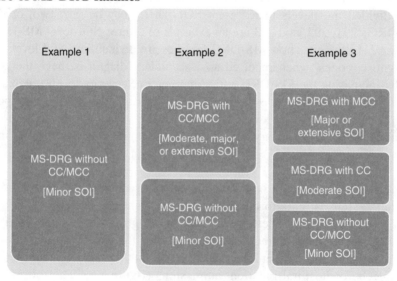

Figure 5.5.   Excerpt of MS-DRG decision tree for surgical MDC 06

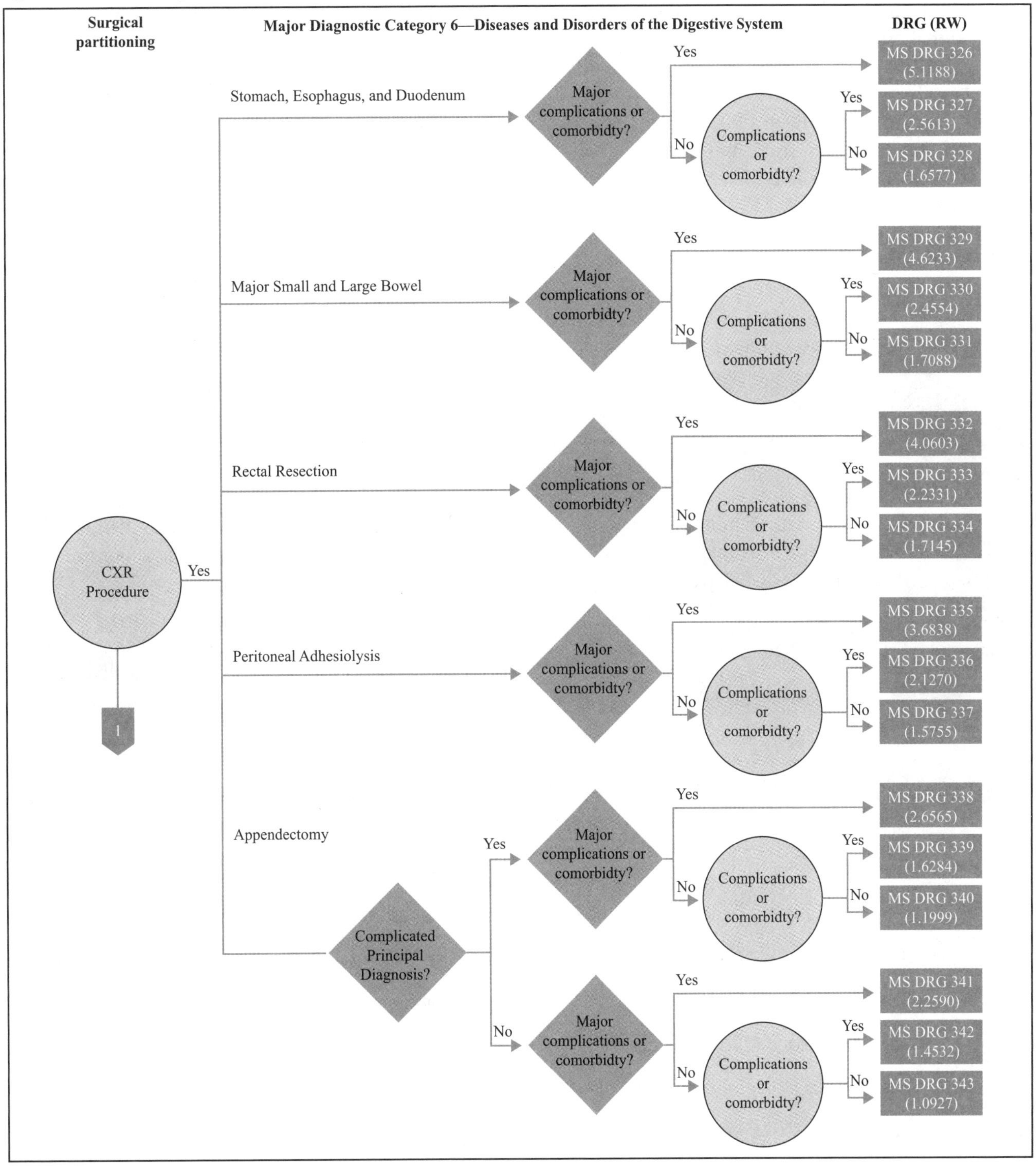

Source: CMS 2023c; HHS 2022.

Step 1: Pre-MDC Assignment

The pre-MDC assignment step was added during the version 8 revision of MS-DRGs. A set of procedures was identified that crosses all MDCs. Therefore, the **principal diagnosis** is not considered for MS-DRG assignment; rather, a defined set of ICD-10-PCS procedures is used to assign the MS-DRG. The principal diagnosis is the reason "established after study to be chiefly responsible for occasioning the admission of the patient to the hospital for care" (Hazelwood 2020, 228). The pre-MDC procedures, transplants, and tracheostomies can be performed for diagnoses from multiple MDCs. Once the admission has been determined to qualify for pre-MDC assignment, the MS-DRG is assigned and the process is complete. No other steps are taken to assign the payment group. The 15 MS-DRGs that qualify for pre-MDC assignment are displayed in table 5.4. If the MS-DRG assignment is made during step 1, all other steps are ignored. Example 5.2 provides an example of pre-MDC assignment.

Table 5.4.   Pre-MDC assignment MS-DRGs v40.1

MS-DRG	Title
001	Heart Transplant or Implant of Heart Assist System with MCC
002	Heart Transplant or Implant of Heart Assist System without MCC
003	Extracorporeal Membrane Oxygenation (ECMO) or Tracheostomy with Mechanical Ventilation 96+ Hours or Principal Diagnosis Except Face, Mouth, and Neck Diagnoses with Major OR Procedure
004	Tracheostomy with Mechanical Ventilation 96+ Hours or Principal Diagnosis Except Face, Mouth, and Neck Diagnoses without Major OR Procedure
005	Liver Transplant with MCC or Intestinal Transplant
006	Liver Transplant without MCC
007	Lung Transplant
008	Simultaneous Pancreas/Kidney Transplant
010	Pancreas Transplant
011	Tracheostomy for Face, Mouth & Neck Diagnoses or Laryngectomy with MCC
012	Tracheostomy for Face, Mouth & Neck Diagnoses or Laryngectomy with CC
013	Tracheostomy for Face, Mouth & Neck Diagnoses or Laryngectomy without CC/MCC
014	Allogenic Bone Marrow Transplant
016	Autologous Bone Marrow Transplant with CC/MCC
017	Autologous Bone Marrow Transplant without CC/MCC
018	Chimeric Antigen Receptor (CAR) T-cell and Other Immunotherapies
019	Simultaneous Pancreas and Kidney Transplant with Hemodialysis

Source: HHS 2022, table 5.

Example 5.2. Step 1: Pre-MDC assignment

A pancreas transplant can be performed for a variety of clinical conditions, including diabetes with renal, ophthalmic, neurological, or peripheral circulatory manifestations (MDC 10); hypertensive renal disease (MDC 05); chronic pancreatitis (MDC 06); chronic renal failure (MDC 11); and complications of transplanted organs (MDC 21). The diagnoses that warrant a pancreas transplant can be found in multiple MDCs. There is only one MS-DRG for all pancreas transplants regardless of the principal diagnosis to maintain a manageable number of MS-DRGs and to adhere to the concept of like-resource consumption groupings. Thus, the patient who received a pancreas transplant would be assigned to MS-DRG 010 regardless of the principal diagnosis.

Step 2: Major Diagnostic Category Determination

The principal diagnosis is used to place the admission into one of the 25 MDCs. MDCs are the highest level in the hierarchical structure of MS-DRGs. The 25 MDCs are primarily based on body system involvement, with a few categories based on disease etiology (see table 5.2). Example 5.3 provides an example of MDC determination. After the MDC is established for the admission, step 2 is complete, and the case moves on to step 3.

Example 5.3. Step 2: MDC determination

Patient A presents and is treated for pneumonia caused by *Streptococcus*, Group A. Group A streptococcus pneumonia is a respiratory disease. Therefore, the ICD-10-CM code for Group A streptococcus pneumonia is assigned to MDC 04, Diseases and Disorders of the Respiratory System.

Step 3: Medical/Surgical Determination

The next step is to determine whether an OR procedure was performed. The procedures considered in this step may be the principal procedure or a secondary procedure. The MS-DRG Definitions Manual identifies which procedures are qualifying OR procedures and therefore allows an admission to be classified as surgical. Additionally, many ICD-10-PCS codebooks provide a flag or indicator for procedure codes that qualify as valid or nonvalid OR procedures. Minor procedures and testing are not qualifying procedures. If a qualifying OR procedure was not performed, the case is assigned a medical status. Example 5.4 provides an illustration of medical or surgical determination.

Once the medical or surgical status is assigned, step 3 is complete, and the case proceeds to step 4.

Example 5.4. Step 3: Medical or surgical determination

Patient A presents and is treated for an acute myocardial infarction of the anterolateral wall, initial episode (heart attack). The ICD-10-CM code for this diagnosis is assigned to MDC 05, Diseases and Disorders of the Circulatory System (step 2). During the hospital stay, a percutaneous transluminal coronary angioplasty (PTCA) is performed on the right coronary artery. The PTCA code is a valid OR procedure. Thus, this case is a surgical case in MDC 05.

Like Patient A, Patient B is also evaluated for an acute myocardial infarction of the anterolateral wall, initial episode (heart attack). The ICD-10-CM code for this diagnosis is assigned to MDC 05, Diseases and Disorders of the Circulatory System (step 2). However, no procedures were performed for this patient during the hospital stay. This case is a medical case in MDC 05.

Step 4: Refinement

Step 4 uses various refinement questions to isolate the correct MS-DRG. This refinement process allows the MS-DRG system to group clinically similar patients with like resource consumption. The following are examples of refinement questions:

- Is an MCC present?

- Is a CC present?

- Did the patient have an acute myocardial infarction, heart failure, or shock?

- Did the patient's coma last less than or greater than one hour?

- Was the procedure performed for a neoplasm?

- What is the patient's sex?

- What is the patient's discharge status code (alive or expired)?

The refinement process may include one question or multiple questions before the final MS-DRG is assigned. The most common pathways are those that identify CC and MCC conditions. The presence of a CC or MCC diagnosis code as a secondary condition represents an expected increase in resource consumption for an admission and, therefore, is part of the refinement process. Examples 5.5 and 5.6 illustrate how the refinement questions are utilized in the MS-DRG assignment process. In example 5.5 there are two refinement questions required to determine the final MS-DRG, and in example 5.6 only one question is required.

Example 5.5. Step 4: Refinement process for a surgical admission

Patient A is 67 years old and is admitted for a duodenum fistula closure procedure. The patient also has osteomyelitis of vertebra of the cervical region. The duodenum fistula code (principal diagnosis) is assigned to MDC 06, Diseases and Disorders of the Digestive System (step 2). The fistula closure procedure code is a valid OR procedure (step 3). Therefore, the case is a surgical MDC 06 case. There are two applicable pathway questions for this admission. First, is there an MCC present? No, the osteomyelitis of vertebra is not on the MCC list (ICD-10-CM MS-DRGs v40.1). Second, is there a CC present? Yes, osteomyelitis of vertebra is a comorbidity. Now that all refinement questions have been answered, the MS-DRG can be assigned. The MS-DRG for this case is 327, Stomach, Esophageal, and Duodenal Procedures with CC.

Example 5.6. Step 4: Refinement process for a medical admission

Patient B is 68 years old and is admitted for cellulitis of the right ankle. Nonexcisional debridement is performed on the right ankle. The patient also has chronic obstructive pulmonary disease (COPD). The cellulitis (principal diagnosis) code is assigned to MDC 09, Diseases and Disorders of the Skin, Subcutaneous Tissue, and Breast (step 2). Nonexcisional debridement is not a valid OR procedure (step 3), so the case is a medical MDC 09 case. There is one applicable pathway question for this admission. Is an MCC present? No, COPD is not an MCC. Now that all refinement questions have been answered, the MS-DRG assignment can be made. The MS-DRG assignment for this case is MS-DRG 603, Cellulitis without MCC.

CC/MCC Exclusion Lists

Each ICD-10-CM code designated as a CC or MCC is assigned exclusion lists. **CC/MCC exclusion lists** consist of principal diagnoses that take away the refinement power from the CC or MCC code. The principal diagnoses included in the exclusion list are often very closely related to the CC or MCC code. When the two conditions are so closely related, the CC/MCC condition is not expected to increase the LOS or resource consumption and, therefore, should not be utilized to assign the admission to a higher-weighted MS-DRG.

For example, ICD-10-CM code I25.3, Aneurysm of the Heart, is a CC. The CC exclusion list for code I25.3 includes principal diagnosis ICD-10-CM code I25.41, Coronary Artery Aneurysm. When code I25.41 is the principal diagnosis and code I25.3 is a secondary diagnosis during the same admission, code I25.3 (CC) will not trigger the refinement pathway for an MS-DRG with CC. Instead, because of the CC exclusion, the admission would follow a without-CC pathway if no other CC or MCC codes are reported for the admission. Essentially, code I25.3 has lost its refinement power for this MS-DRG assignment.

Invalid Coding and Data Abstraction

Accurate diagnosis and procedure coding and healthcare information abstracting are vital to MS-DRG assignment. When invalid codes or data are submitted on the patient claim form, one of two MS-DRGs is assigned. MS-DRG 998, Principal Diagnosis Invalid as Discharge Diagnosis, is assigned when the principal diagnosis reported is not specific enough for MS-DRG assignment. MS-DRG 999, Ungroupable, is assigned when an invalid diagnosis code, age, sex, or discharge status code is reported. Payment for each of these MS-DRGs is zero dollars. The claim is returned to the provider and should be corrected, then resubmitted to Medicare.

Payment System Provision

IPPS uses provisions to provide additional payments for specialized programs and unusual admissions that historically have added significant cost to patient care. Without the additional payments associated with these provisions, it may not be feasible for acute-care facilities to provide all services to Medicare beneficiaries. The following section discusses high-cost outlier admissions, the new medical services and technologies adjustment, and transfer cases.

High-Cost Outlier

Because the Medicare payment for inpatient services is prospective, hospitals will experience profit or loss for individual cases when reimbursements exceed or fall short of their cost. The payment provided to facilities is an average amount, meaning some cases will result in a profit and some a loss. Normally, costs are covered if the facility performs reasonable cost management. However, there are extreme cases, outliers, for which the costs are very high when compared with the average costs for cases in the same MS-DRG. The outlier payment provision provides some financial relief for these individual cases.

For an admission to qualify for an outlier payment, the hospital's Medicare-approved charges reported on the claim are converted to estimated costs using the cost-to-charge ratio (CCR). The CCR is derived from the hospital's cost report. The estimated costs are compared with the fixed-loss cost threshold. The fixed-loss cost threshold is the sum of the MS-DRG case rate, the outlier threshold established for that FY, and any adjustments applicable to the facility or case. There are several adjustments possible. The first is the **indirect medical education (IME)** adjustment. The IME adjustment is a percentage increase in Medicare reimbursement to offset the costs of medical education that a teaching hospital incurs. The second, the **disproportionate share hospital (DSH)** adjustment, is provided for healthcare organizations that meet governmental criteria for percentages of indigent patients. A hospital with an unequally large share of low-income patients is given an adjustment to adjust for the financial burden (CMS 2023d). The third adjustment included in the outlier calculation is **new technology**. New technology is "an advance in medical technology that substantially improves, relative to technologies previously available, the diagnosis or treatment of Medicare beneficiaries" (HHS 2019, 42181). When a hospital uses a new technology during an admission, an additional payment amount is added to the reimbursement for that admission. If the fixed-loss cost threshold is exceeded, additional payment is made. The payment is 80 percent of the difference between the hospital's entire cost for the stay and the fixed-loss cost threshold amount (HHS 2022, 49418). So, the final reimbursement for an outlier case is the MS-DRG payment amount plus the high-cost outlier payment. Even with the high-cost outlier add-on payment amount, the total reimbursement for an outlier admission will still be lower than the actual costs of the admission. The high-cost outlier payment provides some relief but is not intended to cover all the costs for the admission.

It is important to remember that this provision is applied to individual cases when analyzing inpatient data. A data analyst may examine inpatient data by MS-DRG. High-cost outlier admissions will stand out because the reimbursement is higher than the standard MS-DRG amount. See figure 5.6 for a summary of this payment provision.

New Medical Services and New Technologies

New medical services, new technologies, and innovative methods for treating patients are often very costly. Applicants for the status of new technology must submit a formal request, including a full description of the technology's clinical use and the results of any evaluations that demonstrate that the new technology provides a better outcome over current treatment, to demonstrate that the technology should be considered eligible for the high-cost threshold.

Providing these innovative services in a prospective system could, in many cases, lead to inadequate payments. These financial losses may prohibit a facility from offering new and innovative services to patients because they are simply not affordable. Therefore, to ensure new and innovative services and technologies are provided to Medicare beneficiaries, the IPPS allows additional payments to be made for new medical services and new technologies. The add-on reimbursement amount is applied to the individual admissions where the new medical service or technology is used. Again, much like the high-cost outlier policy, it is important to remember that this policy will result in a higher-than-expected reimbursement amount for the impacted admissions. Data analysts examining MS-DRG inpatient data will see individual admissions with higher reimbursement amounts than the standard rate. A portion of those admissions may be due to new medical services and new technology policy. See figure 5.6 for a summary of this payment provision.

Transfer Cases

A **transfer** is an admission where the patient is moved to a different healthcare facility to complete their course of care. There are two types of transfer cases under the IPPS. The first category is a patient transfer between two IPPS hospitals. A type 1 transfer occurs when a patient is discharged from an acute IPPS hospital and is admitted to another acute IPPS hospital on the same day. If a patient leaves an acute IPPS hospital against medical advice and is admitted to another acute IPPS hospital on the same day, this situation is treated as a transfer between two IPPS hospitals.

Payment is altered for the transferring hospital and is based on a per diem rate methodology. The MS-DRG is established for the case and the full payment rate is calculated. This payment rate is divided by the GMLOS established for the MS-DRG, creating a per diem rate. The transferring facility receives double the per diem rate for the first day, plus the per diem rate for each day thereafter for the patient's LOS. DSH, IME, and outlier adjustments are applied after the per diem rate is established. The receiving facility receives full PPS payment for the case. The only exception to this rule is MS-DRG 789, Neonates Died or Transferred to Another Acute Care Facility. The payment and GMLOS established for MS-DRG 789 are based on historical data; no reduction is necessary because it is a transfer-related MS-DRG.

A transfer that occurs from an IPPS hospital to a hospital or unit excluded from IPPS is known as a type 2 transfer. For this type of transfer case, the full PPS payment is made to the transferring hospital, and the receiving hospital or unit is paid based on its respective payment system (CMS 2023e). The type 2 transfer policy applies to the following facility types, which are excluded from IPPS:

- Inpatient rehabilitation facilities or units

- Long-term care hospitals

- Psychiatric hospitals and units

- Children's hospitals

- Cancer hospitals

However, there are exceptions to the payment policy, known as the **post-acute-care transfer (PACT)** policy, for type 2 transfer cases. Under the PACT policy, CMS applies the type 1 transfer methodology to designated MS-DRGs. When conditions are met for a type 1 transfer, a per diem amount, which is lower than the standard MS-DRG reimbursement rate, is paid. This special payment policy better reimburses facilities in the PACT situation while ensuring that there is no incentive for hospitals to discharge patients early to reduce costs while

Figure 5.6.   Summary of payment system provisions

High-Cost Outlier	New Medical Services and Technologies	Transfer Cases
• Actual costs for the case exceed threshold • Additional reimbursement amount is paid • Total reimbursement will never be greater than cost for an high-cost outlier admission • This provision is executed for individual admissions	• CMS's approach to ensuring that new technologies are available to Medicare beneficiaries • Add-on additional reimbursement • This provision is executed for individual admissions	• Patient is transferred from one facility to another • PACT – post-acute-care transfer policy • Reduces reimbursement amount because patient LOS is less than the average LOS • This provision is executed for individual admissions

still receiving full MS-DRG payment. The policy reduces the MS-DRG reimbursement amount because the patient was discharged too early. In addition, this policy allows for proper reimbursement levels when the full course of treatment is divided across two healthcare settings.

When data analysts review MS-DRG inpatient data, they may see individual admissions with a lower-than-expected reimbursement amount. These admissions are PACT cases. The payment rate is reduced via the PACT policy. See figure 5.6 for a summary of this payment provision.

Payment Workflow

The components of the IPPS work together to compute the final payment for an acute-care inpatient admission. Figure 5.7 shows the foundation for an IPPS payment. The process is completed by a MAC, an entity that process claims on behalf of Medicare.

A base payment rate is established for each Medicare-participating hospital for each FY. The **base payment rate** is a per-admission amount that is adjusted for each hospital. It is based on historic national claims data and is updated each year by a fixed percentage to account for inflation.

Each year, the national standardized amount is divided into a labor-related share and a nonlabor share. The **labor-related share** represents the facilities' relative proportion of wages and salaries, employee benefits, professional fees, and other labor-intensive services. Labor-related share is typically 70 to 75 percent of healthcare facilities' costs. The **nonlabor share** is the facilities' operating costs not related to labor. The labor-related share is adjusted by the **wage index** for the hospital's geographic location based on core-based statistical areas (CBSAs). The wage index is a ratio that represents the relationship between the average wages in a healthcare setting's geographic area and the national average for that healthcare setting. The wage-index formula is provided in figure 5.8.

Wage indexes are adjusted annually and published in the *Federal Register*. If the hospital is located in Alaska or Hawaii, the nonlabor share is modified by a **cost-of-living adjustment (COLA)**. COLA reflects a change in the consumer price index (CPI), which measures purchasing power between time periods. The CPI is based on a market basket of goods and services that a typical consumer buys. The COLA formula is provided in figure 5.9.

Wage-index adjustment and COLA are the first steps of changing the national standardized amount to a hospital-specific base rate and are found in the IPPS final rule each year. These adjustments establish the base payment rate adjusted for geographic factors for the effective FY.

The next step in customizing the base rate involves applying the IPPS adjustments of DSH and IME. Effective for discharges occurring on or after May 1, 1986, DSH status was enacted for facilities with a high percentage of low-income patients (CMS 2023d). These hospitals receive additional payment because they experience a financial hardship by providing treatment for patients who are unable to pay for the services rendered.

Approved teaching hospitals are provided an IME adjustment. The hospitals must have residents in an approved graduate medical education program. Teaching hospitals experience higher patient care costs compared to nonteaching hospitals. Thus, Medicare provides IME hospitals with additional reimbursement to help offset the

Figure 5.7.   Foundation of inpatient prospective payment system

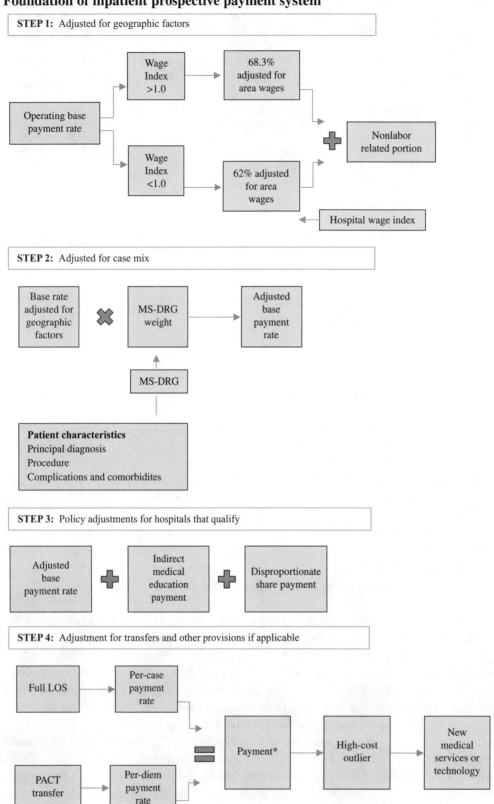

Note: Capital payments are determined by a similar system.
*Additional payment made for certain rural hospitals.
Source: Adapted from MedPAC 2022.

Figure 5.8.   **Wage-index adjustment formula**

> (Federal per diem base rate × Labor percent × Wage index) + (Federal per diem base rate × Nonlabor percentage)

Figure 5.9.   **COLA formula**

> (Federal per diem base rate × Labor percent) + (Federal per diem base rate × Nonlabor percent × COLA)

costs of providing education to new physicians. The IME payment adjustment is hospital specific. The adjustment factor is based on the hospital's ratio of residents to beds and a multiplier established by Congress.

If the hospital has DSH status, the established percentage for that year for that facility is added into the hospital adjusted base payment rate. Likewise, if the hospital qualifies for IME payments, then the established percentage for that year for that facility is incorporated into the base rate value as well. Once the applicable adjustments have been applied, the base rate is then considered to be the fully adjusted, hospital-specific base payment rate.

As shown in figure 5.7, the exact calculation for each admission is complex. Therefore, some revenue cycle professionals perform a basic IPPS calculation to get a reimbursement estimate for inpatient cases. For the calculation, two pieces of information are required: (1) the fully adjusted, hospital-specific base rate and (2) the MS-DRG RW. The fully adjusted, hospital-specific base rate is multiplied by the MS-DRG RW to estimate reimbursement. Examples 5.7 and 5.8 illustrate this calculation.

Example 5.7

Patient A was treated for hip fracture, and an OR procedure was performed. MS-DRG 470 is assigned for the admission. The RW for MS-DRG 470 is 1.9119. The fully adjusted base rate for this hospital is $7,325. The RW is multiplied by the hospital base rate to calculate the estimated payment rate. The estimated payment rate for this case is $14,004.67 (1.9119 × $7,325).

Example 5.8

Patient B was treated for congestive heart failure, and non-OR procedures were performed. MS-DRG 293 is assigned for the admission. The RW for MS-DRG 293 is 0.5603. The fully adjusted base rate for this hospital is $7,325. The RW is multiplied by the hospital base rate to calculate the estimated payment rate. The estimated payment rate for this case is $4,104.20 (0.5603 × $7,325).

Check Your Understanding 5.1

1. Describe CMS's quality reporting program.

2. List the steps of MS-DRG assignment.

3. List two examples of refinement questions used in the fourth step of MS-DRG assignment.

4. What does the labor-related share of the standardized amount represent?

5. What is the formula for the basic IPPS payment calculation?

CMS Value-Based Purchasing Programs for the Hospital Acute Inpatient Setting

Establishing the need to collect data on quality measures led to the need to reward providers with incentive payments for high-quality performance. CMS investigated value-based programs through several demonstration projects, including the Premier Hospital Quality Incentive Demonstration. The success of this demonstration project was reported to Congress in 2007. In this report, CMS supports the introduction of a broad VBP payment policy for hospitals, which includes payment for quality performance (CMS 2009, 8). CMS continues to expand the breadth of the value-based programs across the continuum of healthcare provided to Medicare beneficiaries. Figure 5.10 is from the "Value-Based Programs" section of the CMS website. It provides an excellent overview of the various programs adopted over the last 10-plus years.

Hospital Value-Based Purchasing Program

Section 3001(a)(1) of the Affordable Care Act of 2010 (ACA) requires CMS to implement a Hospital VBP program that rewards hospitals for the quality of care they provide (CMS 2011a, 26493). In April 2011, CMS released the final rule for a Hospital VBP program. The Hospital VBP program takes the Hospital Inpatient Quality Reporting (IQR) program to the next level by providing incentive payments for performance achievement and performance improvement. Implementing this program was a significant VBP step for CMS because hospital payments accounted for the largest share of Medicare spending in 2009, with more than 12.4 million inpatient hospitalizations (CMS 2011b). This program uses a withhold amount to fund the incentive payments. A **withhold** is a portion of facility payments that is held back and then redistributed based on a facility's performance for the designated quality measures. Initially, the MS-DRG base operating payment amounts were reduced by 1 percent in FY 2013. The withhold amount rose to 2 percent by FY 2017 to fund the incentive payments. Since 2017, the

Figure 5.10.   CMS's value-based programs timeline

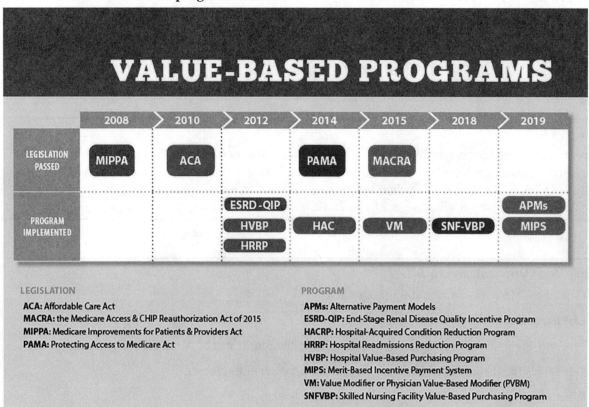

withhold amount has remained at 2 percent (CMS 2021). One hundred percent of the reduction of MS-DRG base amounts is redistributed among participating providers based on their **total performance score (TPS)**. The TPS is a measure of a facility's overall performance for the clinical domain quality measures and other requirements included in the VBP program.

Not all providers are eligible for participation in the incentive program. Providers that are excluded are providers that are the following:

- Subject to payment reductions under the hospital IQR program

- Cited for deficiencies during the performance period that pose immediate jeopardy to the health or safety of patients

- Hospitals without a minimum number of cases, measures, or surveys

It is important to note that hospitals excluded from the incentive program will not have the 2 percent withhold amount taken from their operating base MS-DRG amount.

The Hospital VBP program will measure hospital performance using four domains:

1. Clinical outcomes

2. Person and community engagement

3. Safety

4. Efficiency and cost reduction (HHS 2022, 49113)

Each domain includes a number of measures that must be reported by participating hospitals and are evaluated to determine if a hospital will earn an incentive each year. Measures are added and removed from each of these domains annually when CMS updates the IPPS. For each measure, hospitals are scored based on their performance achievement as well as their performance improvement. **Performance achievement** compares a facility's performance with all other facilities' performance. **Performance improvement** compares a facility's current performance with the facility's baseline performance. When calculating a facility's TPS, each domain is weighted at 25 percent. These weights apply to the 2018 reporting year and beyond.

The measures within each domain are scaled to determine a score for the domain. The domain scores are combined based on their weights, resulting in a TPS. A facility's TPS determines what portion of the withhold amount the facility will earn back. For every point increase in the TPS, the provider will increase payment by a portion of the withhold dollars, so in this VBP, a higher TPS score is desired. An example TPS calculation is displayed in figure 5.11.

The VBP adjustment is expressed as the percentage of the IPPS payment that the hospital will receive. CMS calibrates the VBP adjustment so that the distribution is centered at 100 percent, meaning that the typical hospital will earn back the 2 percent withhold amount and be paid at their full MS-DRG payment. Figure 5.12 shows the distribution of VBP adjustments for FY 2020. Notice that adjustments range from 98 percent (hospital receives none of the 2 percent withhold amount) to 103 percent (hospital receives more than the 2 percent withhold amount).

Hospital-Acquired Conditions Present on Admission Indicator Reporting Provision

Section 5001(c) of Public Law 109-171, the DRA, required the secretary of Health and Human Services to implement the hospital-acquired conditions present on admission indicator (HAC POA) program to IPPS. This provision was added to IPPS in 2002. This additional component of value-based programs uses reported ICD-10-CM diagnosis codes and the **present on admission (POA) indicator** to identify quality issues. The POA indicator identifies if the condition or disease was present before the admission or developed during the hospital admission. If the condition developed during the hospital admission, then it is considered a **hospital-acquired condition (HAC)**.

Figure 5.11.   Example hospital total performance score calculation

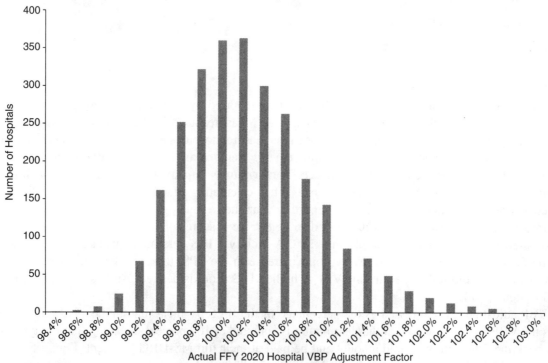

Domain	Unweighted Domain Score		Domain Weight		Weighted Domain Score
✚ Clinical Outcomes	75.00	X	25%	=	18.750
👤 Person and Community Engagement	62.00	X	25%	=	15.500
⚠ Safety	55.00	X	25%	=	13.750
$ Efficiency and Cost Reduction	100.00	X	25%	=	25.000

}73

Source: Quality Reporting Center 2020.

Figure 5.12.   Distribution of VBP payment adjustment factors for FY 2020

Source: CMS 2020, table 16.

The secretary of Health and Human Services included conditions that fall within the following criteria in the provision:

- High cost or high volume
- Result in the assignment of a case to an MS-DRG that has a higher payment when present as a secondary diagnosis
- Could reasonably have been prevented through the application of evidence-based guidelines

Under this program, IPPS payment is adjusted when HAC conditions are reported as occurring during the hospitalization—that is, the condition(s) was(were) not POA. MS-DRG payments are made based on the MS-DRG that the case would be assigned if the HAC secondary diagnosis was not present. Hospitals are required to submit a POA indicator for reportable diagnoses on the UB-04/837I unless the diagnosis is on an exclusion list on or after October 1, 2007.

In the annual IPPS final rule, CMS finalizes the conditions that are included in the HAC POA. CMS recognizes 14 categories of HACs:

1. Foreign object retained after surgery

2. Air embolism

3. Blood incompatibility

4. Stage III and IV pressure ulcers

5. Falls and trauma

6. Catheter-associated urinary tract infection

7. Vascular catheter-associated infection

8. Surgical site infection, mediastinitis, following coronary artery bypass graft

9. Manifestations of poor glycemic control

10. Deep vein thrombosis (DVT)/pulmonary embolism (PE) with total knee or hip replacement

11. Surgical site infection following bariatric surgery

12. Surgical site infection following certain orthopedic procedures of spine, shoulder, and elbow

13. Surgical site infection following cardiac implantable electronic device

14. Iatrogenic pneumothorax with venous catheterization (CMS 2022b)

The HAC POA provision applies only when the selected conditions are the only MCC or CC present on the claim. Figure 5.13 provides a flowchart of the HAC POA process. If additional MCC or CC conditions are present on the claim along with the HAC diagnosis, then the case will continue to be assigned to the higher-paying MS-DRG, and there will be no savings to Medicare from the case.

Hospital-Acquired Condition Reduction Program

Section 3008 of the ACA added Section 1886(p) to the Social Security Act of 1935, which implemented a new initiative titled Hospital-Acquired Condition Reduction Program (HACRP). The HACRP provides payment incentives to facilities for the reduction in HAC conditions beginning October 1, 2014. Hospitals with HACRP scores in the lowest-performing quartile will have payments for all encounters reduced by 1 percent. Unlike the Hospital VBP program and the Hospital Readmissions Reduction Program (HRRP), the payment reduction under the HACRP is the payment amount after the application of program adjustments such as outlier, DSH, and IME. Although both the HACRP and HAC POA are focused on the reduction in HACs, they are actually two separate programs, each with its own controlling laws and regulations.

A total HACRP score is calculated for each hospital based on inpatient claims submitted for Medicare payment. There are two domains included in the total HACRP score:

1. CMS Recalibrated Patient Safety Indicator 90 (CMS PSI 90)

2. Measures maintained by the Centers for Disease Control and Prevention (CDC) and National Healthcare Safety Network (NHSN) used for tracking healthcare-associated infections (HAIs)

Figure 5.13.   Flowchart of the HAC POA process

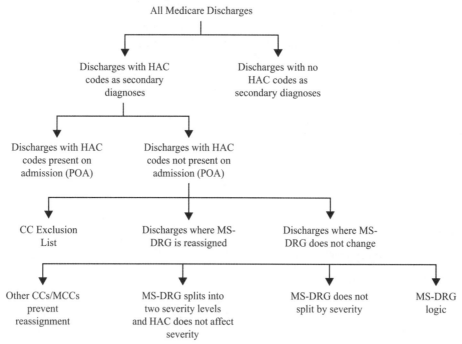

Source: HHS 2014.

Measures included in the program are discussed each year during the rulemaking process. Final measures are reported in the IPPS final rule. Table 5.5 indicates the domains and measures for 2020. Domain I is weighted at 15 percent and domain II is weighted at 85 percent of the total HAC score.

Each facility receives a confidential HACRP report providing the facility's measure scores, domain scores, and total HACRP score. Facilities have an opportunity to review the report and to submit changes to the report prior to the data being posted for public viewing on the Hospital Compare website.

Table 5.5.   HAC domains and measures

Domain	Measure
I	CMS Recalibrated Patient Safety Indicator 90 (CMS PSI 90)
II	Central line-associated bloodstream infection (CLABSI)
	Catheter-associated urinary tract infection (CAUTI)
	Surgical site infection (SSI) – colon and hysterectomy
	Methicillin-resistant Staphylococcus aureus (MRSA) bacteremia
	Clostridium difficile infection (CDI)

Source: CMS 2022c.

Hospital Readmission Reduction Program

Section 3025 of the ACA amended by Section 10309 of the ACA added Section 1886(q) of the act to establish the HRRP beginning October 1, 2012. Under the HRRP, IPPS base operating MS-DRG payment amounts are reduced by a hospital-specific adjustment factor that accounts for the hospital's excess readmissions. For each applicable year, CMS determines which types of admissions will be included in the readmission measurement. An encounter is counted as a readmission when the patient returns to an IPPS hospital for the focus conditions within 30 days of discharge from the original admission, and the admission is not a planned readmission. CMS has established exclusions to the formula to account for planned readmissions for the focus admissions.

Base operating MS-DRG payments (payment rate prior to application of outlier, IME, DSH, and so on) are reduced by the hospital-specific adjustment amount for the floor adjustment amount. Hospital-specific adjustment amounts are released each year in the IPPS final rule. The adjustment amount reported by CMS is actually the proportion of the full IPPS base operating payment that the provider will receive. Example 5.9 illustrates the HRRP adjustment calculation.

Example 5.9

Hospital A has a readmission adjustment factor of 0.9850 and will receive 98.5% (0.9850 × 100) of the full IPPS payment. This may also be expressed as a reduction in payment using the following calculation:

$$1.0000 - 0.9850 = 0.015 \times 100 = 1.5\% \text{ adjustment (reduction)}$$

Base operating payment will be reduced by 1.5% for the applicable payment year.

Thus, hospitals that have excess readmissions may have up to 3 percent of their base MS-DRG operating amount reduced for all admissions during the applicable payment year. Reduction adjustments are recalculated for each federal FY. CMS may change the particular clinical areas subject to the HRRP. For federal FY 2023, the focus areas are as follows:

1. Acute Myocardial Infarction (AMI)

2. Chronic Obstructive Pulmonary Disease (COPD)

3. Heart Failure (HF)

4. Pneumonia

5. Coronary Artery Bypass Graft (CABG) Surgery

6. Elective Primary Total Hip Arthroplasty and/or Total Knee Arthroplasty (THA/TKA) (CMS 2023f)

Although the excess readmission ratio is based only on the six procedures and conditions listed, the reduction in payment is assessed on the IPPS base operating payment for all Medicare inpatient discharges.

The Medicare hospital acute inpatient services payment system demonstrates that payment systems are often extraordinarily complex and include provisions based on healthcare policy. While the reimbursement methodology may be a foundational component, the payment systems are more than a simple reimbursement methodology. The classification system, provisions, and adjustment allow Medicare to reimburse hospitals based on a combination of the beneficiary's health condition and facility-specific circumstances. For this payment system, CMS operates four VBP programs to ensure that high-quality care is provided while incentivizing facilities to achieve operational efficiency.

Patient Connection

Malakai has played basketball his whole life, and he spent 20 years coaching high school boys' basketball. Over the past couple of years, Malakai's right knee pain has been becoming more intense. A couple of months ago, he started to show a significant limp. Last month he saw his primary care physician, Dr. Lewis, to see if he needed to see an orthopedic physician. Malakai saw Dr. Shah, his orthopedic physician, and the news was not good. Dr. Shah indicated that, due to significant and worsening osteoarthritis, Malakai needed a knee replacement. Malakai was admitted to Memorial Hospital, and Dr. Shah performed a right knee arthroplasty. His admission was six days long. A six-day LOS is about double the average LOS for this type of surgery. Malakai had significant issues during recovery and was unable to pass in-hospital physical therapy requirements. He was transferred to a skilled nursing facility upon discharge to help with his recovery.

The MS-DRG assigned for his admission was MS-DRG 470, Major Hip and Knee Joint Replacement or Reattachment of Lower Extremity without MCC. The RW for the MS-DRG is 1.9119. Memorial Hospital's hospital base rate is $6,685. Referring to examples 5.7 and 5.8, we know the basic reimbursement calculation is the MS-DRG RW times the hospital base rate. Therefore, the basic reimbursement calculation for Malakai's admission is: 1.9119 × $6,685. The estimated reimbursement for this admission equals $12,781.05. But how does this compare to the cost of the admission, since Malakai's LOS was six days? The cost of Malakai's visit was $18,673.27. However, since Medicare uses a prospective case-rate reimbursement methodology, Memorial Hospital is responsible for the loss. Medicare will not reimburse Memorial Hospital over the $12,781.05 amount.

Olivia is ready to deliver her baby. She is admitted to Memorial Hospital and has a vaginal delivery. She has a healthy baby boy. She does not have any complications and is discharged after two days, along with her son. Olivia has commercial insurance through Super Payer. Super Payer uses the MS-DRG classification system as the basis for their case-rate methodology negotiated with Memorial Hospital. Their payment system uses MS-DRGs but does not use any of the Medicare-associated provisions. This is a common methodology for non-government-sponsored insurance companies. In these payment systems, the payer uses the MS-DRG RW but replaces the Medicare hospital base rate with its own internally determined base rate.

Olivia's MS-DRG for the admission was 807, Vaginal Delivery without Sterilization or Dilation and Curettage, without CC/MCC. The RW for MS-DRG 807 is 0.6314. The base rate negotiated between Super Payer and Memorial Hospital is $10,125.50. Let's calculate the estimated reimbursement amount using the basic reimbursement calculation we have been using. The calculation is 0.6314 × $10,125.50. The estimated reimbursement for this admission equals $6,393.24.

Chapter 5 Review Quiz

1. Which reimbursement methodology is used in IPPS?

2. Which SOI level is reflected by CC codes? Which SOI level is reflected by MCC codes?

3. Fatima is calculating the MS-DRG for an inpatient admission. She has determined that the encounter does not quality for pre-MDC assignment. What is the next step in the MS-DRG assignment process?

   a. Determine the MDC for the principal diagnosis

   b. Determine the MDC for the principal procedure

   c. Determine if the case is medical or surgical

   d. Determine if there is a CC in the secondary diagnosis position

4. Eli is calculating the MS-DRG for an inpatient admission. He is determining if the encounter is medical or surgical. Which of the following should he do?

   a. Determine if the physician dictated an operative report for the principal procedure; if so, then the encounter is surgical

   b. Determine if the principal procedure is an OR procedure in the MS-DRG Definitions Manual

   c. Determine if any procedure reported, principal or secondary, is an OR procedure in the MS-DRG Definitions Manual

   d. Look at the encounter charges and see if there are any OR charges.

5. Which payment system provision provides additional reimbursement for new technologies that enhance beneficiary outcomes?

6. Why does the IME adjustment add reimbursement for teaching facilities?

7. What are the four domains used in the Hospital VBP program?

8. Discuss the importance of the present on admission (POA) data element in the HAC POA program.

9. Review table 5.5. In the HAC reduction program, domain II tracks healthcare-associated infections (HAIs). Name two measures used in this domain.

10. List a focus area of the Hospital Readmissions Reduction Program (HRRP).

References

AHIMA (American Health Information Management Association). 2017. *Pocket Glossary of Health Information Management and Technology*, 5th ed. Chicago: AHIMA.

Averill, R. F., N. I. Goldfield, J. Eisenhandler, J. S. Hughes, and J. Muldoon. 2001. "Clinical Risk Groups and the Future of Healthcare Reimbursement." In *Reimbursement Methodologies for Healthcare Services* [CD-ROM], edited by L. M. Jones. Chicago: AHIMA.

CMS (Centers for Medicare and Medicaid Services). 2023a. "Cost Reports." https://www.cms.gov/Research-Statistics-Data-and-Systems/Downloadable-Public-Use-Files/Cost-Reports/.

CMS (Centers for Medicare and Medicaid Services). 2023b. "What Is the CMS National Quality Strategy?" https://www.cms.gov/Medicare/Quality-Initiatives-Patient-Assessment-Instruments/Value-Based-Programs/CMS-Quality-Strategy.

CMS (Centers for Medicare and Medicaid Services). 2023c. "ICD-10 MS-DRG Definitions Manual Files V40." https://www.cms.gov/medicare/medicare-fee-for-service-payment/acuteinpatientpps/ms-drg-classifications-and-software.

CMS (Centers for Medicare and Medicaid Services). 2023d. "Disproportionate Share Hospital (DSH)." https://www.cms.gov/medicare/medicare-fee-for-service-payment/acuteinpatientpps/dsh.

CMS (Centers for Medicare and Medicaid Services). 2023e. Medicare Claims Processing Manual. Chapter 3, "Inpatient Hospital Billing," Section 20.1.2.4 – Transfers. https://www.cms.gov/Regulations-and-Guidance/Guidance/Manuals/Internet-Only-Manuals-IOMs-Items/CMS018912.

CMS (Centers for Medicare and Medicaid Services). 2023f. "Hospital Readmissions Reduction Program (HRRP)." https://www.cms.gov/medicare/medicare-fee-for-service-payment/acuteinpatientpps/readmissions-reduction-program.

CMS (Centers for Medicare and Medicaid Services). 2022a. "Value-Based-Programs." https://www.cms.gov/Medicare/Quality-Initiatives-Patient-Assessment-Instruments/Value-Based-Programs/Value-Based-Programs.

CMS (Centers for Medicare and Medicaid Services). 2022b. "ICD-10 HAC List." https://www.cms.gov/Medicare/Medicare-Fee-for-service-payment/hospitalacqCond/icd10_hacs.

CMS (Centers for Medicare and Medicaid Services). 2022c. "Hospital-Acquired Condition Reduction Program (HACRP)." https://www.cms.gov/Medicare/Quality-Initiatives-Patient-Assessment-Instruments/Value-Based-Programs/HAC/Hospital-Acquired-Conditions.

CMS (Centers for Medicare and Medicaid Services). 2021. "The Hospital Value-Based Purchasing (VBP) Program." https://www.cms.gov/Medicare/Quality-Initiatives-Patient-Assessment-Instruments/Value-Based-Programs/HVBP/Hospital-Value-Based-Purchasing.

CMS (Centers for Medicare and Medicaid Services). 2020. "FY2020 Final Rule and Correction Notice Tables." Table 16. https://www.cms.gov/Medicare/Medicare-Fee-for-Service-Payment/AcuteInpatientPPS/IPPS-Regulations-and-Notices-Items/CMS-1716.

CMS (Centers for Medicare and Medicaid Services). 2011a. Medicare program: Hospital inpatient value-based purchasing program; Final rule. *Federal Register* 76(88):26490–26547.

CMS (Centers for Medicare and Medicaid Services). 2011b (April 29). Press Release: CMS Issues Final Rule for First Year of Hospital Value-Based Purchasing Program. https://www.cms.gov/newsroom/fact-sheets/cms-issues-final-rule-first-year-hospital-value-based-purchasing-program.

CMS (Centers for Medicare and Medicaid Services). 2009. Roadmap for Implementing Value Driven Healthcare in the Traditional Medicare Fee-for-Service Program. https://www.cms.gov/Medicare/Quality-Initiatives-Patient-Assessment-Instruments/QualityInitiativesGenInfo/downloads/VBPRoadmap_OEA_1-16_508.pdf.

CMS (Centers for Medicare and Medicaid Services). n.d. "Medicare Fee-for-Service Payment." Accessed June 20, 2023. https://www.cms.gov/Medicare/Medicare.

Hazelwood, A. 2020. "Reimbursement Methodologies." Chapter 7 in *Health Information Management Concepts, Principles, and Practice*, 6th ed., edited by P. Oachs and A. Watters. Chicago: AHIMA.

HHS (Department of Health and Human Services). 2022. Medicare program: Hospital inpatient prospective payment systems for acute-care hospitals and the long-term care hospital prospective payment system and policy changes and fiscal year 2023 rates; quality programs and Medicare promoting interoperability program requirements for eligible hospitals and critical access hospitals; costs incurred for qualified and non-qualified deferred compensation plans; and changes to hospital and critical access hospital conditions of participation. *Federal Register* 87(153):48780–49499.

HHS (Department of Health and Human Services). 2019. Medicare program: Hospital inpatient prospective payment systems for acute-care hospitals and the long-term care hospital prospective payment system and policy changes and fiscal year 2020 rates; quality reporting requirements for specific providers; Medicare and Medicaid promoting interoperability programs requirements for eligible hospitals and critical access hospitals. *Federal Register* 84(159):42044–42701.

HHS (Department of Health and Human Services). 2014. Medicare program: Prospective payment system for acute care hospitals and long-term care hospital prospective payment system and fiscal year 2015 rates; quality reporting requirements for specific providers; reasonable compensation equivalents for physician services in excluded hospitals and certain teaching hospitals; provider administrative appeals and judicial review; enforcement provisions for organ transplant centers; and electronic health record (EHR) incentive program; Final rule. *Federal Register* 79(163):49877.

HHS (Department of Health and Human Services). 2007. Medicare program: Changes to the hospital inpatient prospective payment systems and fiscal year 2008 rates; Final rule with comment period. *Federal Register* 72(162):47130–48175.

Law.com. n.d. "Legal Terms and Definitions: Regulations." Accessed January 17, 2023. https://dictionary.law .com/Default.aspx?selected=1771.

MedPAC (Medicare Payment Advisory Commission). 2022. Payment Basics: Hospital Acute Inpatient Services Payment System. https://www.medpac.gov/wp-content/uploads/2021/11/MedPAC_Payment_Basics_22_hospital _FINAL_SEC.pdf.

MedPAC (Medicare Payment Advisory Commission). 2016. Report to the Congress: Medicare Payment Policy. https://www.medpac.gov/document/march-2016-report-to-the-congress-medicare-payment-policy/.

Quality Reporting Center. 2020. "Step-by-Step Calculations for Value-Based Purchasing." https://www.quality reportingcenter.com/globalassets/iqr_resources/july-2019/vbp_fy2020_ppsrrelease_scoring_qrg_vfinal508.pdf.

Chapter 6
Medicare Skilled Nursing Facility Services Payment System

Learning Objectives

- Describe the Medicare skilled nursing facility services payment system
- Explain the patient-driven payment model
- Illustrate the variable per diem adjustment included in the payment model
- Describe the skilled nursing facility value-based purchasing program

Key Terms

Case-mix group (CMG)
Patient-driven payment model (PDPM)
Skilled nursing facility (SNF)

Skilled nursing facility value-based purchasing program (SNF VBP)
Variable day adjustment

Nursing homes are healthcare facilities that are licensed by a state to offer, on a 24-hour basis, both skilled nursing care and personal care services (ASPE n.d.) One type of nursing home is a **skilled nursing facility (SNF)**. On an inpatient basis, SNFs provide *short-term* skilled nursing care and rehabilitation services to Medicare beneficiaries after an acute-care inpatient hospitalization. In the SNF setting, patients are referred to as residents. Therefore, this chapter uses the term *resident* instead of *patient* or *beneficiary*.

SNFs can be freestanding facilities, hospital-based units, or swing beds in acute-care hospitals. In acute-care hospitals, swing beds are beds that may be used for both acute inpatient care and skilled nursing care. Typically, these acute-care hospitals are small, rural hospitals or critical access hospitals. CMS must approve the dual use of the beds (MedPAC 2022, 1). About 97 percent of SNF admissions are in freestanding facilities (MedPAC 2022, 1).

Medicare Part A covers the cost of SNF services for Medicare beneficiaries. Medicare beneficiaries are eligible for SNF services immediately after an acute-care inpatient hospitalization of at least three days. They may receive up to 100 days of SNF-covered services per benefit period (see chapter 3, "Government-Sponsored Healthcare Programs"). As described in chapter 3, Medicare beneficiaries pay cost sharing for their SNF services. Residents are assessed for activities of daily living (ADLs). ADLs are basic personal activities that include bathing, eating, dressing, mobility, transferring from bed to chair, and using the toilet. ADLs are used to measure how dependent a person may be on requiring assistance in performing any or all of these activities (ASPE n.d.). The types of care provided to Medicare residents include the following:

- Skilled nursing care: Daily nursing and rehabilitative care that can be performed only by or under the supervision of skilled medical personnel. This includes care such as injections, catheterizations, and dressing changes. This type of care is provided by trained medical professionals, such as physicians, nurses, and physical therapists.

- Rehabilitation services: Services designed to improve or restore a person's functioning. Services include physical, occupational, and speech therapy.

- Personal care: Assistance with ADLs as well as with self-administration of medications and preparing special diets. Typically, these are services that individuals would accomplish themselves if they did not have a disability, such as bathing, toileting, and light housekeeping. (ASPE n.d.)

The SNF services payment system was mandated by Section 4432 of the Balanced Budget Act of 1997 and was effective in 1998. The SNF payment system utilizes a per diem reimbursement methodology. Therefore, it pays a daily rate for each day of care. The SNF payment system covers the costs of skilled nursing care, rehabilitation services, ancillary services, capital costs, and other goods and services (MedPAC 2022, 1). The costs included in the daily rate are for services that would be expected for an SNF to efficiently deliver routine services. High-cost, low-probability services are excluded from the daily rate and are paid separately (MedPAC 2022, 1).

Patient-Driven Payment Model

In 2019 a revised case-mix-based payment model was adopted. The **patient-driven payment model (PDPM)** was designed to assign residents to payment categories based on individual patient characteristics rather than reimbursing facilities based on therapy minutes. The previous SNF reimbursement classification system was Resource Utilization Groups (RUGs). RUGs based most reimbursement categories on the number of therapy minutes provided to residents. The change in philosophy to pay reimbursement categories for individual patient characteristics used in PDPM is based in concerns regarding thresholding. Thresholding is providing just enough therapy for residents to surpass the relevant therapy thresholds to achieve a higher reimbursement level. Several Office of Inspector General (OIG) reports between 2010 and 2015 expressed concerns about thresholding in SNFs. Therefore, the Centers for Medicare and Medicaid Services (CMS) developed and implemented PDPM for fiscal year (FY) 2019.

SNFs have data reporting requirements related to medical necessity and development and maintenance of patient care plans. The Resident Assessment Instrument (RAI) is used for Medicare. This instrument has three components: the Minimum Data Set (MDS) Version 3.0, the Care Area Assessment (CAA) process, and the RAI Utilization Guidelines. These three components provide information about the resident's functional status, strengths, weaknesses, and preferences (CMS 2019a, 1–6). Throughout the SNF section the MDS will be referenced when data elements from this instrument contribute to reimbursement determination.

Patient-Driven Payment Model Structure

The PDPM model uses six components to determine the per diem rate for SNF resident stays. The six components of care are as follows:

1. Nursing

2. Physical therapy (PT)

3. Occupational therapy (OT)

4. Speech-language pathology services (SLP)

5. Nontherapy ancillary services and supplies (NTA)

6. Non-case-mix category (includes room and board services)

Adjustments based on resident and facility circumstance are made at the component level. At each case-mix-adjusted component level a **case-mix group (CMG)** is assigned. The CMG is a classification system used in PDPM to place residents into groups of similar clinical reason for stay and function levels. CMGs are assigned for nursing, PT, OT, SLP, and NTA components. CMGs are not assigned for the non-case-mix category because this component is not case-mix adjusted. In the next sections the six PDPM components are discussed in detail.

Physical Therapy and Occupational Therapy Components

There are two factors that drive classification for the PT and OT components. First, the resident's clinical reason for stay, and second, the resident's functional status. There are four clinical categories for PT and OT:

1. Major joint replacement or spinal surgery

2. Non-orthopedic surgery and acute neurologic

3. Other orthopedic

4. Medical management

Some of the categories include surgeries. These categories indicate that the resident had the surgery in an acute-care inpatient facility directly prior to admission to the SNF. Types of conditions included in the medical management category include acute infections, cancer, pulmonary conditions, and cardiovascular diagnoses. In addition to the resident's clinical reason for stay, the resident's functional score is also considered. The functional score is reported in section GG of the MDS. Example measures included in determining the functional score are toileting hygiene, oral hygiene, sit to stand, walk 10 feet, and walk 50 feet with two turns. When clinical categories are combined with functional status, the result is 16 possible PT and OT PDPM CMGs, as shown in table 6.1.

The CMG established for PT and OT is used in the final SNF payment determination. For PT and OT, an adjustment is applied to the CMG. CMS research identified that the cost of providing PT and OT is not constant throughout a resident's stay (CMS 2019c, 1). Therefore, a **variable day adjustment** is applied for the PT and OT components. This adjustment may result in a different per diem amount to be paid on various payment days during the resident's stay. The cost of PT and OT services remains constant for the first 20 days of the stay, and then slowly decreases through the remainder. The PT and OT components' variable per diem adjustment schedule is shown in table 6.2.

The adjustment is applied during the final SNF payment determination. In an upcoming section, final SNF payment determination is discussed in detail.

Speech-Language Pathology Component

Like PT and OT, the clinical reason for the visit is the major contributing factor to the SLP component. There are two clinical categories applicable to SLP:

1. Acute neurologic

2. Non-neurologic

The non-neurologic category includes surgeries and conditions such as major joint replacement, orthopedic surgery, acute infections, cancer, and cardiovascular conditions. The other contributing factors to determining the SLP component level are as follows:

• Presence of a swallowing disorder (item K0100 on MDS)

• Mechanically altered diet (item K0510C2 on MDS)

• Comorbidity conditions

• Cognitive impairment

Table 6.1. **PT and OT case-mix classification groups**

Clinical Category	Section GG Function Score	PT/OT Case-Mix Group (CMG)	PT Case-Mix Index	OT Case-Mix Index
Major Joint Replacement or Spinal Surgery	0–5	TA	1.53	1.49
Major Joint Replacement or Spinal Surgery	6–9	TB	1.70	1.63
Major Joint Replacement or Spinal Surgery	10–23	TC	1.88	1.69
Major Joint Replacement or Spinal Surgery	24	TD	1.92	1.53
Other Orthopedic	0–5	TE	1.42	1.41
Other Orthopedic	6–9	TF	1.61	1.60
Other Orthopedic	10–23	TG	1.67	1.64
Other Orthopedic	24	TH	1.16	1.15
Medical Management	0–5	TI	1.13	1.18
Medical Management	6–9	TJ	1.42	1.45
Medical Management	10–23	TK	1.52	1.54
Medical Management	24	TL	1.09	1.11
Non-Orthopedic Surgery and Acute Neurologic	0–5	TM	1.27	1.30
Non-Orthopedic Surgery and Acute Neurologic	6–9	TN	1.48	1.50
Non-Orthopedic Surgery and Acute Neurologic	10–23	TO	1.55	1.55
Non-Orthopedic Surgery and Acute Neurologic	24	TP	1.08	1.09

Source: CMS 2019b, 3.

Table 6.2. **PT and OT components' variable per diem adjustment schedule**

Medicare Payment Days	Adjustment Factor	Medicare Payment Days	Adjustment Factor
1–20	1.00	63–69	0.86
21–27	0.98	70–76	0.84
28–34	0.96	77–83	0.82
35–41	0.94	84–90	0.80
42–48	0.92	91–97	0.78
49–55	0.90	98–100	0.76
56–62	0.88		

Source: CMS 2019c.

There are 12 SLP-related comorbidities that were found to increase the cost of therapy. These comorbidities are shown in table 6.3.

When the clinical categories are combined with the SLP-related comorbidities, the result is 12 possible SLP CMGs, as shown in table 6.4.

The CMG established for the resident for the SLP component is used in the final SNF payment determination, which is discussed in an upcoming section.

Table 6.3.   SLP-related comorbidities

SLP-Related Comorbidities	
Aphasia	Laryngeal cancer
CVA (cerebrovascular accident), TIA (transient ischemic attack), or stroke	Apraxia
Hemiplegia or hemiparesis	Dysphagia
Traumatic brain injury	ALS (amyotrophic lateral sclerosis)
Tracheostomy care (while SNF resident)	Oral cancers
Ventilator or respirator (while SNF resident)	Speech and language deficits

Source: CMS 2019b, 4.

Table 6.4.   SLP case-mix classification groups

Present of Acute Neurologic Conditions, SLP-Related Comorbidity, or Cognitive Impairment	Mechanically Altered Diet or Swallowing Disorder	SLP-CMG	SLP Case-Mix Index
None	Neither	SA	0.68
None	Either	SB	1.82
None	Both	SC	2.67
Any one	Neither	SD	1.46
Any one	Either	SE	2.34
Any one	Both	SF	2.98
Any two	Neither	SG	2.04
Any two	Either	SH	2.86
Any two	Both	SI	3.53
All three	Neither	SJ	2.99
All three	Either	SK	3.70
All three	Both	SL	4.21

Source: CMS 2019b, 4–5.

Nursing Component

The nursing component uses five categories to determine the component CMG:

1. Use of extensive services (tracheostomy, ventilator, infections)

2. Clinical conditions

3. Depression

4. Number of restorative nursing services

5. Functional score (section GG MDS)

The clinical conditions category covers a variety of conditions. It is broken into two groups: serious medical conditions and conditions requiring complex medical care. There are two levels for serious medical conditions. Examples of conditions that are included in the first level of serious conditions are coma, septicemia, and respiratory therapy. Second level examples include radiation therapy and dialysis. Examples of conditions requiring complex medical care include pneumonia, surgical wounds, and burns. There are 25 nursing component CMGs based on these five categories. Table 6.5 lists the 25 nursing component CMGs.

Table 6.5 illustrates how the five nursing categories work together to determine the final nursing CMG. There is an HIV/AIDS adjustment for the nursing component. CMS conducted an analysis that determined that the NTA costs per day were 151 percent higher for residents with AIDS. Additionally, wage-weighted nursing staff time was 18 percent greater for AIDS residents (CMS 2019d, 2). Therefore, AIDS—reported with *International Classification of Diseases, Tenth Revision, Clinical Modification* (ICD-10-CM) diagnosis code B20—is awarded eight points in the NTA scoring system (discussed in the next section). Additionally, the nursing component is adjusted by 18 percent (1.18) for residents with AIDS to account for the additional nursing required for these residents. An upcoming section will discuss how the nursing CMG and this HIV/AIDS adjustment is used in the final SNF payment determination.

Nontherapy Ancillary Component

The NTA component represents ancillary services and supplies, such as drugs, laboratory tests, respiratory therapy, and other medical supplies. The use of extensive services and resident comorbid conditions are evaluated to determine the final CMG for this component. CMS assigned points to services and conditions that impact the cost of care for SNF residents. For example, lung transplant status is three points, and endocarditis is one point. The points are totaled to determine the NTA score. Table 6.6 provides the NTA CMGs.

The NTA component has a variable per diem adjustment. Through analysis, NTA costs were found to be concentrated at the beginning of a resident's stay (CMS 2019c, 2). Therefore, an adjustment is made for payment days 1 through 3, as shown in table 6.7.

Like the other components, the NTA CMG is used in the final PDPM reimbursement determination formula.

Non-Case-Mix Component

The sixth component of PDPM is the non-case-mix component. The non-case-mix component is simply a base rate (dollar value) that represents room and board services. It is not case-mix adjusted; rather, it is a constant that is applied for every resident.

Wage-Index Adjustment

Each component of PDPM is wage-index adjusted to account for varying geographic differences in the cost of labor. The formula for wage-index adjustment can be found in figure 5.8 of chapter 5, "Medicare Hospital Acute Inpatient Payment System." The labor portion is 70.8 percent for FY 2023. This portion is adjusted with the hospital wage index.

Table 6.5. Nursing case-mix classification groups

Extensive Services	Clinical Conditions	Depression	Number of Restorative Nursing Services	Function Score	PDPM Nursing CMG	Nursing Case-Mix Index
Tracheostomy & Ventilator				0–14	ES3	4.06
Tracheostomy & Ventilator				0–14	ES2	3.07
Infection				0–14	ES1	2.93
	Serious medical conditions I	Yes		0–5	HDE2	2.40
	Serious medical conditions I	No		0–5	HDE1	1.99
	Serious medical conditions I	Yes		6–14	HBC2	2.24
	Serious medical conditions I	No		6–14	HBC1	1.86
	Serious medical conditions II	Yes		0–5	LDE2	2.08
	Serious medical conditions II	No		0–5	LDE1	1.73
	Serious medical conditions II	Yes		6–14	LBC2	1.72
	Serious medical conditions II	No		6–14	LBC1	1.43
	Conditions requiring complex medical care	Yes		0–5	CDE2	1.87
	Conditions requiring complex medical care	No		0–5	CDE1	1.62
	Conditions requiring complex medical care	Yes		6–14	CBC2	1.55
	Conditions requiring complex medical care	Yes		15–16	CA2	1.09
	Conditions requiring complex medical care	No		6–14	CBC1	1.34
	Conditions requiring complex medical care	No		15–16	CA1	0.94
	Behavioral or cognitive symptoms		2 or more	11–16	BAB2	1.04
	Behavioral or cognitive symptoms		0–1	11–16	BAB1	0.99

(continued)

Table 6.5. *(continued)*

Extensive Services	Clinical Conditions	Depression	Number of Restorative Nursing Services	Function Score	PDPM Nursing CMG	Nursing Case-Mix Index
	Assistance with daily living and general supervision		2 or more	0–5	PDE2	1.57
	Assistance with daily living and general supervision		0–1	0–5	PDE1	1.47
	Assistance with daily living and general supervision		2 or more	6–14	PBC2	1.22
	Assistance with daily living and general supervision		2 or more	15–16	PA2	0.71
	Assistance with daily living and general supervision		0–1	6–14	PBC1	1.13
	Assistance with daily living and general supervision		0–1	15–16	PA1	0.66

Source: CMS 2019b, 5–7.

Table 6.6. **NTA case-mix classification groups**

NTA Score Range	NTA Case-Mix Group	NTA Case-Mix Index
12+	NA	3.24
9–11	NB	2.53
6–8	NC	1.84
3–5	ND	1.33
1–2	NE	0.96
0	NF	0.72

Source: CMS 2019b, 8.

Table 6.7. **Variable per diem adjustment factors and schedule for NTA component**

Medicare Payment Days	Adjustment Factor
1–3	3.0
4–100	1.0

Source: CMS 2019c, 2.

Determining PDPM Reimbursement

The six components are combined to determine the per diem PDPM payment rate. Figure 6.1 shows the foundation of the SNF payment system.

Each year in the SNF payment system final rule, an urban and rural base rate for each of the six components is published in the *Federal Register*. The final rule and associated tables can be found on the CMS website under the section "Medicare Fee-for-Service Payment." Table 6.8 displays the urban and rural base rates for FY 2020.

Figure 6.1 outlines the steps for payment determination. First, the facility determines if the urban or rural base rate is used. Next, the base rate is wage-index adjusted. Third, the CMI for the appropriate CMG is multiplied by the adjusted base rate. The next step is to determine if a variable per diem adjustment is made based on the payment day. The last step is to total the payment amounts for the six SNF components. The result is the per diem payment rate. Remember, not every day of the stay will have the same payment amount. Depending on the payment day, the payment rate may be different because the PT, OT, or NTA adjustment may be applied. Examples 6.1 and 6.2 illustrate determination of SNF reimbursement.

Figure 6.1.   **Foundation of SNF payment system**

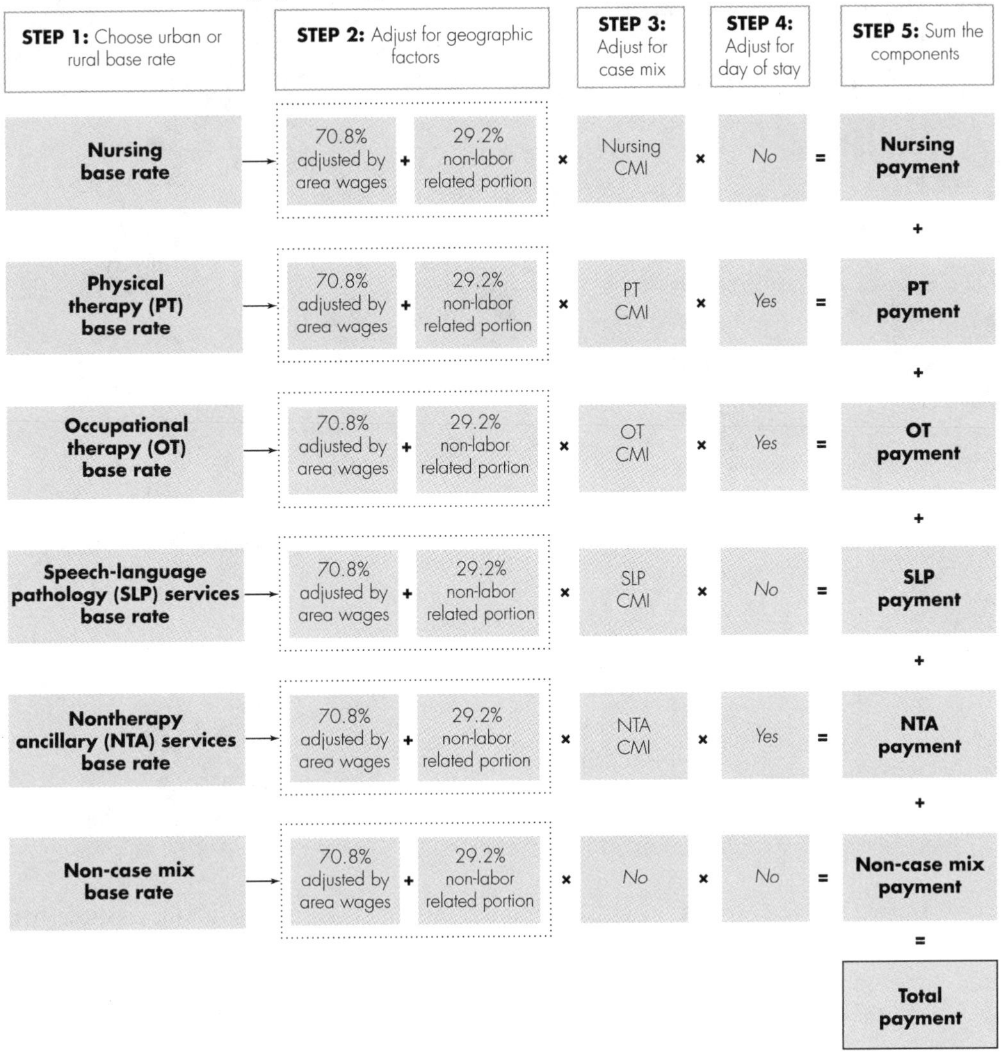

Source: MedPAC 2022, 2.

Table 6.8.   FY 2020 unadjusted urban and rural SNF base rates

	PT	OT	SLP	Nursing	NTA	Non-Case Mix
Urban	$66.06	$61.49	$24.66	$115.15	$86.88	$103.12
Rural	$75.30	$69.16	$31.07	$110.02	$83.00	$105.03

Source: MedPac 2022, 3.

Example 6.1

Jose is a resident at Community SNF, which is classified as an urban facility. He had a 10-day stay with a clinical category of acute neurologic condition. His PT and OT function score was 10, and his nursing function score was 7. He has moderate cognitive impairment. He receives a mechanically altered diet for SLP-related comorbidity of dysphagia, which is a swallowing disorder. His nursing level is assistance with daily living and general supervision, and he receives two restorative nursing services. His NTA comorbidity score was 7.

Component	Urban Base Rate	Wage-Index Adjusted Rate (1.241*)	CMG	CMG CMI	Adjusted for CMI	Adjusted for Variable Day Factors/AIDS	Component Payment
PT	$66.06	$77.33	TO	1.55	$119.86	1.0 All days	$119.86
OT	$61.49	$71.99	TO	1.55	$111.58	1.0 All days	$111.58
SLP	$24.66	$28.87	SL	4.21	$121.54	--	$121.54
Nursing	$115.15	$134.79	PBC2	1.22	$164.44	--	$164.44
NTA	$86.88	$101.71	NC	1.84	$187.15	3.0 Days 1–3 1.0 Days 4–10	$561.45 $187.15
Non-Case Mix	$103.12	$120.71	--	--	--	--	$120.71
Total per diem rate days 1–3 ($119.86 + $111.58 + $121.54 + $164.44+ $561.45 + $120.71)							**$1,199.58**
Total per diem rate days 4–10 ($119.86 + $111.58 + $121.54 + $164.44+ $187.15 + $120.71)							**$825.28**

* Wage index of 1.241 is an example wage-index value.

The first step is selecting the correct base rate. Community SNF is classified as urban, so the urban base rates are chosen. In step two, the urban base rate is wage-index adjusted. The labor portion (70.8 percent) is adjusted with the hospital wage index of 1.241. Since the wage-index amount is greater than 1.0, the base rate increases once adjusted. In step three, the adjusted base rate is multiplied by the CMG CMI. The CMG is determined based on the resident characteristics provided in the scenario (use tables 6.1, 6.4, 6.5, and 6.6 in the text).

(continued)

The result is shown in the column labeled "Adjusted for CMI." The fourth step is to apply the variable day adjustments. The PT and OT day adjustment for days 1 through 10 is 1.0 (table 6.2). The NTA day adjustment for days 1 through 3 is 3.0, and for days 4 through 10 it is 1.0 (table 6.7). The last step is to sum the fully adjusted component rates to determine a total per diem. The total per diem rate for days 1 through 3 equals $1,199.58; this accounts for the increase in payment for NTA during the first three days of the stay. The total per diem rate for days 4 through 10 equals $825.28. The total reimbursement for the entire stay equals $9,375.70 [($1,199.58 × 3) + ($825.28 × 7)].

Example 6.2

Victoria is a resident at Memorial SNF, which is classified as a rural facility. She had a 22-day stay with a clinical category of medical management. Victoria has lung cancer and is receiving radiation therapy. Her PT and OT function score was 6 and her nursing function score was 6. Her nursing level was "serious medical conditions" due to the radiation therapy. Victoria has AIDS and depression. Her NTA comorbidity score was 9.

Component	Rural Base Rate	Wage-Index Adjusted Rate (0.9871*)	CMG	CMG CMI	Adjusted for CMI	Adjusted for Variable Day Factors / AIDS	Component Payment
PT	$75.30	$74.61	TJ	1.42	$105.94	1.0 Days 1–20 0.98 Days 21–22	$105.94 $103.82
OT	$69.16	$68.52	TJ	1.45	$99.36	1.0 Days 1–20 0.98 Days 21–22	$99.36 $97.37
SLP	$31.07	$30.78	SA	0.68	$20.93	--	$20.93
Nursing	$110.02	$109.02	LBC2	1.72	$187.51	1.18	$221.26
NTA	$83.00	$82.24	NB	2.53	$208.06	3.0 Days 1–3 1.0 Days 4–10	$624.17 $208.06
Non-Case Mix	$105.03	$104.07	--	--	--	--	$104.07
Total per diem rate days 1–3 ($105.94 + $99.36 + $20.93 + $221.26 + $624.17 + $104.07)							**$1,175.73**
Total per diem rate days 4–20 ($105.94 + $99.36 + $20.93 + $221.26 + $208.06 + $104.07)							**$759.62**
Total per diem rate days 21–22 ($103.82 + $97.37 + $20.93 + $221.26 + $208.06 + $104.07)							**$755.51**

* Wage index of 0.9871 is an example wage-index value.

(continued)

Example 6.2 *(continued)*

The first step is selecting the correct base rate. Memorial SNF is classified as rural, so the rural base rates are chosen. In step two, the rural base rate is wage-index adjusted. The labor portion (70.8 percent) is adjusted with the hospital wage index of 0.9871. Since the wage-index amount is less than 1.0, the base rate decreases once adjusted. In step three, the adjusted base rate is multiplied by the CMG CMI. The CMG is determined based on the resident characteristics provided in the scenario (use tables 6.1, 6.4, 6.5, and 6.6 in the text). The result is shown in the column labeled "Adjusted for CMI." The fourth step is to apply the variable day adjustments and AIDS adjustment. The PT and OT day adjustment for days 1 through 20 is 1.0, and for days 21 through 22 it is 0.98 (table 6.2). The NTA day adjustment for days 1 through 3 is 3.0, and for days 4 through 10 it is 1.0 (table 6.7). Victoria is an AIDS resident; therefore, the nursing component is adjusted by 1.18 (18 percent increase). The last step is to sum the fully adjusted component rates to determine a total per diem. The total per diem rate for days 1 through 3 equals $1,175.73; this accounts for the increase in payment for NTA during the first three days of the stay. The total per diem rate for days 4 through 20 equals $759.62. The total per diem rate for days 21 through 22 equals $755.51; this accounts for the decrease in payment for PT and OT after day 20. The total reimbursement for the entire stay equals $17,951.75 [($1,175.73 × 3) + ($759.62 × 17) + ($755.51 × 2)].

As illustrated in examples 6.1 and 6.2, calculating SNF payment can be complex. The next section focuses on the quality side of the payment system. The SNF value-based purchasing program (SNF VBP) will be discussed in detail.

Check Your Understanding 6.1

1. What are the three therapy components used in the PDPM model for SNF payment?
2. Describe the variable day adjustment for PT and OT components.
3. What are the clinical categories available for the SLP component?
4. List the five categories used to determine the nursing component CMG.
5. What types of services are included in the NTA component?

Skilled Nursing Facility Value-Based Purchasing Program

In accordance with Section 215(b) of the Protecting Access to Medicare Act of 2014 (PAMA), CMS established the **skilled nursing facility value-based purchasing program (SNF VBP)**. The SNF VBP ties facility performance for established quality measures into the SNF services payment system. Currently, there is one measure for this program, which is the skilled nursing facility 30-day all-cause readmission after hospital measures (SNFRM) (CMS 2022). As noted at the beginning of this chapter, Medicare beneficiaries qualify for an SNF admission after an acute-care inpatient stay. This measure determines how often Medicare SNF residents are readmitted to the acute-care setting within 30 days from their original discharge date. There are some exclusions, like when a resident is discharged from the SNF against medical advice or when a resident is admitted to observation instead of an inpatient admission. Additional measures have been approved for FY 2026 and 2027. Beginning in FY 2026 (October 2025), the following measures will be active:

1. Skilled Nursing Facility Healthcare-Associated Infections (SNF HAIs) Requiring Hospitalization
2. Total Nurse Staffing Hours per Resident Day

The SNF HAIs measure estimates the rate of how many SNF residents experience a hospital-acquired infection at the SNF and subsequently need to be admitted for inpatient care. The total nurse staffing hours per resident day tracks how many hours licensed nurses and nursing aides are available to provide care. For FY 2027, the Discharge to Community (DTC)—Post-Acute Care Measure for SNFs will be active (CMS 2023). The DTC measure evaluates how successful the SNF is at discharging residents to home without unplanned readmissions or death occurring within 31 days of the SNF discharge.

There are two components to the total performance score (TPS): achievement score and improvement score. The achievement score compares a facility's performance to all facilities nationwide. The improvement score compares a facility's performance score to the facility's baseline score (CMS 2022). SNFs are ranked by performance from lowest to highest based on the applicable measures. Facilities with the highest ranking will get incentive payments. Facilities ranked in the lowest 40 percent will receive decreased payments. CMS withholds 2 percent of SNF payments to fund the incentive program. CMS redistributes 60 percent of the withholding pool to high-performing SNFs (CMS 2022). The performance of all SNF providers is publicly reported on the Nursing Home Compare website (CMS n.d.).

The Medicare SNF services payment system revision in 2019 to adopt the PDPM is an improvement over the previous version because it establishes reimbursement amounts that are related to the health status of the individual resident. One goal of the new model was to eliminate thresholding and other noncompliant practices. However, it is too early to determine if the implementation of PDPM will improve revenue integrity in this clinical setting. The SNF VBP ensures that quality measures are tied to reimbursement levels through the TPS and withhold amounts.

Patient Connection

In chapter 5's Patient Connection we learned that Malakai had a knee replacement and had difficulty with his recovery at Memorial Hospital. Therefore, case management arranged for him to be transferred to an SNF. Malakai was transferred to Neighborhood SNF and had a six-day stay, where he received the therapy services and nursing care he needed. In this Patient Connection, let's figure out how much reimbursement Neighborhood SNF will receive for Malakai's stay.

To determine the OT and PT CMG, we need Malakai's clinical category and function score from the MDS. Malakai had a knee replacement (knee arthroplasty), so the clinical category for his admission is major joint replacement or spinal surgery. Malakai can still perform activities of daily living at a high level, and his function score is 22. Referencing table 6.1, we can see that the CMG is TC. The PT CMI value for TC equals 1.88 and the OT CMI value to TC equals 1.69. Since Malakai was a resident for six days, the variable day adjustment is 1.0 for all six days, as shown in table 6.2. Let's add the PT and OT information to the applicable rows in our payment calculation table.

Component	Urban Base Rate	Wage-Index Adjusted Rate (1.241*)	CMG	CMG CMI	Adjusted for CMI	Adjusted for Variable Day Factors/AIDS	Component Payment
PT	$66.06	$77.33	TC	1.88	$145.38	1.0 All days	$145.38
OT	$61.49	$71.99	TC	1.69	$121.66	1.0 All days	$121.66

* Wage index of 1.241 is an example wage-index value.

(*continued*)

Patient Connection   *(continued)*

For SLP, Malakai's clinical category is non-neurologic. He doesn't have any SLP comorbidities, he didn't have an altered diet, he doesn't have a swallowing disorder, and he doesn't have cognitive impairment. Referencing table 6.4, we can determine that the SLP CMG is SA. The CMI value for SA equals 0.68. Let's add this to our table.

Component	Urban Base Rate	Wage-Index Adjusted Rate (1.241*)	CMG	CMG CMI	Adjusted for CMI	Adjusted for Variable Day Factors/AIDS	Component Payment
PT	$66.06	$77.33	TC	1.88	$145.38	1.0 All days	$145.38
OT	$61.49	$71.99	TC	1.69	$121.66	1.0 All days	$121.66
SLP	$24.66	$28.87	SA	0.68	$19.63	--	$19.63

* Wage index of 1.241 is an example wage-index value.

Malakai had some issues with his surgical wound. It started to become infected and was treated. Therefore, his clinical conditions category for the nursing component is conditions "requiring complex medical care." Although he was discouraged by his slow recovery, Malakai did not have depression documented in his health record. Malakai's nursing function score was 15. Referencing table 6.5, the nursing CMG is CA1, which had a CMI of 0.94. Let's add this to our payment table.

Component	Urban Base Rate	Wage-Index Adjusted Rate (1.241*)	CMG	CMG CMI	Adjusted for CMI	Adjusted for Variable Day Factors/AIDS	Component Payment
PT	$66.06	$77.33	TC	1.88	$145.38	1.0 All days	$145.38
OT	$61.49	$71.99	TC	1.69	$121.66	1.0 All days	$121.66
SLP	$24.66	$28.87	SA	0.68	$19.63	--	$19.63
Nursing	$115.15	$134.79	CA1	0.94	$126.70	--	$126.70

* Wage index of 1.241 is an example wage-index value.

Because of his surgical wound infection, Malakai has an NTA score of 2. Referencing table 6.6, we can determine that his NTA CMG is NE, which has a CMI equal to 0.96. Since his admission is greater than three days, the variable day adjustment for NTA applies for payment days 1 through 3. Let's enter this into our payment table.

(continued)

Component	Urban Base Rate	Wage-Index Adjusted Rate (1.241*)	CMG	CMG CMI	Adjusted for CMI	Adjusted for Variable Day Factors/AIDS	Component Payment
PT	$66.06	$77.33	TC	1.88	$145.38	1.0 All days	$145.38
OT	$61.49	$71.99	TC	1.69	$121.66	1.0 All days	$121.66
SLP	$24.66	$28.87	SA	0.68	$19.63	--	$19.63
Nursing	$115.15	$134.79	CA1	0.94	$126.70	--	$126.70
NTA	$86.88	$101.71	NE	0.96	$97.64	3.0 Days 1–3 1.0 Days 4–10	$292.92 $97.64

* Wage index of 1.241 is an example wage-index value.

The final steps are to add in the non-case-mix adjusted component and to sum the dollar amounts for the six PDPM components per payment day. Let's complete our table.

Component	Urban Base Rate	Wage-Index Adjusted Rate (1.241*)	CMG	CMG CMI	Adjusted for CMI	Adjusted for Variable Day Factors/AIDS	Component Payment
PT	$66.06	$77.33	TC	1.88	$145.38	1.0 All days	$145.38
OT	$61.49	$71.99	TC	1.69	$121.66	1.0 All days	$121.66
SLP	$24.66	$28.87	SA	0.68	$19.63	--	$19.63
Nursing	$115.15	$134.79	CA1	0.94	$126.70	--	$126.70
NTA	$86.88	$101.71	NE	0.96	$97.64	3.0 Days 1–3 1.0 Days 4–10	$292.92 $97.64
Non-Case Mix	$103.12	$120.71	--	--	--	--	$120.71
Total per diem rate days 1–3 ($145.38 + $121.66 + $19.63 + $126.70 + $292.92 + $120.71)							**$827.00**
Total per diem rate days 4–6 ($145.38 + $121.66 + $19.63 + $126.70 + $97.64 + $120.71)							**$631.72**
TOTAL REIMBURSEMENT FOR THE ADMISSION *($827.00 × 3) + ($631.72 × 3)*							*$4,376.16*

* Wage index of 1.241 is an example wage-index value.

(continued)

Patient Connection *(continued)*

Neighborhood SNF received $4,376.16 for Malakai's six days of care. Malakai recovered from his wound infection and made progress with PT during his stay. He was discharged home and instructed to continue with PT until he fully recovers from this knee replacement.

Chapter 6 Review Quiz

1. Which reimbursement methodology is used in the SNF services payment system?

2. List the six components used in PDPM. Which components are case-mix adjusted?

3. Regina is a resident at Community SNF. Her clinical reason for admission is major joint replacement. Her function score is 8. Use table 6.1 to determine the CMG and CMI for the PT component of PDPM.

4. Rashaun is a resident at Memorial SNF. His nursing category is "condition requiring complex medical care." Rashaun has depression and his function score is 15. Use table 6.5 to determine the CMG and CMI for the nursing component of PDPM.

5. How are PDPM components adjusted for residents that are living with HIV/AIDS?

6. Why does the NTA variable day adjustment impact the first three days of the resident's admission?

7. What services or supplies are included in the non-case-mix component?

8. List the steps for SNF payment determination.

9. Review example 6.2. Explain why there are three different total per diem rates for this admission.

10. What percentage of the withhold does CMS pay back to providers in incentive payments under SNF VBP?

References

ASPE (Assistant Secretary for Planning and Evaluation). n.d. "Glossary of Terms." Accessed February 21, 2023. https://aspe.hhs.gov/glossary-terms.

CMS (Centers for Medicare and Medicaid Services). 2023. "The Skilled Nursing Facility Value-Based Purchasing (SNF VBP) Program." https://www.cms.gov/Medicare/Quality-Initiatives-Patient-Assessment-Instruments/Value-Based-Programs/SNF-VBP/SNF-VBP-Page.

CMS (Centers for Medicare and Medicaid Services). 2022. "The Skilled Nursing Facility Value-Based Purchasing (SNF VBP) Program FY 2023 Program Year Fact Sheet." https://www.cms.gov/files/document/fy-2023-snf-vbp-fact-sheet.pdf.

CMS (Centers for Medicare and Medicaid Services). 2019a. Long-Term Care Facility Resident Assessment Instrument 3.0 User's Manual, Version 1.17.1. https://downloads.cms.gov/files/mds-3.0-rai-manual-v1.17.1_october_2019.pdf.

CMS (Centers for Medicare and Medicaid Services). 2019b. "Fact Sheet: PDPM Patient Classification." https://www.cms.gov/Medicare/Medicare-Fee-for-Service-Payment/SNFPPS/Downloads/PDPM_Fact_Sheet_Template_Payment-Overview_v5.zip.

CMS (Centers for Medicare and Medicaid Services). 2019c. "Fact Sheet: Variable Per Diem Adjustment." https://www.cms.gov/Medicare/Medicare-Fee-for-Service-Payment/SNFPPS/Downloads/PDPM_Fact_Sheet _VPD_v3_508.pdf.

CMS (Centers for Medicare and Medicaid Services). 2019d. "Fact Sheet: PDPM Payments for SNF Patients with HIV/AIDS." https://www.cms.gov/Medicare/Medicare-Fee-for-Service-Payment/SNFPPS/Downloads/PDPM _Fact_Sheet_AIDS_v3_508.pdf.

CMS (Centers for Medicare and Medicaid Services). n.d. "Nursing Home Compare." Accessed June 20, 2023. https://www.medicare.gov/nursinghomecompare/.

MedPAC (Medicare Payment Advisory Commission). 2022. Payment Basics: Skilled Nursing Facility Services Payment System. https://www.medpac.gov/wp-content/uploads/2021/11/MedPAC_Payment_Basics_22_SNF _FINAL_SEC.pdf.

Resource

CMS (Centers for Medicare and Medicaid Services). n.d. "Medicare." https://www.cms.gov/medicare/medicare.

Chapter 7
Medicare Hospital Outpatient Payment System

Learning Objectives

- ❖ Define bundling
- ❖ Define packaging
- ❖ Describe how payment status indicators represent reimbursement methodologies
- ❖ Illustrate how packaging is utilized in OPPS reimbursement
- ❖ Describe the OPPS provisions

Key Terms

Ambulatory payment classification (APC)	Packaging
Bundling	Partial hospitalization program (PHP)
Conversion factor (CF)	Pass-through
National unadjusted payment	Payment status indicator (SI)
Outpatient Code Editor (OCE)	Sole-community hospital (SCH)

Before the implementation of the Medicare hospital outpatient payment system, Medicare payment for hospital outpatient services was based on an estimate of the cost incurred by the provider. The estimated cost of services was calculated by converting total charges for each encounter to cost by using department-specific cost-to-charge ratios (CCRs) developed from cost report statistics. However, as healthcare costs continued to rise, the Centers for Medicare and Medicaid Services (CMS) moved toward a prospective payment system (PPS) to encourage a more efficient delivery of care for outpatient beneficiaries (CMS 2004, 50450). The Medicare hospital outpatient payment system was implemented in August 2000 and is the payment system used for hospital-based outpatient encounters. The Medicare Payment Advisory Commission (MedPAC) and others use this name on webpages and documents. However, this payment system is also referred to as the hospital outpatient prospective payment system (OPPS) throughout CMS webpages, CMS documents, and the *Federal Register*. In this chapter, the initialism OPPS is used for this payment system. Most Medicare reimbursement systems utilize one reimbursement methodology to determine payment rates for services and supplies. However, OPPS is unique in that the system incorporates multiple reimbursement methodologies. In the following section we discuss this approach.

Reimbursement for Outpatient Hospital Services

CMS uses three reimbursement methods to reimburse facilities for hospital outpatient services: fee schedule payment, prospective payment, and reasonable cost payment. The primary standard that distinguishes a PPS from a fee schedule system is that, in the PPS, the costs for certain items and secondary services associated with a primary procedure are packaged into the payment for that procedure, which is determined before the service is provided (prospectively). A fee schedule system establishes a separate payment amount for each item or service, and no packaging occurs (CMS 2004, 50505). Since most of the services in the OPPS are paid via a prospective methodology, the overall system is considered prospective even though there are a few services reimbursed under fee-scheduled arrangements or by reasonable cost. The third methodology, cost-based, is used for specified services and certain pharmaceutical items. Pharmaceutical items are paid based on the average sales price (ASP) plus 6 percent. The addition of the so-called ASP plus 6 percent methodology is designed to pay providers for the cost of the drug (ASP) and the added cost required for processing and administration (plus 6 percent). The other services assigned the reimbursement methodology are determined by multiplying the facility charge times the hospital CCR.

Ambulatory Payment Classification System

Most ambulatory services under OPPS are paid via **ambulatory payment classification (APC)**. The APC system combines procedures or services that are clinically comparable, with respect to resource use, into groups called APCs. All procedures or services assigned to an APC group must meet the "two-times rule," which establishes that the median cost of the most expensive item or service within a group cannot be more than two times greater than the median cost of the least expensive item or service within the same group (CMS 2004, 50454). CMS can propose exceptions to the two-times rule based on the following criteria:

- Resource homogeneity

- Clinical homogeneity

- Hospital concentration (few hospitals provide the service)

- Frequency of service (low volume)

- Opportunity for upcoding and code fragments (CMS 2004, 50463)

Violations of the two-times rule are reviewed by the APC Advisory Panel. After analysis of each situation, the panel makes recommendations for each group that violated the rule. CMS uses the recommendations proposed by the panel and makes the final determination. The following section will explore characteristics and components of the APC system including the level of packaging and the use of payment status indicators (SIs).

Partially Packaged System Methodology

Packaging and bundling concepts are used in OPPS to combine payment for multiple services. In the 2008 OPPS final rule, CMS defines packaging and bundling as follows:

- **Packaging** occurs when reimbursement for minor ancillary services associated with a significant procedure is combined into a single payment for the procedure.

- **Bundling** occurs when payment for multiple significant procedures or multiple units of the same procedure related to an outpatient encounter or to an episode-of-care is combined into a single unit of payment. (CMS 2007, 66610)

The concepts of packaging and bundling allow CMS to provide financial incentives for healthcare facilities to improve their efficiency by avoiding unnecessary ancillary services, supplies, and pharmaceuticals, and by substituting less expensive, but equally effective, options.

Packaging is extensive in OPPS. Ancillary and supportive services are packaged with significant, surgical, and evaluation procedures. When packaging occurs, the reimbursement for the ancillary and supportive services is automatically combined into the significant procedure, surgical service, or evaluation APC payment rate. Example 7.1 illustrates packaging in OPPS.

Example 7.1

A patient is seen in radiology for an MRI of the lumbar spine with contrast (Current Procedural Terminology [CPT] code 72149). The contrast utilized during the MRI is an iron-based magnetic resonance contrast agent that is reported with CPT code Q9953. Under OPPS packaging, the contrast medium is considered a supportive service and is included in the reimbursement for the MRI of the lumbar spine. A separate payment is not made for the contrast agent.

Service	CPT Code	APC	Reimbursement (2023)
MRI lumbar spine with contrast	72149	APC 5572	$368.43
Iron-based magnetic resonance contrast agent	Q9953	No APC	Packaged ($0.00)

Source: CMS 2023a.

Various levels of packaging are executed under OPPS, some of which are activated based on combinations of services performed during the encounter.

Bundling takes a predetermined set of services that, when performed together during an encounter, result in the reimbursement for all services being combined into one payment amount. Examples of bundling include critical care services, imaging, and mental health services. Example 7.2 illustrates bundling in OPPS.

Example 7.2

A patient is seen by her primary care physician for continued neck and back pain. The physician orders MRIs to be performed at the cervical, thoracic, and lumbar regions. The MRI of each region is an individual component (in other words, cervical, thoracic, and lumbar). When these three components are provided during the same encounter, the payment for the components is combined into one APC.

APC	Components	Reimbursement (2023)
8007 – MRI and MRA without Contrast Composite	• 72141, MRI cervical • 72146, MRI thoracic • 72148, MRI lumbar	$527.17

Source: CMS 2023b.

This example shows how the component procedures are bundled together into one service. Most bundling occurs within component APCs, which will be discussed in the next section of this text.

The APC system is a partially packaged system. Services or items, such as recovery room, anesthesia, and some pharmaceuticals, are packaged or bundled into a single payment. Although most ancillary and supportive services are packaged or bundled, other services are not. Thus, this system is partially packaged as opposed to fully packaged, like the inpatient prospective payment system (IPPS). For the inpatient setting, it is easier to predict which resources a patient will consume for a given clinical issue. However, in the outpatient setting, treatment pathways vary greatly from patient to patient, making it much more difficult to determine the resources that will be consumed for a clinical issue. Therefore, a partially packaged system was created to provide adequate reimbursement and to allow the treatment flexibility that is needed to appropriately care for patients in the outpatient setting. The partially packaged nature of the OPPS implies that each claim may be assigned more than one APC, while in the fully packaged IPPS, each claim is assigned only one Medicare severity diagnosis-related group (MS-DRG).

Although OPPS has been a partially packaged system since its inception in 2000, CMS has been moving toward a fully packaged case-rate system over the past several years. Each year, CMS has increased packaging of ancillary and supportive services, which were previously payable separately. The OPPS packages payments for multiple and interrelated items and services to promote effective and efficient care in the following ways:

- Encourage hospitals to provide efficient care and to manage resources with maximum flexibility

- Incentivize hospitals to choose the most cost-efficient option when a variety of devices, drugs, items, and supplies could be utilized to meet the patient's needs

- Encourage hospitals to effectively negotiate with manufacturers and suppliers to reduce the purchase price for supplies and items

- Influence hospitals to establish protocols to ensure the necessary services are provided, but scrutinize practitioner orders to maximize the efficient use of hospital resources (CMS 2017, 52390)

Each year, CMS continues to examine payment for services under OPPS to determine if further services can be packaged. CMS's goal is to advance the OPPS into a fully packaged case-rate system.

Payment Status Indicators

OPPS requires that facilities use Healthcare Common Procedure Coding System (HCPCS) codes to report services and procedures performed and items and supplies provided for beneficiaries. Each code in HCPCS has been assigned a **payment status indicator (SI)**. The SI is a code that identifies how a service, procedure, or item is paid in OPPS (for example, fee schedule, APC, reasonable cost, not paid). Table 7.1 provides a listing of the SI codes and their definitions for 2023.

Interpreting SIs is the foundation of determining OPPS reimbursement. SIs are assigned to all HCPCS codes. HCPCS codes are displayed in Addendum B of the OPPS final rule. Addendum B is updated quarterly and is available on the CMS website. Since multiple HCPCS codes are reported for a single encounter, there will be multiple SIs per claim. Due to the extensive amount of packaging utilized in OPPS, all of the SIs for an encounter must be critically examined together to determine the reimbursement outcome for the claim. To assist with the complex packaging executed under OPPS, individuals can use the **Outpatient Code Editor (OCE)** software from CMS. In addition to editing the claim for billing requirements, the OCE performs the packaging and bundling logic of OPPS. The output is the final APC and reimbursement determinations for an encounter. The desktop version of the OCE can be downloaded from the CMS website under the Medicare tab. The editing component of the OCE is discussed further in chapter 13 of this text, "Revenue Compliance."

Each HCPCS code is assigned to only one APC group, and that group is assigned an SI. The APC assignment for a procedure or service does not change based on the patient's medical condition or the severity of illness. There may be an unlimited number of APCs per encounter for a single patient. The number of APC assignments is based on the number of covered procedures or services provided for that patient.

Each APC contains a title, SI, relative weight, national unadjusted payment amount, national unadjusted copayment amount, and code range. These components are shown in figure 7.1.

The relative weight is a measure of the resource intensity of a procedure or service. The **national unadjusted payment** amount is the product of the conversion factor (CF) multiplied by the relative weight, unadjusted for geographic differences. This is the unadjusted amount a hospital will receive for a procedure or service in that APC. The national unadjusted payment amount is divided into two components: Medicare facility amount and beneficiary copayment amount. Both the Medicare facility component and the beneficiary copayment components are adjusted for differences in wage indexes. This is the only adjustment made to APC payment rates to account for differences among hospitals. Sixty percent of the facility amount is wage-index adjusted. The wage-index amount for the facility location based on core-based statistical area (CBSA) is determined in the IPPS update for the corresponding rate year.

Table 7.1.   Payment status indicators for 2023

Payment Status Indicator	Reimbursement Method	Procedure or Service Example
A	Fee schedule payment	Ambulance, separately payable clinical diagnostic laboratory, physical, occupational, and speech therapy, non-implantable prosthetics and orthotics, diagnostic mammogram, screening mammogram, and unclassified drugs and biologicals
B	Not reimbursed under OPPS	Service not appropriate for Part B claim
C	Not reimbursed under OPPS	Inpatient-only services
D	Not reimbursed under OPPS	Code is discontinued
E1	Not reimbursed under OPPS	Not covered by any Medicare outpatient benefit category, is statutorily excluded by Medicare, or is not reasonable and necessary
E2	Not reimbursed under OPPS	Items and services for which pricing information and claims data are not available
F	Reasonable cost payment	Acquisition of corneal tissue and certain certified registered nurse anesthetist (CRNA) services
G	APC Payment	Pass-through drugs and biologicals
H	Reasonable cost payment	Pass-through device categories No copayment
J1	Comprehensive APC payment	All services are packaged with the primary J1 service except services with SI F, G, H, L, and U; ambulance services; diagnostic and screening mammography; rehabilitation therapy services; self-administered drugs; all preventive services; certain Part B inpatient services; services assigned to a new technology APC; and FDA-authorized or approved drugs and biologicals that are authorized or approved to treat or prevent COVID-19.
J2	Services may be paid through a comprehensive APC payment	All services on the claim are packaged into a single payment for specific combinations of services except services with SI F, G, H, L, and U; ambulance services; diagnostic and screening mammography; rehabilitation therapy services; self-administered drugs; all preventive services; certain Part B inpatient services; services assigned to a new technology APC; and FDA-authorized or approved drugs and biologicals that are authorized or approved to treat or prevent COVID-19. Packaged APC payment if billed on the same claim as an HCPCS code assigned status indicator J1
K	APC payment	Non-pass-through drugs and nonimplantable biologicals, including therapeutic radiopharmaceuticals

(continued)

Table 7.1. *(continued)*

Payment Status Indicator	Reimbursement Method	Procedure or Service Example
L	Reasonable cost payment	Influenza vaccine; pneumococcal pneumonia vaccine; Hepatitis B vaccines; COVID-19 vaccine; monoclonal antibody therapy product No copayment or deductible amount
M	Not reimbursed under OPPS	Services not billable to the Medicare administrative contractor (MAC) Pharmacy dispensing fee, chemo assessment of nausea, pain, fatigue, and such
N	Packaged payment	Payment is packaged into payment for other services
P	Per diem APC payment	Partial hospitalization
Q1	Conditional APC payment	STV conditionally packaged services. Packaged on same claim as a code with S, T, or V
Q2	Conditional APC payment	T conditionally packaged services. Packaged on same claim as a code with T
Q3	Composite APC payment	Services that may be paid through a composite APC
Q4	Conditional APC payment	Conditionally packaged laboratory tests. Packaged on same claim as a code with SI J1, J2, S, T, V, Q1, Q2, or Q3 If not packaged, SI is A and service is paid via the Clinical Lab Fee Schedule
R	APC payment	Blood and blood products
S	APC payment	Procedure or service, multiple procedure reduction does not apply
T	APC payment	Procedure or service, multiple procedure reduction applies
U	APC payment	Brachytherapy sources
V	APC payment	Clinic or emergency department visits
Y	Not reimbursed under OPPS	Nonimplanted durable medical equipment (DME) that must be billed directly to the DME MAC

Source: Adapted from CMS 2022a.

Payment Status Reimbursement Methods

Understanding how an encounter is reimbursed under OPPS requires that the various categories of SI be correctly applied. However, when determining encounter reimbursement, each category cannot be assessed in isolation. Instead, all SIs must be used in combination to correctly determine reimbursement under OPPS. There are nine SI reimbursement methods currently used in the OPPS:

- APC payment
- Per diem APC payment

- Comprehensive APC (C-APC) payment
- Conditional APC payment
- Composite APC payment
- Packaged payment
- Fee schedule payment
- Reasonable cost payment
- Services not reimbursed under OPPS

In the sections that follow, each of the SI reimbursement methods is discussed in detail.

Ambulatory Payment Classification Payment: Status Indicators G, K, R, S, T, U, and V

There are seven SIs in the APC payment reimbursement methods. They represent services or procedures that are reimbursed by prospective payment methodology through APCs. Following are the SIs and their descriptions:

- G: Pass-through drugs and biologicals
- K: Non-pass-through drugs and nonimplantable biologicals, including radiopharmaceuticals
- R: Blood and blood products
- S: Significant procedures for which multiple procedure reduction does not apply
- T: Surgical procedures for which multiple procedure reduction applies
- U: Brachytherapy services
- V: Clinic and emergency department visits

When services with one of these SIs are performed, associated ancillary and supportive items are packaged into the payment for the service. Example 7.3 illustrates OPPS reimbursement for APC payment SIs.

Figure 7.1. **APC components**

APC 5021 Title: Level 1 Type A ED Visits	
Payment Status Indicator	V
Relative Weight	0.8774
National Unadjusted Payment Amount	$75.09
National Unadjusted Copayment Amount	N/A
Minimum Copayment Amount	$15.02
HCPCS Procedure Code(s) 99281 Emergency Department Visit	

Source: CMS 2023b.

Example 7.3

A patient is seen for wound care after she fell and sustained a scalp laceration. During the wound care visit the physician treated her for wound dehiscence (split wound) (CPT code 12020). The physician gave the patient an injection of lidocaine to numb the area prior to starting the closure procedure. The injection of lidocaine and supplies required to perform the closure are packaged into the payment for the procedure. Only the service with SI T, the simple closure, is payable separately.

CPT Code and/or Service Description	SI	APC	Reimbursement
12020 – Closure of split wound	T	5053	$580.95
J2001 – Lidocaine injection	N (packaged)	0000	$0.00
Supplies and drugs reported without HCPCS Codes	Packaged	0000	$0.00

Source: CMS 2023a.

Multiple surgical procedures with payment SI T performed during the same operative session are discounted. Discounting is a reimbursement policy where the highest-weighted procedure is fully reimbursed and all other procedures with payment SI T are reimbursed at 50 percent. This reduction is made to account for resource saving that hospitals experience by performing multiple procedures together. For example, operating room surgical instruments are prepped only once, anesthesia is administered once, and the recovery room is used once for all the procedures performed.

Although many services assigned to these APC payment SIs are payable separately in most circumstances, they can be packaged with C-APCs, which are discussed later in this section. The only exception is pass-through drugs and biologicals (SI G), which are exempt from packaging policies. A **pass-through** is a high-cost supply that is reimbursed under a different reimbursement methodology than other supplies. The pass-through policy for drugs, biologicals, and devices is discussed in the Provisions of OPPS section later in this chapter.

Within the APC payment SI category are new technology APCs. New technology APCs are a special group of APCs created to allow new procedures and services to enter OPPS quickly, even though their complete cost and payment information are not known. New technology APCs house modern procedures and services until enough data are collected to properly place the new procedure in an existing APC or to create a new APC for the service or procedure. A procedure or service can remain in a new technology APC for an indefinite amount of time. The APC system contains 82 new technology APCs. Forty-one groups have SI S and are not subject to multiple-procedure discounting. The remaining 41 groups have SI T and are subject to the multiple-procedure discount provision. Placement into new technology APCs is based on cost bands. For example, APC 1491, New Technology–Level IA, contains procedures that have an average cost of $0 to $10. The payment for the group is $5.

Per Diem Ambulatory Payment Classification Payment: Status Indicator P

The **partial hospitalization program (PHP)** is an intensive outpatient program of psychiatric services provided as an alternative to inpatient psychiatric care to patients who have an acute mental illness (CMS 2004, 50543). Partial hospitalization may be provided by hospital outpatient departments and Medicare-certified community mental health centers (CMHCs). Patients who receive psychiatric services and who have a diagnosis of an acute mental health disorder are grouped into APC 5853, partial hospitalization (three or more services) for CMHCs, or APC 5863, partial hospitalization (three or more services) for hospital-based PHPs. The unit of service for partial hospitalization is one day. Therefore, the APC payment rate for APCs 5853 and 5863 is based on a per diem amount. For 2023, the APC payment rate for APC 5853 is $142.70, of which $28.54 is the beneficiary copayment amount. The APC payment rate for APC 5863 is $268.22, of which $53.65 is the beneficiary copayment amount (CMS 2022a).

Comprehensive Ambulatory Payment Classification Payment: Status Indicatorss J1 and J2

With the goal of moving toward a fully packaged outpatient PPS, CMS created C-APCs. C-APCs are all-inclusive APC categories where a primary procedure is identified for the encounter and then most other procedures, services, and supplies are packaged into the C-APC payment amount. Services that are packaged are adjunctive, integral, ancillary, supportive, or dependent services that are provided to support the primary service (CMS 2017, 52363). C-APCs were first introduced in 2015. Since then, the number of C-APCs has grown from 25 to 70 in 2023. Figure 7.2 is an example of a claim that includes a C-APC.

In figure 7.2, code 26607 is assigned as the primary service and, therefore, is assigned as the C-APC for the encounter. Even though code 26720 has an SI T and is often separately payable, here, the service is packaged because it is part of a C-APC encounter. This is shown after final adjudication by the SI changing from T to N. *Adjudication* is the determination of the reimbursement amount based on the beneficiary's insurance plan benefits. Adjudication is performed by Medicare and uses the Medicare OCE and pricing logic to determine reimbursement amounts. Hospitals also use the Medicare OCE and pricing logic to determine the expected reimbursement amount they will receive from Medicare. Adjudication is discussed in detail in chapter 11, "Revenue Cycle Back-End Processes—Claims Production and Revenue Collection."

For some encounters there will be more than one C-APC. However, there can only be one primary service for the encounter. CMS ranks C-APC procedures each year in Addendum J of the final rule. Whichever procedure is ranked highest is deemed the primary C-APC for the encounter. All other J1 procedures are then packaged.

There is one caveat to C-APCs. Some combinations of procedures are costlier than others. Therefore, CMS developed the C-APC complexity adjustment. The complexity adjustment allows for a higher payment when established criteria are met.

Figure 7.2.   Example of C-APC encounter

Claim Services with SI Information from Addendum B (2023)		
CPT Code	**Description**	**SI (from Addendum B, before packaging logic)**
26607	Closed treatment of metacarpal fracture	J1 (C-APC)
26720	Closed treatment of phalangeal shaft fracture	T (Surgical procedure; discount applies)
99284	Emergency department visit	J2 (C-APC)
73120	X-ray hand	Q1 (Conditionally packaged)
Claim Services with Final APCs		
CPT Code	**APC with description**	**SI (after adjudication)**
26607	5113, Level 3 Musculoskeletal Procedures	J1 (C-APC)
26720	0000, No APC	N (packaged)
99284	0000, No APC	N (packaged)
73120	0000, No APC	N (packaged)

Source: CMS 2023a.

Conditional Ambulatory Payment Classification Payment: Status Indicators Q1, Q2, and Q4

Conditional APC payment services are assigned SIs Q1, Q2, and Q4. These services are conditionally packaged only when certain criteria are met. There are three types of conditionally packaged services. First are Q1 or STV-packaged items. When an ancillary service with SI Q1 is reported on the same encounter as a service with an SI of S, T, or V, then the ancillary service is packaged. But if the ancillary service is performed without any service with an SI of S, T, or V, then payment is provided for the ancillary service. The example provided in figure 7.3 illustrates how Q1 packaging is executed.

In this example (figure 7.3), Claim 1 shows how the ankle x-ray is packaged when it is performed during the same encounter as the ankle strapping. When performed independently of another procedure, as shown in Claim 2, the x-ray is reimbursed separately, and the SI changes from Q1 to S.

The second type of conditional packaging is Q2 or T-packaged codes. The concept is like the STV-packaged codes, but only SI T affects whether the ancillary service is separately paid or not. Example 7.4 illustrates conditional packing in OPPS.

Example 7.4

A patient is admitted to the emergency department for a possible hip dislocation. A hip x-ray with contrast is performed and shows a hip dislocation. Therefore, treatment is provided to return the hip to proper alignment. The hip x-ray is assigned SI Q2. The dislocation treatment is assigned SI T. Because the hip x-ray is conditionally packaged and performed with a T procedure, payment is only made for dislocation treatment.

Conditionally packaged laboratory tests are the third type and are assigned SI Q4. Laboratory tests are packaged if billed on the same claim as SIs J1, J2, S, T, V, Q1, Q2, or Q3. In OPPS, laboratory services are packaged most of the time. However, if the laboratory service is present on a claim without one of the designated SIs, then the service is SI A and is reimbursed via the Medicare Clinical Lab Fee Schedule (CLFS).

Figure 7.3.   Example of SI Q1 packaging

Claim Services with SI Information from Addendum B (2023)		
CPT Code	**Description**	**SI (from Addendum B, before packaging logic)**
29540	Strapping of ankle/foot	T
73610	X-ray ankle	Q1
Claim 1 – Services with Final APC		
CPT Code	**APC with description**	**SI (after adjudication)**
29540	5101, Level 1 Strapping and Cast Application	T – surgical procedure
73610	0000, No APC	N – packaged
Claim 2 – Only Radiology Service Provided, No Strapping Performed – Final APC		
CPT Code	**APC with description**	**SI (after adjudication)**
73610	5521, Level 1 Imaging without Contrast	S

Source: CMS 2023a.

Composite APC Payment: Status Indicator Q3

Composite APCs are created by bundling individual components of a larger service into one payment group. Composite APCs are formed by grouping services that are always performed together into a single payment. Currently, there are six composite APCs included in OPPS; they are listed in table 7.2.

Each composite APC includes parameters for when the composite APC will be assigned rather than individual APC assignments for each component. The APC 8004, Ultrasound, composite is activated when more than one of the designated ultrasound procedures are reported for the same encounter. The services included in table 7.3 are included in the ultrasound composite. Example 7.5 shows a composite APC in action.

Table 7.2.   Composite APCs for 2023

APC Number	APC Title
5041	Critical Care
5045	Trauma Response with Critical Care
8004	Ultrasound
8005	CT and CTA without Contrast
8006	CT and CTA with Contrast
8007	MRI and MRA without Contrast
8008	MRI and MRA with Contrast
8010	Mental Health Services

Source: CMS 2022a, addendum A.

Table 7.3.   APC 8004, ultrasound composite

CPT Code	Code Description
76700	Ultrasound exam of abdomen, complete
76705	Ultrasound exam of abdomen, limited
76770	Ultrasound, retroperitoneal, complete
76776	Ultrasound, transplanted kidney, with Doppler
76831	Saline infusion sonohysterography (SIS)
76856	Ultrasound exam of pelvis, complete
76857	Ultrasound exam of pelvis, limited
76981	Ultrasound, elastography; parenchyma
76982	Ultrasound, elastography; first target lesion

Source: CMS 2022a, addendum B.

Example 7.5

A patient with abdominal and pelvic pain is sent to radiology to receive several ultrasound services. The physician has ordered ultrasounds of the abdomen, retroperitoneal, and pelvis at the local hospital. Because all the radiology services performed for this patient are part of composite APC 8004, the facility will receive one APC payment for all three services.

Code with description	SI	APC	Reimbursement
76700, ultrasound exam of abdomen, complete	Q3	8004	$302.65
76770, ultrasound of retroperitoneal, complete	Q3		
76856, ultrasound of pelvis, complete	Q3		

Source: CMS 2022a.

Packaged Payment: Status Indicator N

As discussed earlier in this section, the use of packaging and bundling is a major component of the OPPS. SI N is assigned to identify procedures, services, and supplies that have been packaged into the cost and reimbursement for APC services with which they are most often performed. These items are always packaged. It is important to note that these services are covered under OPPS, but a separate payment is not provided for the individual service or supply. Examples of packaged services that are assigned SI N are provided in table 7.4.

As can be seen from the packaged service listing, anesthesia services, add-on procedures (except drug administration add-ons), and vaccinations are all packaged in OPPS. Identifying all packaged services by CPT code is done by examining the most current Addendum B located on the "Hospital Outpatient PPS" page on the CMS website. Additionally, any OPPS services and supplies that do not have an HCPCS code are packaged.

Fee Schedule Payment: Status Indicator A

Services such as ambulance transportation, physical therapy, and mammography are reimbursed based on a fee schedule amount. Various fee schedules are used for the reimbursement rates. For example, the Medicare physician fee schedule (MPFS) is used for the physical therapy payments. Fee schedule amounts are exempt from many of the

Table 7.4.   Sample of packaged services with SI N in OPPS

00102	Anesthesia repair of cleft lip
11045	Debridement of subcutaneous tissue add-on
23350	Injection for shoulder x-ray
35500	Harvest vein for bypass
49427	Injection abdominal shunt
58110	Biopsy done with colposcopy add-on
64832	Repair nerve add-on
90632	Hepatitis vaccine adult intramuscular

Source: CMS 2022a.

OPPS adjustments and provisions. For example, fee schedule reimbursement rates are not wage-index adjusted via the OPPS methodology because the fee schedule amount has already been adjusted for geographical differences.

Reasonable Cost Payment: Status Indicators F, H, and L

There is a small subset of services and supplies that are reimbursed at reasonable cost. In the cost-based payment calculation, the hospital-specific outpatient CCR is utilized. Reasonable cost is calculated by multiplying the charge for the service times the CCR developed from cost report statistics.

Not Reimbursed under OPPS: Status Indicators B, C, D, E1, E2, M, and Y

There are numerous procedures, services, and supplies that are not reimbursed under OPPS. There are services that are statutorily excluded from the Medicare benefit package, procedures that are not reasonable or necessary, and services that are not appropriate for the outpatient setting.

SI C is used for inpatient-only (IPO) procedures. Because Level I HCPCS codes (CPT codes) were originally designed to report physician services in all healthcare settings, the coding system contains codes for inpatient and outpatient procedures. OPPS covers only outpatient services. Each year, CMS reviews claims data and determines which procedures are IPO procedures and creates the IPO list. All procedures on the IPO list are assigned SI C. To move off the IPO list, a procedure must be performed in outpatient settings at least 60 percent of the time. To be reimbursed, procedures with SI C must be provided to Medicare beneficiaries in an inpatient setting, and payment is made under the IPPS.

Check Your Understanding 7.1

1. Define packaging and bundling as they pertain to OPPS.

2. List a way that packaging promotes effective and efficient care.

3. Match the SI to APC category.

   a. Q3   1. APC payment
   b. K   2. C-APC
   c. J1   3. Composite APC payment
   d. Q4   4. Conditional APC payment

4. A claim is produced for an outpatient ambulatory surgery encounter. There are three codes on the claim. One code has SI J1, the second code has SI T, and the third code has SI S. Which codes are separately payable and which are packaged?

5. Describe discounting as it applies to payment SI T.

OPPS Provisions

The OPPS uses provisions to provide additional payments for high-cost items and unusual admissions that historically have added significant cost to patient care. Without the additional payments associated with these provisions, it may not be feasible for hospital outpatient facilities to provide all services to Medicare beneficiaries. OPPS has numerous provisions, which include the following:

- Interrupted services

- High-cost outlier

- Rural hospital adjustment

- Cancer hospital adjustment

- Pass-through payment policy

Each of the OPPS provisions and the related payment adjustments is discussed in detail in the sections that follow.

Interrupted Services

Interrupted services are reported with modifiers. When modifiers are applied to the surgical codes, a reduction in payment may be applied. Procedures reported with modifier 73, surgery discontinued for a patient who has been prepared for surgery (that requires anesthesia) and taken to the operating room but before the administration of anesthesia, will be reduced by 50 percent. A procedure reported with modifier 74, surgery discontinued after administration of anesthesia or initiation of the procedure, will be reimbursed at 100 percent of the APC rate. Procedures and services that do not require anesthesia but that are reduced or discontinued at the physician's discretion should be reported with modifier 52. For these procedures, the payment rate will be reduced by 50 percent.

High-Cost Outlier

This provision is intended to provide financial assistance for unusually high-cost services. The outlier provision is based on the cost of individual services rather than the cost for the entire encounter (all services). Therefore, there may be multiple outlier calculations per claim. The equations for case qualification and additional payment levels are adjusted each year. Medicare limits the percentage of total payments that can be attributed to outlier payments to 1 percent. There are two types of outlier calculations: one for CMHCs' partial hospitalization services and one for all other facilities and services.

Rural Hospital Adjustment

Public Law 108-173, better known as the Medicare Prescription Drug, Improvement, and Modernization Act of 2003, allowed for a payment adjustment to be applied for rural hospitals if warranted after study. CMS presented the results of its study in the 2006 final rule. Regression analysis showed that overall, the cost of treating Medicare beneficiaries at rural hospitals was only 2.4 percent greater than at urban hospitals and did not warrant an adjustment. However, further analysis showed that the cost to rural **sole-community hospitals** (SCHs) was 7.1 percent greater than that of urban hospitals. SCHs are hospitals that, by reason of factors such as isolated location, weather conditions, travel conditions, or absence of other hospitals, are the sole source of patient hospital services reasonably available to Medicare beneficiaries in a geographic area. SCH status is determined by the secretary of the Department of Health and Human Services. Because the cost at SCHs is significantly higher than the cost at other facilities, an adjustment is warranted. Therefore, beginning in the 2006 OPPS, a rural adjustment of 7.1 percent was provided to SCHs, including essential access community hospitals (EACHs).

Cancer Hospital Adjustment

The Affordable Care Act of 2010 (Public Law 111-148) provides for an adjustment to dedicated cancer hospitals to address the higher costs incurred by this type of facility. CMS first proposed an adjustment in the 2011 proposed rule, but the proposed methodology was disputed by many in the healthcare community. One cause of dispute was that the copayment amounts for beneficiaries would be significantly higher at the cancer hospitals. Based on the numerous comments received by CMS, the proposed methodology was not adopted.

In the 2012 final rule, CMS adopted a new methodology for the cancer hospital adjustment. This methodology allows for aggregate payments to be made to each cancer hospital at cost report settlement rather than at the APC level on each claim. This allows the adjustment to be provided to the cancer hospitals without negatively impacting the beneficiary copayments.

Additional payments are provided to each of the 11 specified cancer hospitals so that each cancer hospital's payment-to-cost ratio (PCR) is equal to the weighted average PCR for all other OPPS facilities. The weighted average PCR is also known as the target PCR. For 2023, the target PCR is 0.89. A target PCR of 0.89 means that for each dollar in cost, the payment for OPPS services is 89 cents. Specified cancer facilities' payments are increased so that they equal 89 cents for each dollar of cost.

Pass-through Payment Policy

Pass-throughs are exceptions to the Medicare PPSs. These exceptions exist for high-cost supplies. Pass-throughs are not included in the packaging component of PPS and are passed through to other payment mechanisms that attempt to adjust for the high cost of items. Therefore, pass-throughs minimize the negative financial effect of combining all services into one lump-sum payment. Pass-throughs occur in both IPPS and OPPS.

Drugs, biological agents, and devices qualify for pass-through status if they were not being paid for as a hospital outpatient drug as of December 31, 1996, and their cost is "not insignificant" in relation to the OPPS payment for the procedures or services associated with their use (CMS 2004, 50502). The pass-through status application process is described on the CMS website (CMS 2022b).

Figure 7.4.   Foundation of hospital OPPS

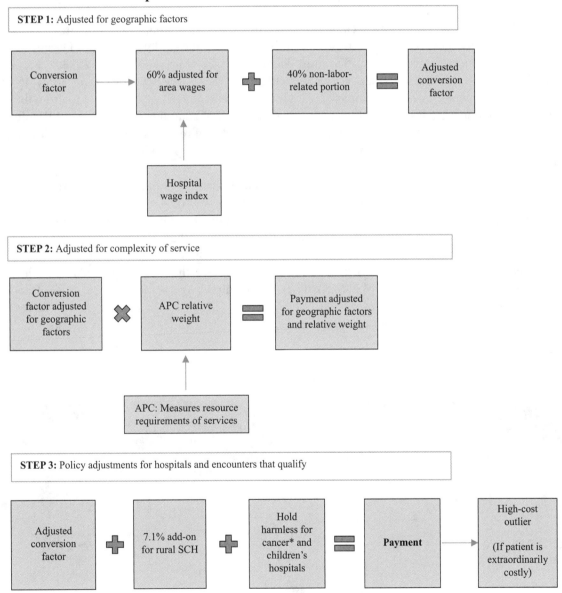

*Medicare adjusts outpatient prospective payment system payment rates for 11 cancer hospitals so the payment-to-cost ratio (PCR) for each cancer hospital is equal to the weighted average PCR for all hospitals.
Source: MedPAC 2022.

Pass-through device APCs (SI H) are paid on a reasonable cost basis less the device offset amount. The device offset amount is the portion of the payment amount that CMS has determined is associated with the cost of the device (CMS 2004, 50501). This amount is deducted from the pass-through payment because it is already reimbursed as part of the surgical APC payment.

OPPS Payment Workflow

Hospitals submit a claim to Medicare for payment. Claims are sent electronically to the designated Medicare administrative contractor (MAC). Each claim contains visit information, patient information, facility information, detailed charges by procedure code, and diagnosis codes. The MAC performs an audit of the claim to ensure the claim contains complete and accurate information based on the edits found in the OCE. The OCE is discussed in greater detail in chapter 13, "Revenue Compliance." During the editing process, APCs are assigned using grouper software as appropriate, based on the HCPCS codes submitted. The foundation of OPPS payment is displayed in figure 7.4.

The OPPS payment calculation uses **conversion factor (CF)**—a national dollar multiplier that sets the allowance for the relative values—to convert the APC relative weight into a dollar amount. During step one, the CF is adjusted to account for geographic differences. The CF for 2023 is $85.58 (CMS 2023a). Pricer software released by CMS completes the steps necessary to calculate the claim payment, including applying the OPPS provisions. When the payment steps are completed, payment is made to the facility, and the data from the encounter are included in the national claims history file. The outpatient standard analytical file and the OPPS file, extracted from the national claims history file, are used for statistical analysis and research. Figure 7.5 provides an example of a simple payment calculation for a Level II emergency department visit provided in a facility with a wage index of 0.9775.

Figure 7.6 provides an example of a more complex calculation for a shoulder repair surgery performed in a facility with a wage index of 0.9775. This example highlights the use of packaging through C-APCs. Prior to adjudication, codes 23430, 29824, and 93005 are eligible for separate APC payments (Addendum B SI). However, using the C-APC logic associated with SI J1, only one procedure can be the primary procedure for the encounter. According to the C-APC hierarchy, code 23430 is indicated as the primary C-APC for this encounter. All other procedures, because of their SI, are then packaged into the payment for the primary procedure. Their SI changes from the Addendum B SI to the Final SI of N (packaged). The result is payment for APC 5114 (CPT code 23430).

OPPS is one of the more complex payment systems used by Medicare. It is also one of the few payment systems without a value-based program component. Currently, organizations that provide hospital outpatient

Figure 7.5.   Example of simple calculation of OPPS payment

2020 CF	Wage-index Adjustment	CPT Code	Addendum B SI	APC	APC RW	Final SI (after adjudication)	Reimbursement
$85.58	(85.58 × 0.60 × 0.9775) + (85.58 × 0.40) 50.19 + 34.23 = $84.42	99282	V	5022	1.6322	V	
Multiply the wage-index adjusted CF times the APC RW to calculate the reimbursement level $84.42 × 1.6322							$137.79

Source: CMS 2022a.

Figure 7.6. Example of complex calculation of OPPS payment

2020 CF	Wage-index Adjustment	CPT Code	Addendum B SI	APC	APC RW	Final SI (after adjudication)	Reimbursement
$85.58	(85.58 × 0.60 × 0.9775) + (85.58 × 0.40)	23430	J1	5114	77.2872	J1	
		29824	J1	5113	34.7802	N	
	50.19 + 34.23 = $84.42	29826	N	0000	0.000	N	
		93005	Q1	5733	0.6716	N	
Multiply the wage-index adjusted CF times the APC RW for the payable APC to calculate the reimbursement level. $84.42 × 77.2872							$6,524.58

Source: CMS 2022a.

services only participate in the hospital quality reporting program, as discussed in the first sections of chapter 5, "Medicare Hospital Acute Inpatient Payment System."

Patient Connection

It's September, and Malakai is due to get his flu and pneumonia vaccines. Malakai goes to the flu shot clinic at Memorial Hospital to receive his shots. The flu shot clinic makes it easy for Medicare beneficiaries because no appointment is necessary; walk-ins can arrive between 10 a.m. and 3 p.m. to be vaccinated. The claim submitted for Malakai's visit includes the following charges:

42 REV CD	43 DESCRIPTION	44 HCPCS/ RATES	45 SERV. DATE	46 SERV. UNITS	47 TOTAL CHARGES	
0771	Admin influenza virus vaccine	G0008	9/12/2X	1	100	00
0771	Admin pneumococcal vaccine	G0009	9/12/2X	1	100	00
0636	Influenza virus vaccine, IM	90662	9/12/2X	1	75	00
0636	Pneumococcal polysaccharide vaccine, IM	90732	9/12/2X	1	125	00

Let's calculate the reimbursement for this encounter. Using OPPS Addendum B, we identify that the APC for both code G0008 and code G0009 is 5691, which has an unadjusted payment rate of $42.37. Further, the copayment amount is $0. The payment SI for APC 5691 is S. Codes 90662 and 90732 both have the SI of L and are not assigned to APCs. Referencing table 7.1, let's determine which lines are separately payable and which lines, if any, are packaged or bundled.

The payment SI for APC 5691 is S. HCPCS codes with payment SI S are paid via the APC rate. Further, S represents procedures or services for which the multiple procedure reduction does not apply. But remember, to determine bundling we must consider all payment SIs for the claim. So, let's look at payment SI L for the vaccines. HCPCS codes with payment SI L are paid via reasonable cost methodology. To calculate reasonable cost, we multiply the facility charge by the facility CCR, which for Memorial Hospital is 0.35. Further, table

(continued)

Patient Connection   (continued)

7.1 indicates that the beneficiary does not have to pay a deductible amount or copayment amount for the influenza and pneumococcal vaccines. According to table 7.1, no packaging or bundling is involved when only payment SIs S and L are included on a claim.

But before we finalize reimbursement, we need to perform a wage-index adjustment to the payment rate for APC 5691. The wage-index amount for Memorial Hospital is 1.0014. The formula for wage-index adjustment can be found in figure 5.8 of chapter 5, "Medicare Hospital Acute Inpatient Payment System." The wage-index adjustment calculation is as follows:

$$(\$42.37 \times 0.60 \times 1.0014) + (\$42.37 \times 0.40)$$

The wage-index adjustment payment amount is $42.41. Remember that when the wage-index amount is greater than 1.0, the payment rate will be higher after it is wage-index adjusted. Pulling all our information together, we can calculate the final reimbursement. The reimbursement rates are as follows:

- $21.00 for code G0008 ($42.41 × 0.4951)
- $21.00 for code G0009 ($42.41 × 0.4951)
- $26.25 for code 90662 [$75 × 0.35 (hospital CCR)]
- $43.75 for code 90732 [$125 × 0.35 (hospital CCR)]

The total payment to Memorial Hospital equals $112.00 ($21.00 + $21.00 + $26.25 + $43.75). However, Malakai owes nothing. These vaccines are provided to Medicare beneficiaries free of deductible and cost sharing.

Chapter 7 Review Quiz

1. Which reimbursement methodologies are used in OPPS?

2. Which SI is used to identify services that are packaged?

3. Which SIs are used to identify services that are paid using a reasonable cost-based methodology?
   a. F, T, S
   b. H, P, L
   c. J1, L, M
   d. F, H, L

4. Which of the following SIs is the highest-ranked SI and causes all other services to be packaged on a claim?
   a. T
   b. S
   c. J1
   d. J2

5. Which classification system is used in OPPS to combine procedures or services that are clinically comparable and have similar resource use together into groups?

(continued)

6. Which type of service includes an APC per diem methodology that includes payment for all services provided on a single day of service under OPPS?

   a. Clinic visits

   b. Partial hospitalization

   c. Emergency department visits

   d. Same-day surgery

7. Which type of APCs did CMS establish in order to support access for Medicare beneficiaries to receive new and innovative drugs, biologicals, and devices in the hospital outpatient setting?

8. Comprehensive APCs (C-APCs) have SIs J1 and J2. They are CMS's first step in moving OPPS from a partially packaged system to a _____ packaged system.

9. What is the purpose of the cancer hospital adjustment provision?

10. Why do sole-community hospitals receive a rural hospital adjustment under OPPS?

References

CMS (Centers for Medicare and Medicaid Services). 2023a. "Addendum B, January 2023." https://www.cms.gov/medicare/medicare-fee-service-payment/hospitaloutpatientpps/addendum-and-addendum-b-updates/january-2023.

CMS (Centers for Medicare and Medicaid Services). 2023b. "Addendum A, January 2023." https://www.cms.gov/medicare/medicare-fee-service-payment/hospitaloutpatientpps/addendum-and-addendum-b-updates/january-2023-0.

CMS (Centers for Medicare and Medicaid Services). 2022a. Medicare program: Hospital outpatient prospective payment and ambulatory surgical center payment systems and quality reporting programs; organ acquisition; rural emergency hospitals: payment policies, conditions of participation, provider enrollment, physician self-referral; new service category for hospital outpatient department prior authorization process; overall hospital quality star ration; COVID-19. *Federal Register* 87(225):71748–72310.

CMS (Centers for Medicare and Medicaid Services). 2022b. "Pass-Through Payment Status and New Technology Ambulatory Payment Classification (APC)." https://www.cms.gov/Medicare/Medicare-Fee-for-Service-Payment/HospitalOutpatientPPS/passthrough_payment.

CMS (Centers for Medicare and Medicaid Services). 2017. Medicare program; Hospital outpatient prospective payment and ambulatory surgical center payment systems and quality reporting programs; Final rule with comment period. *Federal Register* 82(217):52356–52637.

CMS (Centers for Medicare and Medicaid Services). 2007. Medicare program: Changes to the Hospital Outpatient Prospective Payment System and CY 2008 payment rates, ambulatory surgical center payment system and CY 2008 payment rates, hospital inpatient prospective payment system and FY 2008 rates and payments for graduate medical education for affiliated teaching hospitals in certain emergency situations. *Federal Register* 72(227):66610.

CMS (Centers for Medicare and Medicaid Services). 2004. Medicare program; Proposed changes to the Hospital Outpatient Prospective Payment System and calendar year 2005 payment rates; Proposed rule. *Federal Register* 69(157):50447–50546.

MedPAC (Medicare Payment Advisory Commission). 2022. Payment Basics: Outpatient Hospital Services Payment System. https://www.medpac.gov/wp-content/uploads/2022/10/MedPAC_Payment_Basics_22_OPD _FINAL_SEC_v3.pdf.

Resources

CMS (Centers for Medicare and Medicaid Services). Medicare Outpatient Code Editor. https://www.cms.gov /medicare/coding/outpatientcodeedit.

Chapter 8
Medicare Physician and Other Health Professional Payment System

Learning Objectives

❖ Describe how the two parts of the Medicare physician and other health professional payment system, RBRVS and MPFS, work together to determine payment

❖ Define the three elements of the RBRVS relative value unit

❖ Describe how the geographic practice cost index is used to adjust for cost differences across the US

❖ Discuss the provisions of the Medicare physician and other health professional payment system

❖ Describe the Quality Payment Program (QPP)

Key Terms

Alternative payment model (APM)
Assignment of benefits
Geographic practice cost index (GPCI)
Health professional shortage areas (HPSAs)
Incident to
Malpractice (MP) element
Medicare physician fee schedule (MPFS)

Nonparticipating physician (nonPAR)
Participating physician (PAR)
Physician work (WORK) element
Practice expense (PE) element
Quality Payment Program (QPP)
Relative value unit (RVU)
Resource-based relative value scale (RBRVS)

The Medicare physician and other health professional payment system provides reimbursement to physicians and other health professionals. The services of physicians and other health professionals provided to Medicare beneficiaries are covered under Part B Medicare. These services include office visits, diagnostic and surgical procedures, and other therapies, and may be delivered in a wide range of settings, such as in offices, ambulatory surgery centers, inpatient acute-care hospitals, outpatient dialysis facilities, skilled nursing facilities, and hospice. Providers of these services are physicians, such as audiologists, chiropractors, clinical social workers, optometrists, podiatrists, psychologists, nurse midwives, nurse practitioners, nutritionists, physician assistants, physical and occupational therapists, and speech-language pathologists. Approximately 56 percent of the clinicians in Medicare's registry are physicians; the remainder are either health professionals practicing independently or practicing under the supervision of a physician (MedPAC 2022, 1).

The payment system is divided into two parts: the resource-based relative value scale and the Medicare physician fee schedule (MPFS). To develop payment rates, the Centers for Medicare and Medicaid Services (CMS) uses the **resource-based relative value scale (RBRVS)**, a resource measurement system that assigns values to services performed by physicians and other health professionals based on the cost of furnishing services in different settings, the skill and training levels required to perform the services, and the time and risk involved. RBRVS permits comparisons of the resources needed or appropriate prices for various units of service. It considers labor, skill, supplies, equipment, space, and other costs for each procedure or service. Under RBRVS, each service is assigned a **relative value unit (RVU)**. An RVU is the unit of measure. Like relative weights, it represents the physician skill level, costs of providing care, and cost for supplies and equipment. A conversion factor (CF), an across-the-board multiplier, is used to convert the RVUs into reimbursement amounts. The result is the **Medicare physician fee schedule (MPFS)**. The reimbursement methodology for this payment system is a fee schedule. While the fees are predetermined, the MPFS is *not* a prospective payment system. A physician can increase reimbursements by increasing the volume of individual services provided to a patient. The Medicare Payment Advisory Commission (MedPAC) and others refer to this payment system as the Medicare physician and other health professional payment system. However, throughout CMS documents and webpages the acronym MPFS is used. In practice, RBRVS and MPFS are often used interchangeably, which can be confusing. It is important to remember that RBRVS is a resource measurement system and the MPFS is the reimbursement methodology platform. This chapter uses both acronyms, RBRVS and MPFS, when applicable. When discussing payments to physicians and other health professionals, the term *physician* is used as a global term for all providers paid with the MPFS. Any differences in the payment system based on the type of profession are noted when needed. The MPFS became effective January 1, 1992. For health personnel, it is important to understand this payment system because 77 percent of public and private payers, including Medicaid, have adopted its various components (AAP 2020, 1).

Structure of Payment

Payments to physicians are based on three components: (1) an RVU, (2) its geographic adjustment, and (3) a CF. In the following sections we will explore the structure of payment by examining the RVU, geographic practice cost index (GPCI), and CF. We conclude with performing a reimbursement calculation.

Relative Value Unit and Geographic Practice Cost Index

The Healthcare Common Procedure Coding System (HCPCS), which includes Current Procedural Terminology (CPT), is used by physicians to report procedures, services, and supplies. Each HCPCS code has been assigned an RVU. Each RVU is subdivided into three elements. Each element has a unique weight. The weights of these three elements are summed to calculate the total RVU weight:

- Physician work (WORK)—at 51 percent of the total RVU weight
- Practice expense (PE)—at 45 percent of the total RVU weight
- Malpractice (MP)—at 4 percent of the total RVU weight

National averages for these three elements are available on the CMS website.

The **physician work (WORK) element** is the element that covers the physician's salary. This work is the time the physician spends providing a service and the intensity with which that time is spent. The four aspects of intensity are as follows:

1. Mental effort and judgment
2. Technical skill
3. Physical effort
4. Psychological stress

The **practice expense (PE) element** represents the overhead costs of running a health professional or physician practice. CMS conducts a survey entitled the Socioeconomic Monitoring System (SMS) to obtain data to calculate the overhead costs of a practice. The SMS includes six categories of PE costs:

1. Clinical payroll (including fringe benefits) for nonphysician clinical personnel (such as physician assistants and nurse practitioners)

2. Administrative payroll (including fringe benefits) for nonphysician administrative personnel (for example, administrators, secretaries, and clerks)

3. Office expenses for rent, mortgage interest, depreciation on medical buildings, utilities, telephones, and other related costs

4. Medical material and supply expenses for drugs, x-ray films, disposable medical products, and other related costs

5. Medical equipment expenses, including depreciation, leases, and rentals for medical equipment used in the diagnosis or treatment of patients

6. All other expenses, such as legal services, accounting, office management, professional association memberships, and any professional expenses

PE is categorized as either facility or nonfacility (table 8.1). According to CMS experts, PEs differ for physicians when they perform services in facilities, such as hospitals, versus when they perform services in nonfacilities, such as their own offices and clinics.

- Facilities: Organization incurs the overhead costs of personnel, supplies, and equipment, among other costs.

- Nonfacilities: Physician incurs the overhead costs of personnel, supplies, and equipment, among other costs.

Thus, the PE is generally higher for nonfacilities than for facilities because physicians in nonfacilities incur more costs. Some procedural codes do not have separate facility and nonfacility PEs. In these procedural codes, the description includes the setting, such as evaluation and management and initial hospital care, or the nature of the procedure restricts it to a particular site, such as major surgical procedures that must be performed in hospitals.

The **malpractice (MP) element** represents the cost of the premiums for MP insurance. Because the services of nonphysicians may also be reimbursed under the RBRVS, this element also contains data for professional liability insurance premiums. CMS collects data from both commercial and physician-owned MP and professional liability insurance carriers from all 50 states, the District of Columbia, and Puerto Rico.

Table 8.1.   **Facility and nonfacility settings for physician PEs**

Facility	**Nonfacility**
Ambulatory service (land, air, or water)	Clinic
Ambulatory surgical center	Dialysis center
Community mental health center	Independent laboratory
Comprehensive inpatient rehabilitation facility	Nonskilled nursing facility
Emergency department	Patient's home
Inpatient hospital setting	Physician's office
Inpatient psychiatric facility	Urgent care facility
Military treatment facility	All other settings
Outpatient hospital setting	
Psychiatric facility partial hospital	
Psychiatric resort treatment center	
Skilled nursing facility	

RVUs are routinely maintained to ensure up-to-date information. Annually, as new health services are implemented or existing health services are revised, the Relative Value Scale Update Committee (RUC) of the American Medical Association recommends appropriate RVUs for these health services to CMS. In addition, CMS analysts review the RVUs at least every five years to ensure the accuracy of the weights. The update includes a review of changes in medical practice, coding changes, and new data (MedPAC 2022, 3).

Each of the three elements is adjusted to local costs through the **geographic practice cost indexes (GPCIs)**. A geographic adjustment is necessary because costs vary in different areas of the country. To reflect local costs, CMS defines about 90 payment areas, known as localities. Localities reflect differences in the cost of resources (CMS 2013, 74230). Localities can be large metropolitan areas, such as Boston or San Francisco, portions of states ("rest-of-state areas"), or entire states. The GPCI for the locality is based on relative variations in the cost of a market basket of goods across different geographic areas. In that way, different localities have GPCIs that match the costs in that geographic area. Each element of the RVU—WORK, PE, and MP—has its own unique GPCI as shown in figure 8.1. The GPCIs can be found on the CMS website. Through the GPCIs, each element of an RVU is adjusted for the geographic cost differences.

Conversion Factor

The CF is an across-the-board multiplier. Unlike the GPCIs, the CF is a constant that applies to the entire RVU. The CF transforms the geographic-adjusted RVU into a fee schedule amount. The CF is the government's most direct control on Medicare payments to physicians and other professionals. CMS raises or lowers the CF to raise or lower physician and professional payments. CMS updates the CF annually and publishes the amount in the *Federal Register*.

Calculation

RVUs are converted to reimbursement amounts and published in the MPFS. The MPFS is the maximum amount of reimbursement that Medicare will allow for a service. The MPFS consists of a list of payments for services by HCPCS code. The MPFS is calculated using the following formula:

$$[(RVU_w) (GPCI_w) + (RVU_{pe}) (GPCI_{pe}) + (RVU_{mp}) (GPCI_{mp})] \times CF = MPFS$$

Table 8.2 shows the formula in action for a sample service. Reimbursement specialists should understand the generic formula to determine how proposed changes in components of the formula will affect the revenues of their healthcare entity.

Finally, as covered in chapter 3, "Government-Sponsored Healthcare Programs," the Medicare beneficiary is responsible for an annual deductible and a 20 percent coinsurance amount for each covered service. The provider receives 80 percent of the MPFS amount from Medicare. Using the payment example from table 8.2, figure 8.2 shows the percentage of $56.90 that is the responsibility of the beneficiary and that of CMS.

Figure 8.1.   Example of GPCI application

	RVU	GPCI	Product of RVU and GPCI
WORK	0.93	1.00	0.93
PE	1.14	0.912	1.0396
MP	0.08	1.063	0.0850
SUM			2.0546

*MAC locality 1520200 (Ohio). CPT code 99202.
Source: CMS 2023.

Table 8.2.   **Example of calculation of nonfacility payment**

Element	RVU	GPCI	Result
Work value (WORK)	0.70	1.017	0.7119
Practice expense (PE)	0.92	1.017	0.9357
Malpractice (MP)	0.06	0.711	0.0427
Sum		=	1.68
× CF		×	$33.8872
Adjusted payment		=	$56.93

*MAC locality 0441211 (Dallas, TX). CPT code 99212.
Source: CMS 2023.

Figure 8.2.   **Example of Medicare beneficiary coinsurance portion**

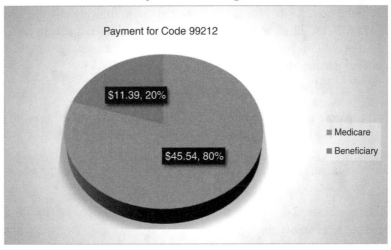

Source: CMS 2023.

Check Your Understanding 8.1

1. Define RBRVS.

2. In the RBRVS, which element comprises the largest portion of the total RVU?

3. List three of the six categories of PE.

4. What does GPCI stand for?

5. What portion of the MPFS is paid by Medicare?

Medicare Physician and Other Health Professional Payment System Provisions

Reimbursement under the RBRVS may be adjusted for several reasons, such as the type of clinician providing the service, special circumstances, additional geographic considerations, and other factors. The provisions of the Medicare physician and other health professional payment system are discussed in the next sections.

Clinician Type

Medicare's reimbursement may be adjusted by the type or characteristics of the provider. There are three categories of providers for whom the payment system adjusts. The adjustment is applied to the MPFS amount. The categories include participation status for physicians, anesthesiologists, and nonphysician providers (NPPs).

Participating Physician versus Nonparticipating Physician

Physicians that participate in Medicare are referred to as **participating physicians (PARs)**. Physicians who opt out of Medicare participation are referred to as **nonparticipating physicians (nonPARs)**. PARs have signed a contract with Medicare to accept an **assignment of benefits**. An assignment of benefits is a contract between a physician and Medicare in which the physician agrees to bill Medicare directly for covered services, to bill the beneficiary only for any coinsurance or deductible that may be applicable, and to accept the Medicare payment as payment in full. Medicare pays the physician directly rather than sending the check to the Medicare beneficiary. Physicians who do not participate in Medicare are nonPARs. There are two types of nonPAR providers: providers who accept assignment and providers who do not accept assignment. Medicare payments to nonPAR physicians that accept assignment are reduced by 5 percent (95 percent of what a PAR receives). This is called the nonPAR MPFS amount. NonPAR physicians who do not accept assignment are reduced by the 5 percent but are granted permission to collect reimbursement above the nonPAR MPFS at a level of the claim limiting charge, which is 115 percent of the nonPAR MPFS amount (AMA 2015, 82). The nonPAR provider who does not accept assignment may balance bill the patient the difference between 95 percent of the MPFS and the limiting charge. Table 8.3 provides an example of the three levels of physician participation.

Anesthesiologists

Anesthesia services have a separate payment method. The following elements are used to calculate a payment for anesthesia services:

- Base units for anesthesia services from a uniform relative value guide based on anesthesia CPT codes (RVUs)

- Base units for CPT anesthesia codes range from 3 (anesthesia services for needle biopsy of thyroid) to 30 (anesthesia services for liver transplant)

- Time units in 15-minute intervals (personal performance of anesthesia services) or in 30-minute intervals (medically directing the performance of others, such as certified nurse anesthetists) and reduced for the number of concurrent procedures

- Separate CF adjusted for locality (because there is no GPCI)

The generic formula is:

$$[\text{Base Unit} + \text{Time (in units)}] \times \text{CF} = \text{MPFS for Anesthesiologists}$$

Nonphysician Providers

NPPs practicing within their scope of practice and within state laws may receive MPFS payment. Examples of NPPs include audiologists; certified nurse midwives; certified registered nurse anesthetists; clinical nurse specialists; clinical psychologists; nurse practitioners; physician assistants; registered dietitians; and occupational, physical, and speech therapists. For the purposes of Medicare payment, these NPPs generally receive 85 percent of the full MPFS amount.

NPPs may only submit claims for reimbursement when their services are neither "**incident to**," nor under the direct supervision of a physician. "Incident to" services are those services that nonphysician clinicians, such as

Table 8.3. Example of reimbursement differences between PAR and nonPAR physicians

Reimbursement Arrangement	Total Reimbursement	Reimbursement Amount from Medicare	Reimbursement Amount from Beneficiary
PAR Physician	100% MPFS $50.00	MAC reimburses physician $40.00 (80%)	Beneficiary reimburses physician $10.00 (20%)
NonPAR Physician accepting assignment	95% MPFS $47.50	MAC reimburses physician $38.00 (80%)	Beneficiary reimburses physician $9.50 (20%)
NonPAR Physician nonaccepting assignment	Claim limiting charge of 115% of 95% MPFS $54.63	MAC does not reimburse physician	MAC reimburses beneficiary $38 (80% of nonPAR amount) Beneficiary reimburses physician $9.50 (20% of nonPAR amount) Beneficiary reimburses physician $7.13 (the balance of the bill since the provider does not accept assignment)

a nurse or physician assistant, provide to patients in a physician's office under the physician's supervision. For services that are not "incident to," the NPP bills for the service using their Medicare provider number, and Medicare reimburses the NPP.

If the services are "incident to" or under the physician's direct supervision, Medicare pays the full MPFS amount to the physician. For "incident to" services, the physician bills for the service using their provider number. The reimbursement is provided to the physician. The physician pays the NPP based on their employment contract.

Special Circumstances

Medicare can adjust payments for special circumstances using modifiers. Sometimes services or procedures are altered in some way (see chapter 10, "Revenue Cycle Middle Processes—Resource Tracking"). Modifiers provide information about this alteration so Medicare and other payers can process the claim (MedPAC 2022, 2). The following are examples of modifiers:

- *Bilateral procedures.* For bilateral procedures, Medicare will pay the lower of (a) the total actual charge for both sides or (b) 150 percent of the MPFS amount for the single code.

- *Multiple procedures.* When multiple procedures are performed on the same day, Medicare reimburses the physician for the first procedure at 100 percent; subsequent procedures through the fifth procedure are reimbursed at 50 percent (sixth and more require review).

- *Physicians assisting in surgery.* When physicians assist in surgery, they are reimbursed at 16 percent of the MPFS amount for the primary surgeon.

Other common modifiers represent preoperative or postoperative management only or surgery only.

Underserved Area

Through the Medicare physician and other health professional payment system, CMS provides an incentive for physicians to render services in underserved areas known as **health professional shortage areas (HPSAs)**. The purpose of the incentive is to attract physicians to these areas (MedPAC 2022, 3). CMS makes 10 percent bonus payments to physicians who render medical care services in HPSAs.

The US Health Resources and Services Administration (HRSA) designates certain geographic areas as HPSAs. These areas have a shortage of providers in medical care, dental care, or mental health care, or some combination of these. The CMS website has information about the HPSAs and about the zip codes that qualify for the bonus.

Medicare Physician and Other Health Professional Payment Workflow

The previous sections have explored the payment structure and provisions of the Medicare physician and other health professional payment system. Both components are combined to calculate the final payment, as shown in figure 8.3.

As shown in figure 8.3, the first step has multiple components. The first component is to adjust each RVU element for geographic factors. Then the adjusted RVUs are summed and multiplied by the CF. If any modifiers apply, such as discounting for multiple procedures, the payment adjustment is applied. The result is the adjusted fee schedule payment rate. The second step is to further adjust the fee schedule payment rate if applicable. For example, if reimbursement is being determined for a nonPAR, then the payment is reduced. After all applicable adjustment policies are applied, the result is the final payment. Examples 8.1 and 8.2 provide example calculations.

Figure 8.3. **Foundation of Medicare physician and other health professional payment system**

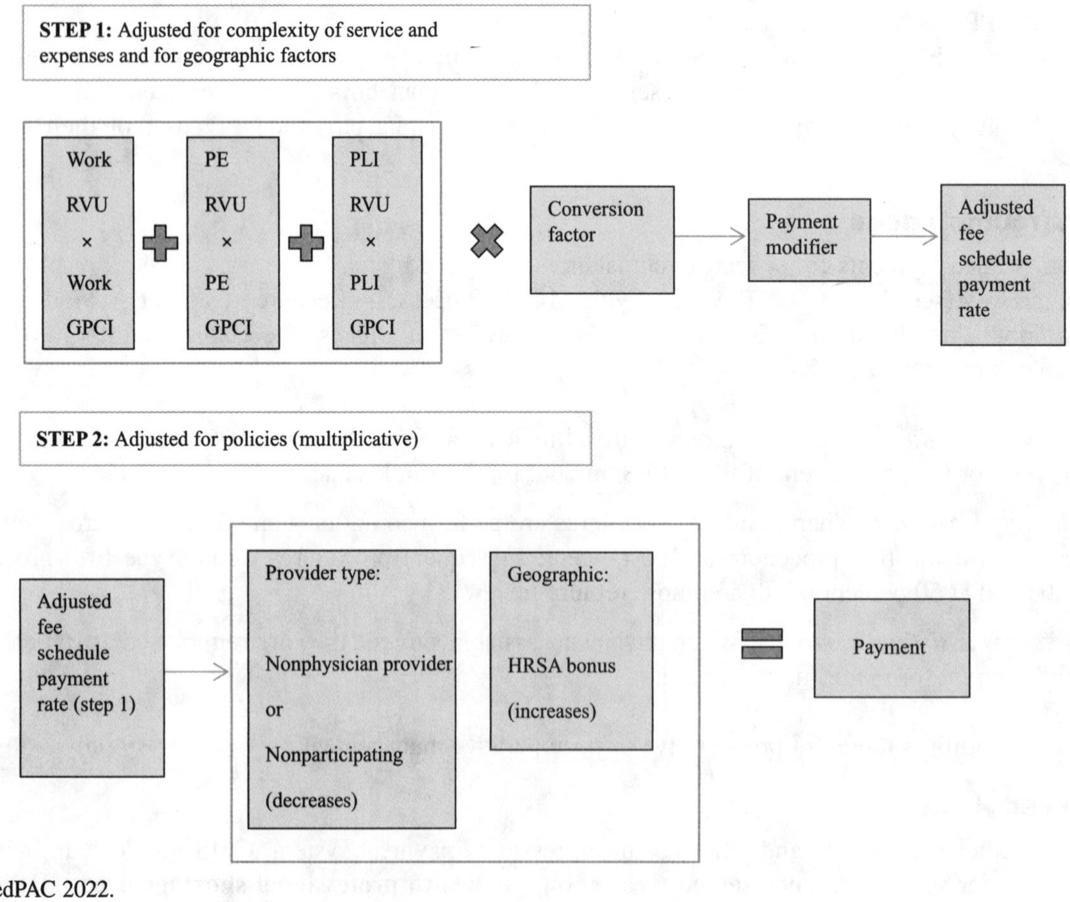

Source: MedPAC 2022.

Example 8.1

Dr. Johansson performed an esophagoscopy. During the esophagoscopy she removed two polyps using a snare technique. Dr. Johansson reported HCPCS code 43217 for the procedure. Dr. Johansson performs outpatient surgery at a facility-based surgery center in Ohio and is a Medicare PAR provider.

Element	RVU	× GPCI	Result
Physician work (WORK)	2.80	1.000	2.80
Practice expense (PE)	1.52	0.915	1.3908
Malpractice (MP)	0.30	1.049	0.3147
Sum		=	4.5055
× CF		×	$33.89
Adjusted payment		=	$152.69

Source: CMS 2023.

In this example, the RVU elements are adjusted for the GPCI applicable to the Ohio locality (1520200). The result is a total RVU of 4.5055. The total RVU is multiplied by the CF of $33.89. The result is an MPFS amount of $152.69. Since Dr. Johansson is a physician and is a Medicare PAR provider and did not provide this service in an HPSA, $152.69 is the final payment amount.

Example 8.2

Ms. Garcia is a nurse practitioner at Sunshine Neighborhood Clinic. She provided a Level I office visit for an established patient. She does not work "incident to" a physician and operates within the scope of duties delineated by the state of Ohio. Ms. Garcia is a Medicare PAR provider.

Element	RVU	× GPCI	Result
Physician work (WORK)	0.18	1.000	0.18
Practice expense (PE)	0.46	0.915	0.4209
Malpractice (MP)	0.01	1.049	0.1049
Sum		=	0.6114
× CF		×	$33.89
Adjusted payment		=	$20.72
Adjusted for NPP			$17.61 ($20.72 × 0.85)

Source: CMS 2023.

(continued)

Example 8.2 *(continued)*

In this example, the RVU elements are adjusted for the GPCI applicable to the Ohio locality (1520200). The result is a total RVU of 0.6114. The total RVU is multiplied by the CF of $33.89. The result is an MPFS amount of $20.72. Ms. Garcia is a nurse practitioner; therefore, her payment is reduced by 15 percent. The result is a reimbursement amount of $17.61. Since Ms. Garcia is a Medicare PAR provider and did not provide this service in an HPSA, $17.61 is the final payment amount.

Quality Payment Program

CMS established the **Quality Payment Program (QPP)** in accordance with Sections 101(c) and 101(d) of the Medicare Access and CHIP Reauthorization Act of 2015 (MACRA). The QPP is a payment incentive program for physicians and eligible clinicians that provide high-value and high-quality services. It reduces payments to clinicians who are not meeting performance standards (QPP n.d.). The strategic objectives for the QPP are as follows:

- To improve beneficiary population health
- To improve the care received by Medicare beneficiaries
- To lower costs to the Medicare program through improvement of care and health
- To advance the use of healthcare information between allied providers and patients
- To educate, engage, and empower patients as members of their care team
- To maximize QPP participation with a flexible and transparent design and easy-to-use program tools
- To maximize QPP participation through education, outreach, and support tailored to the needs of practices, especially those that are small, rural, and in underserved areas
- To expand alternative payment model (APM) participation
- To provide accurate, timely, and actionable performance data to clinicians, patients, and other stakeholders
- To continuously improve QPP, based on participant feedback and collaboration (QPP n.d.)

The program has two tracks: the Merit-Based Incentive Payment System (MIPS) and the advanced APMs.

The MIPS consolidates the Medicare meaningful use incentive, the physician quality reporting system, and the physician value-based payment modifier program into one model that links payment to quality and efficiency. Under MIPS, physicians and clinicians may receive bonuses based on their performance on metrics related to the cost and quality of patient care, improvement to clinical care processes, patient engagement, and physician use of certified health record technology (QPP n.d.).

An **alternative payment model (APM)** is a payment approach that provides incentives for the provider to deliver high-quality and cost-efficient care (QPP n.d.). APMs are developed in conjunction with the clinician community and can be designed for a specific condition, care episode, or population. Advanced APMs are models that have a significant risk for providers and offer a potential for significant rewards. Examples of advanced APMs include Independence at Home Demonstration and Primary Care First Model Options (CMS n.d.). There are two tracks for participation. Practices receive a full or reduced payment for evaluation and management services through MPFS based on track selection. Quarterly, the practice receives care management payments. Therefore, the reimbursement is a blend of traditional MPFS and per beneficiary per month (PBPM) payments. Additionally, incentive payments are provided in advance, and practices either keep the incentive payments or pay them back to Medicare based on their performance for patient experience measures, clinical quality measures, and utilization measures. These measures drive efficiency for the total cost of care.

Patient Connection

Olivia went out for a run, and two blocks from home she sprained her ankle. Her husband took her to a network urgent care facility, Community Urgent Care, for treatment. Dr. McGee evaluated Olivia and determined that she had a grade 2 left ankle sprain. Grade 2 sprains include partial tearing of the ligament, and Dr. McGee told Olivia she would continue to have moderate swelling, tenderness, and possible instability. Dr. McGee gave Olivia a walking boot for phase one of her recovery. In addition, Olivia is to use the RICE method of rest, ice, compression, and elevation.

Dr. McGee submitted a claim to Super Payer for Olivia's encounter. Super Payer uses a fee schedule for physician services. They use Medicare's RBRVS RVUs and then apply their CF of $55. Dr. McGee submitted code 99203, Level III clinic visit for the encounter. The total RVU for code 99203 is 3.33. So, Dr. McGee received $183.15 ($55 × 3.33) for the urgent care encounter.

It's common for commercial insurance companies to reimburse higher than Medicare and Medicaid. While Medicare has a significant patient volume to offer healthcare organizations and providers, often insurance companies must use higher payments during contract negotiations to entice healthcare facilities and providers to join their networks.

Super Payer reimbursed Dr. McGee $183.15 for this encounter. Let's compare that to how much Medicare would pay for the urgent care visit. We already know that the total RVU for code 99203 is 3.33. The 2023 Medicare CF is $33.8872. Medicare would reimburse $112.84 ($33.8872 × 3.33) for the encounter. CMS pays 38 percent less than Super Payer for the same encounter. It's important to understand that there can be significant variability in physician payments among various insurance companies and government payers. The provider charge may be constant, but the reimbursement typically is not.

Chapter 8 Review Quiz

1. Which code set do physicians use to report services and procedures?

2. What are the three elements of the RVU?

3. Juan is preparing a presentation for the office staff at Happy Physicians. He is preparing the slide that discusses the different RVU elements. Which RVU element represents physician mental effort and judgment, technical skill, physical effort, and psychological stress?

4. How are physician payments adjusted for the price differences across various parts of the country?

5. Jordie is practicing calculating MPFS amounts. Which RVU elements are adjusted by the GPCI?

   a. WORK and PE

   b. WORK and MP

   c. PE and MP

   d. WORK, PE, and MP

6. Which GPCI-adjusted RVU results in a higher MPFS payment: 0.985 or 24.32?

7. For which clinicians is RBRVS modified by a formula that includes base units and time?

   a. Anesthesiologists

   b. NonPARs

   c. Physical therapists

   d. Surgeons

(continued)

Chapter 8 Review Quiz   *(continued)*

8. Raphael, who is a Medicare beneficiary, is seen in Dr. Haver's office. The total charge for the office visit is $250. Raphael has previously paid his Medicare Part B deductible. The MPFS amount for the service is $200. The nonparticipating MPFS amount is $190. Dr. Haver is a Medicare PAR. What is the total amount of Raphael's cost sharing for this encounter?

    a. $200

    b. $160

    c. $40

    d. $30

9. Nurse practitioners whose practice is not considered to be "incident to" are reimbursed at which percentage of the MPFS?

10. What type of bonus do physicians who treat patients in underserved areas receive?

References

AAP (American Academy of Pediatrics). 2020. "RBRVS: What Is It and How Does It Affect Pediatrics?" https://downloads.aap.org/AAP/PDF/2020%20RBRVS.pdf.

AMA (American Medical Association). 2015. *The Physicians' Guide to Medicare RBRVS*, edited by S. L. Smith. Chicago: AMA.

CMS (Centers for Medicare and Medicaid Services). 2023. "Physician Fee Schedule Look-Up Tool." https://www.cms.gov/medicare/physician-fee-schedule/search.

CMS (Centers for Medicare and Medicaid Services). 2013. Medicare program; Revisions to payment policies under the physician fee schedule, clinical laboratory fee schedule & other revisions to part B for CY 2014; Final rule. *Federal Register* 78(237):74229–74823.

CMS (Centers for Medicare and Medicaid Services). n.d. "Innovation Models." Accessed April 6, 2023. https://innovation.cms.gov/innovation-models#views=models&stg=accepting%20letters%20of%20intent, accepting%20applications,ongoing.

MedPAC (Medicare Payment Advisory Commission). 2022. Physician and Other Health Professional Payment System. https://www.medpac.gov/wp-content/uploads/2021/11/MedPAC_Payment_Basics_22_Physician _FINAL_SEC.pdf.

QPP (Quality Payment Program). n.d. "Quality Payment Program Overview." Accessed February 24, 2023. https://qpp.cms.gov/about/qpp-overview.

Part III:
Revenue Cycle
Processes

Chapter 9
Revenue Cycle Front-End Processes—Patient Engagement

Learning Objectives

- Describe the processes included in the front end of the revenue cycle component
- Analyze patient financial agreements
- Explore the scheduling and registration process
- Understand the impact of cost sharing on the patient's financial position

Key Terms

Advance beneficiary notification of noncoverage (ABN)

Hospital-issued notices of noncoverage (HINN)

Patient financial responsibility agreement

Patient portal

Patient registration

Price transparency

Chapter 1, "Healthcare Reimbursement and Revenue Cycle Management," introduced the concepts of revenue cycle and revenue cycle management (RCM). As a refresher, revenue cycle is the regular set of tasks and activities that produces reimbursement (revenue). RCM is the supervision of all the administrative and clinical functions that contribute to the capture, management, and collection of patient service reimbursement. This chapter, and chapters 10 and 11 that follow, will discuss the intricate details of the healthcare revenue cycle. It is important to remember that every facility and physician practice is unique and may customize processes to fit their needs or use different terminology to describe the tasks. In this text we discuss the most common revenue cycle processes used by most facilities and practices. Figure 9.1 displays a refresher of the revenue cycle components and highlights the processes for the front end of the revenue cycle, which are discussed in this chapter.

The front-end process is primarily patient-facing and begins when the patient schedules services. It ends when the patient registers at the point of care. Much of this pre-care work is focused on complying with regulations such as the Health Insurance Portability and Accountability Act of 1996 (HIPAA) and ensuring that all parties understand the financial obligations associated with the care that will be provided. Insurance coverage and patient cost sharing are becoming more and more complex. Thus, the front end of the revenue cycle requires careful management.

Scheduling Services

The first step in the healthcare revenue cycle is the scheduling of a service, such as an office visit or a surgical procedure. Typically, the patient starts the process by contacting the healthcare provider via telephone or a patient portal. If the patient is new to the provider, scheduling includes not only selection of an appointment time, but also the collection of basic demographic information, services required, and insurance coverage status.

Patients have a number of methods of contacting providers to make an appointment or schedule a procedure. Most electronic health record (EHR) systems have a patient portal that allows a patient to send and receive

Figure 9.1.   Components of the revenue cycle

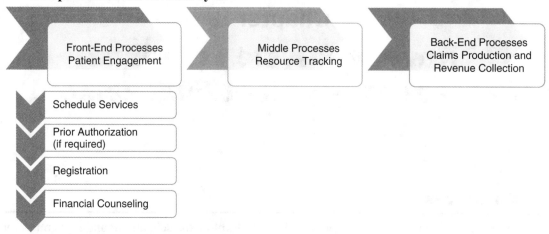

information with a provider electronically. They often allow patients to schedule appointments themselves. Upon entering the portal, the patient is presented with a list of providers and services they may schedule. Upon selecting the provider or service, a list of available appointments and locations is presented. The patient may then schedule and often has the option to add appointments and reminders to their online calendar.

Historically, patients were primarily focused on the convenience of scheduling and accessing the provider of their choice. More recently, the rise of high-deductible health insurance plans and higher cost-sharing amounts are motivating patients to investigate the out-of-pocket cost of care prior to scheduling procedures. According to a 2022 report, one-third of adults in the US say they or a family member has skipped recommended medical services due to cost. Further, 4 out of 10 American adults say they have delayed needed care due to high costs (Montero et al. 2022). Providing pretreatment cost estimates is a challenge for providers and, thus, they are difficult for patients to obtain. This difficulty is due to a combination of factors, including access to a readily available price listing for services as well as uncertainty around exactly which items or procedures may be required to treat a patient before they see a provider.

Price Transparency

Many states and the federal government have **price transparency** regulations that require providers to make their standard or list prices available to the public. The Healthcare Financial Management Association (HFMA) defines price transparency as, "readily available information on the price of healthcare services that, together with other information, helps define the value of those services and enables patients and other care purchasers to identify, compare, and choose providers that offer the desired level of value" (HFMA 2014, 2). The Centers for Medicare and Medicaid Services (CMS) released regulations regarding price transparency that require hospitals to publish the standard charges of 300 "shoppable services" (HHS 2019, 61434). The rule defines shoppable services as services that can be scheduled in advance and are generally not emergency services. Examples of shoppable services include imaging, laboratory tests, or outpatient visits.

In addition to federal price transparency rules, many states enacted laws that require hospitals to post prices online. The information posted varies, but often exceeds the shoppable services requirements. The Source on Healthcare Price and Competition provides a database where users can access state laws related to healthcare costs and quality. There are also state-run websites that allow for price comparisons for that particular state. For example, the New Hampshire Insurance Department's website allows consumers to compare both pricing and quality information for all hospitals in that state. Their website also provides detailed cost-sharing estimates based on the patient's insurance coverage, insurance carrier, and plan type. The website includes data for the three most common carriers in the state as well as a category for other plans and no coverage. Figure 9.2 displays the cost estimate for a patient undergoing a colonoscopy with polyp removal in the outpatient setting. The results are customized for a

Figure 9.2.   Example of New Hampshire procedure cost estimates

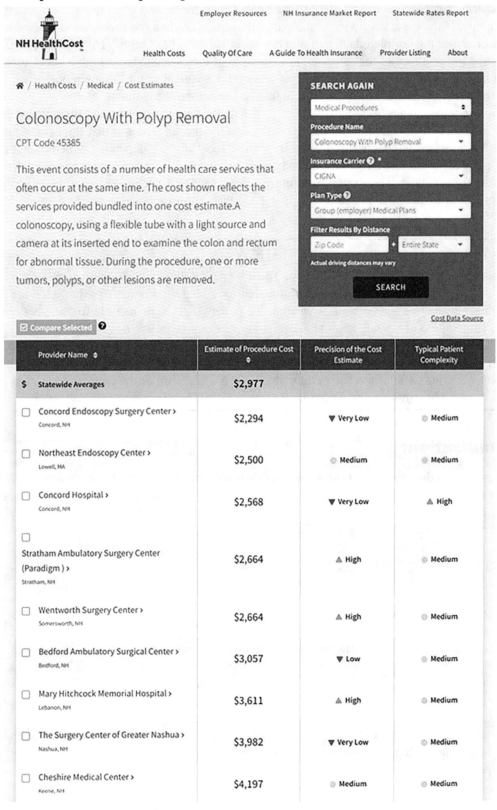

Source: NH HealthCost n.d.

group plan with Cigna as the insurance company. Notice that the cost-sharing amounts vary from $2,294 at a free-standing ambulatory surgery center to $4,197 at a hospital. This website also gives the user an idea of the precision of the cost estimate. If the costs vary widely at a particular provider, then the precision is labeled as "low"; if the cost is consistent across the sampled data, then the precision is labeled as "high." The reported precision helps the patient understand the accuracy of the estimate. For example, if the estimate has a high level of precision, then the patient should be confident that their cost will be as reported. Conversely, an estimate reported with low precision indicates that their actual cost may be a good bit higher or lower than the estimate.

Although price transparency is a good first step in helping patients understand the amount of cost sharing required for a service, it is not enough information to determine the full amount that the patient may need to pay out of pocket. As discussed in chapter 2, "Health Insurance," cost sharing depends on the amount allowed by the insurance company for a service, the required copayment amount or coinsurance percentage, as well as the status of the deductible for a patient. The example in figure 9.2 is close to a useful cost-sharing estimate but does not consider the impact of deductibles or the details of a patient's particular health plan. Example 9.1 illustrates this concept.

Example 9.1

A patient requires an office visit with an allergist. The allergist's office notified the patient that the fee for the office visit is $150. The patient cannot determine their cost-sharing amount based only on the fee. The details of the insurance coverage, as well as whether the patient met the deductible for the year, must all be known to determine the cost-sharing amount. The patient's insurance policy has an allowed amount of $90 for a specialist office visit, a 20 percent coinsurance amount, and a $500 deductible. If the patient satisfied the deductible prior to the allergist visit, then the cost-sharing amount would be 20 percent of $90, or $18. If the patient has only satisfied $400 of the $500 deductible and still has $100 of the deductible to meet prior to the allergist visit, the cost-sharing amount would be $90.

Prior Authorization

An important process in the front end of the revenue cycle involves ensuring that the provider has all of the relevant information to confirm the patient's insurance eligibility and coverage for the service to be provided. During the scheduling of services, the provider's representative typically asks the patient for information about insurance coverage. The relevant data elements include the following:

* Primary insurance company
* Guarantor
* Existence of additional coverage

Many providers validate coverage prior to providing services to patients. This process is often automated and occurs within the EHR either at the registration desk or via preregistration in some settings. The provider may need to obtain a prior authorization (PA) from the insurance company before treatment begins. PA is a process of obtaining approval from a health insurance company before providing healthcare services. Insurance companies use PA as a method to control the cost of care. This managed care concept was discussed in chapter 2, "Health Insurance." PAs are required primarily for higher-cost services, such as expensive diagnostic testing, a surgical procedure, or an inpatient hospital admission. PAs may be submitted via several methods, including direct submission from the EHR, a payer portal, fax, telephone, or email. Most of the PA process is now electronic, but the rules and timing of the process are different for each insurance company and can be a significant administrative burden for providers.

The American Medical Association (AMA) provides several tips to help physician practices reduce the administrative work with respect to PAs. These tips are also relevant for other healthcare settings.

1. Check PA requirements before providing services or sending prescriptions to the pharmacy.

2. Establish a protocol to consistently document data required for PA in the medical record.

3. Select the PA method that will be most efficient, given the particular situation and health plan's PA options.

4. Regularly follow up to ensure timely PA approval.

5. When a PA is inappropriately denied, submit an organized, concise, and well-articulated appeal with supporting clinical information. (AMA 2015, 1–5)

These tips are useful for all types of providers. The key to a successful PA process is a consistent workflow that transmits all required information to the payer and efficiently communicates the results of the PA to the provider.

Patient Intake

Upon the patient's arrival for the service, the **patient registration** process begins. Patient registration includes collecting data regarding the patient's provisional diagnosis and planned treatment, additional insurance details, and an agreement to fulfill any financial obligations. During patient registration, the patient's insurance card is copied or scanned into the EHR. An image of the insurance card is a stopgap to correct any data entry errors on the part of the patient or the registration clerk when inputting the patient's coverage details. If the claim for the service provided will be electronically submitted, then the subscriber identification number, plan identification, and insurance company must all be correct for a successful submission. If a paper submission is needed, then incorrect data can cause a delay in the claims processing and payment. The patient may also be asked to provide a picture ID to confirm their identity. This is to prevent insurance fraud, wherein one person uses another person's insurance card to obtain care.

An important step in the patient intake process is ensuring the patient understands that they are responsible for the cost of any services that may not be covered by their insurance company. This is communicated to the patient via a **patient financial responsibility agreement**. This form outlines an agreement between the provider and the patient. The agreement typically states that the provider will submit a claim for the service to the patient's insurance company, but the patient is responsible to pay any cost-sharing amounts as well as the cost of any procedures that may be denied by the insurance company. This reduces the provider's financial risk and ensures that all parties understand the expectations of payment for services. This agreement is accompanied by a HIPAA authorization form that allows the provider to use the patient's information to submit the claim for the services provided.

If the patient is a Medicare beneficiary and will receive services that may not be covered by Medicare, then the provider must comply with the Medicare beneficiary notices initiative (BNI). This initiative requires providers and facilities to provide Medicare beneficiaries with a notice that communicates financial liability and appeal rights and protections. The forms used to communicate this information vary based on the healthcare setting. For example, outpatient and physician services are communicated with the **advance beneficiary notification of noncoverage (ABN)**, and hospital inpatient services are communicated with the **hospital-issued notices of noncoverage (HINN)**. The ABN and HINN are patient financial responsibility forms specific to Medicare. Beneficiary notice of noncoverage forms must be provided to the patient prior to service using a format that is approved by CMS. The format of the ABN for 2023 is included in figure 9.3 (CMS 2023). Although a notice of noncoverage form may be presented to a patient, Medicare could still pay for the service. CMS requires providers to present the form so that the patient is aware of the potential financial liability of receiving the service. The Medicare Rights Center describes the utility of the ABN process from the patient's point of view as follows:

The ABN allows beneficiaries to decide whether to receive treatment and to pay for the treatment out of pocket if the service is denied by Medicare or not to receive the treatment at that time. In the notice, the provider must include the reason why it expects Medicare will not pay. Doing so helps patients determine if they should accept financial responsibility or refuse the service. For example, an ABN might say, "Medicare only pays for this test once every three years." The beneficiary can then decide if they want to wait for the three-year period to expire or

Figure 9.3.   Medicare advance beneficiary notice of noncoverage

A. Notifier:

B. Patient Name: **C. Identification Number:**

Advance Beneficiary Notice of Non-coverage
(ABN)

<u>**NOTE:**</u> **If Medicare doesn't pay for D._____below, you may have to pay.**

Medicare does not pay for everything, even some care that you or your health care provider have good reason to think you need. We expect Medicare may not pay for the **D._____**below.

D.	E. Reason Medicare May Not Pay:	F. Estimated Cost

WHAT YOU NEED TO DO NOW:

* Read this notice, so you can make an informed decision about your care.
* Ask us any questions that you may have after you finish reading.
* Choose an option below about whether to receive the **D._____**listed above.

Note: If you choose Option 1 or 2, we may help you to use any other insurance that you might have, but Medicare cannot require us to do this.

G. OPTIONS: Check only one box. We cannot choose a box for you.

☐ **OPTION 1.** I want the **D._____**listed above. You may ask to be paid now, but I also want Medicare billed for an official decision on payment, which is sent to me on a Medicare Summary Notice (MSN). I understand that if Medicare doesn't pay, I am responsible for payment, but I can appeal to Medicare by following the directions on the MSN. If Medicare does pay, you will refund any payments I made to you, less co-pays or deductibles.

☐ **OPTION 2.** I want the **D._____**listed above, but do not bill Medicare. You may ask to be paid now as I am responsible for payment. I cannot appeal if Medicare is not billed.

☐ **OPTION 3.** I don't want the **D._____**listed above. I understand with this choice I am **not** responsible for payment, and I cannot appeal to see if Medicare would pay.

H. Additional Information:

This notice gives our opinion, not an official Medicare decision. If you have other questions on this notice or Medicare billing, call **1-800-MEDICARE** (1-800-633-4227/**TTY:** 1-877-486-2048).

Signing below means that you have received and understand this notice. You may ask to receive a copy.

I. Signature:	J. Date:

You have the right to get Medicare information in an accessible format, like large print, Braille, or audio. You also have the right to file a complaint if you feel you've been discriminated against. Visit Medicare.gov/about-us/accessibility-nondiscrimination-notice.

According to the Paperwork Reduction Act of 1995, no persons are required to respond to a collection of information unless it displays a valid OMB control number. The valid OMB control number for this information collection is 0938-0566. The time required to complete this information collection is estimated to average 7 minutes per response, including the time to review instructions, search existing data resources, gather the data needed, and complete and review the information collection. If you have comments concerning the accuracy of the time estimate or suggestions for improving this form, please write to: CMS, 7500 Security Boulevard, Attn: PRA Reports Clearance Officer, Baltimore, Maryland 21244-1850.

Form CMS-R-131 (Exp.01/31/2026)   Form Approved OMB No. 0938-0566

Source: CMS 2023.

if they want the treatment now and will pay for it themselves. Providers are not required to give a patient an ABN for services or items that Medicare never covers, such as hearing aids. Providers are not permitted to give an ABN for every service or treatment, nor may they have a blanket ABN policy (Medicare Rights Center n.d.).

Check Your Understanding 9.1

1. What methods might patients use to schedule an appointment with a provider?

2. Who is responsible for obtaining a PA for services?

3. What types of data are collected at patient registration?

4. How are PAs submitted to an insurance company?

5. When is a provider required to present a patient with an ABN?

Patient Financial Counseling

Many insurance companies offer plans with deductibles of $5,000 or more. Patients are essentially self-insured or self-pay prior to satisfying the deductible. It is common for hospitals and large physician practices to include financial counseling as a service to their patients as they try to manage payment of a deductible while receiving essential healthcare services. This counseling may take many forms, including offering payment plans, healthcare loans, or payment support from manufacturers of high-cost pharmaceuticals.

Although tools like ABNs and patient financial liability agreements are in place, patients are often surprised by the level of out-of-pocket costs and struggle to pay them in a timely manner. The unexpected cost causes financial issues for both the patient and the provider. Financial counseling is one strategy to help both parties. Financial counseling is worth the cost of administering the program to help the patient find a way to pay for their share of the cost of care. Financial counselors can help a patient understand their coverage prior to care to facilitate proactive planning to meet the required cost sharing.

Programs such as drug copayment (copay) cards can help patients pay for drugs that may not be on the insurance company's formulary or may have higher cost-sharing amounts because of the lack of a generic equivalent. These programs are sometimes highlighted in television, magazine, and online advertisements for drugs. Because they are considered an inducement or encouragement to purchase a certain brand-name drug, copay cards are not available to patients with government insurance due to anti-kickback statutes. Still, they are a valuable tool for financial counselors helping commercially insured or uninsured patients, as they often do not have income-based requirements.

Patient Connection

Olivia's husband, Tony, was prescribed a new drug for his asthma. The drug is not on the Super Payer formulary, and therefore the copay amount is 30 percent of the $3,110 price each month. Their pharmacist recommended that they search the manufacturer's website to determine if they have any programs that can reduce that cost. The drug's website had an explanation of the cost that helped Olivia and Tony understand the factors that influenced her copay amount.

Olivia and Tony were able to locate information about a copay card that would reduce the copayment amount to $0 for the drug. Tony instantly signed up for the program and was able to save a significant amount of money.

Chapter 9 Review Quiz

1. In which component of the revenue cycle is a patient's type of insurance coverage and current insurance company determined?

2. Many states and the federal government have price transparency regulations. How does price transparency help patients and guarantors?

3. What is the purpose of a PA?

4. What type of information is collected from the patient during scheduling?

5. What is the purpose of a patient financial responsibility agreement?

6. How is an ABN different from a patient financial responsibility agreement?

7. What is the role of a financial counselor in the revenue cycle?

8. Patients may use programs known as _____ to help offset their out-of-pocket costs for drugs that may not be on their insurance company's formulary or may have a higher cost-sharing amount.

9. Why is knowledge regarding the charge or price of a healthcare service not enough information to determine the cost-sharing amount?

10. Why is a HIPAA authorization form required by a provider prior to treating a patient?

References

AMA (American Medical Association). 2015. "Tips to Help Physicians Reduce the Prior Authorization Burden in Their Practice." Chicago: AMA. https://www.ama-assn.org/media/7411/download.

CMS (Centers for Medicare and Medicaid Services). 2023. "Beneficiary Notices Initiative." https://www.cms .gov/Medicare/Medicare-General-Information/BNI.

HFMA Price Transparency Task Force. 2014. Price Transparency in Health Care. Westchester, IL: HFMA. https://www.hfma.org/payment-reimbursement-and-managed-care/pricing/22274/.

HHS (Department of Health and Human Services). 2019. Requirements for hospitals to make public a list of their standard charges and request for information (RFI): Quality measurement relating to price transparency for improving beneficiary access to provider and supplier charge information. *Federal Register* 84(218):61434.

Medicare Rights Center. n.d. "Advance Beneficiary Notice (ABN)." Accessed February 24, 2023. https://www .medicareinteractive.org/get-answers/medicare-denials-and-appeals/original-medicare-appeals/advance -beneficiary-notice-abn.

Montero, A., A. Kearney, L. Hamel, and M. Brodie. 2022. "Americans' Challenges with Health Care Costs." https://www.kff.org/health-costs/issue-brief/americans-challenges-with-health-care-costs/.

NH HealthCost. n.d. "Compare Health Costs & Quality of Care." Accessed February 24, 2023. https://nhhealthcost.nh.gov/.

Resources

University of California San Francisco Law. n.d. "Source on Healthcare." https://sourceonhealthcare.org/.

Chapter 10
Revenue Cycle Middle Processes—Resource Tracking

Learning Objectives

❖ Describe technology-based charge capture strategies

❖ Identify the components of the charge description master

❖ Differentiate the various code sets approved by the Health Insurance Portability and Accountability Act of 1996

❖ Describe the structure of approved code sets

❖ Illustrate the coding process

Key Terms

AHA Coding Clinic for HCPCS
AHA Coding Clinic for ICD-10-CM and ICD-10-PCS
Category I CPT code
Category II CPT code
Category III CPT code
Charge
Charge capture
Charge code
Charge description
Charge description master (CDM)
Charge status indicator
Classification system
CPT Assistant
Current Procedural Terminology (CPT)
Department code
Hard coding
Health Insurance Portability and Accountability Act of 1996 (HIPAA)

Healthcare Common Procedure Coding System (HCPCS)
Healthcare Common Procedure Coding System (HCPCS) codes
ICD-10-CM/PCS Coordination and Maintenance Committee
International Classification of Diseases, Tenth Revision, Clinical Modification (ICD-10-CM)
International Classification of Diseases, Tenth Revision, Procedure Coding System (ICD-10-PCS)
Line item
Medicare Claims Processing Manual
Modifier
National Center for Health Statistics (NCHS)
Payer identifier
Revenue code
Single path coding
Soft coding
World Health Organization (WHO)

The middle processes of the revenue cycle, where resources are tracked and recorded, include complex and detailed tasks. The processes are guided by copious rules and regulations. Therefore, the middle processes require a significant amount of management and oversight. Figure 10.1 provides a refresher of the revenue cycle components and highlights the processes for the middle of the revenue cycle.

Resource tracking is the identification and recording of all resources a provider uses to treat a beneficiary. Resource tracking allows the healthcare organization to calculate the exact cost of treating a patient. In healthcare, the term for resource tracking is *charge capture*. This chapter begins with a detailed exploration of the charge capture process.

Simply put, reimbursement is payment to healthcare providers and facilities for services rendered to patients. Communication of the services provided is transmitted from the provider to the third-party payer, government-sponsored or commercial, via coded information. Using standardized data sets and administrative coding systems allows for a stable and efficient payment process. Payment methodologies and systems used to determine coverage of services and supplies vary, but the data sets and code sets remain constant across all healthcare settings. Following charge capture, this chapter will explore critical reimbursement code sets approved by the **Health Insurance Portability and Accountability Act of 1996 (HIPAA)** and the coding process. HIPAA is a significant piece of legislation aimed at improving healthcare data transmission among providers and insurers. This act established the designated code sets to be used for electronic transmission of claims. Management strategies used to ensure code reporting aligns with revenue integrity principles are discussed in chapter 12, "Coding and Clinical Documentation Integrity Management."

Charge Capture and Its Structure

Charge capture is the accounting for all reportable services and supplies rendered to a patient. There are numerous services and supplies associated with each patient encounter that can be categorized into three types, as shown in figure 10.2.

The services in the room rate and unit charges categories are the services that are chargeable. For example, facilities may not charge a patient for coding their medical record, but they do charge for performing and evaluating laboratory tests. As discussed in chapter 4, "Healthcare Reimbursement Methodologies," and chapters 5 through 8, which detail Medicare payment systems, individual charges and total charges for an encounter may be a key data point for a reimbursement methodology or may be used to calculate an adjustment or provision. Therefore, it is critical for facilities and providers to capture and submit all reportable charges on the claim.

The introduction of the electronic health record (EHR) allowed the use of several of technology-based charge capture strategies. The traditional approach to charge capture was noting the use of items via a checklist or

Figure 10.1.   Components of the revenue cycle

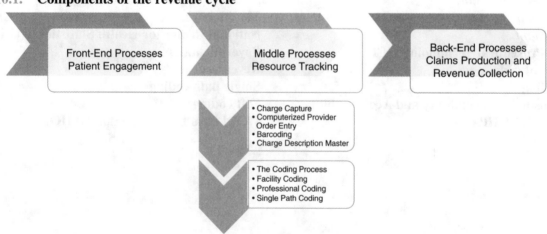

Figure 10.2. Types of patient care services

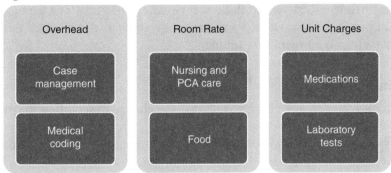

documentation of orders within the paper record. This was a time-consuming task and one that often led to missed charges, especially for inpatient services. Examples of electronic charge capture methods are described in the following sections.

Computerized Provider Order Entry

Computerized provider order entry (CPOE) is a method that allows physicians and other providers to order services for a patient via a computerized system instead of the paper ordering system used historically. CPOE is used in both inpatient and outpatient settings. In the inpatient and ambulatory surgery and emergency department settings, CPOE allows for consistent and efficient communication between the provider, nursing and ancillary departments, and the pharmacy. In outpatient clinic and physician practice settings CPOE allows easily communicating most prescriptions to pharmacies. CPOE has a number of advantages over paper orders:

- Reduce errors and improve patient safety: At a minimum, CPOE can help organizations reduce errors by ensuring providers produce standardized, legible, and complete orders. In addition, CPOE technology often includes built-in clinical decision-support tools that can automatically check for drug interactions, medication allergies, and other potential problems.

- Improve efficiency: By enabling providers to submit orders electronically, CPOE can help organizations get medication, laboratory, and radiology orders to pharmacies, laboratories, and radiology facilities faster, saving time and improving efficiency.

- Improve reimbursements: Some orders require preapprovals from insurance plans. CPOE, when integrated with an electronic practice management system, can flag orders that require preapproval, helping organizations reduce denied insurance claims. (HealthIT.gov n.d.)

CPOE may be used for medications as well as diagnostic tests such as laboratory and radiology orders. When physicians use CPOE to write prescriptions for medications, the prescription is checked against any allergies that are documented in the patient's EHR. During the CPOE process, the prescription may be sent directly to the patient's pharmacy as allowed by state regulations. For example, some states do not allow electronic prescriptions for controlled substances. This makes the process of filling prescriptions both safer and more convenient for the patient. CPOE allows the provider to check that the tests were completed or that the prescription was filled. This computerized approach also ensures accurate charges for the services.

Barcoding

Another common method used in charge capture is barcode scanning to track items and services dispensed to a patient. In healthcare facilities, a patient is issued an identification wristband during the registration process. This wristband typically includes a barcode that uniquely identifies that patient. As items such as pharmaceuticals or supplies are used to evaluate or treat the patient, the provider scans the patient's barcode and then the barcode on the item. The scanning process tracks exactly which items were used, the quantity, and the time of delivery. Barcoding is incredibly important in treatment areas where there are a large number of items used during a short time period, such as an emergency department or urgent care setting.

Charge Description Master

A key tool to ensure complete and accurate charge capture is the **charge description master (CDM)**. The CDM is a data table used by healthcare facilities to manage required billing elements for all services provided to patients. Different facilities use different terminology for the CDM. Some more common synonyms include chargemaster, charge compendium, service master, price list, service item master, and charge list (Casto 2011, 222).

The primary function of the CDM is to enumerate the items and services used to produce hospital claims. It is used to translate the services and supplies provided to the patient into the data elements required for submitting a claim for payment. Using the CDM allows for a consistent method of communication to payers. Traditionally, the CDM is managed in the finance department. However, many clinical and ancillary areas share in the maintenance responsibility. Nonetheless, the CDM coordinator typically reports to a finance management team member. Some facilities have moved the responsibility to the health information management (HIM) department because managing the CDM requires a strong coding background.

The Charge Description Master Team

The size of the CDM unit or team will vary from facility to facility. The number of full-time equivalents (FTEs)—employees who work 40 hours per week—in the unit depends on the size of the CDM as well as how many satellite or off-site areas use the CDM for charge capture. Typically, there is a CDM coordinator who manages the CDM unit. CDM coordinator position requirements vary based on the philosophy and complexity of a facility's or practice's CDM management. In general, CDM coordinators should possess the following:

- Considerable knowledge of the revenue cycle
- Good communication skills, both verbal and written
- Understanding of coding and reimbursement systems
- Management experience

The CDM coordinator position is one of immense importance. Even though it is a very detail-oriented position, the coordinator must also be able to engage others in the maintenance process. Individuals interested in this position must be able to strike a balance between control and delegation—not always an easy task.

Though the CDM has been, and continues to be, housed primarily in the finance department at many facilities, HIM professionals have a key role in the maintenance of the CDM due to their coding and reimbursement expertise. The coding and reimbursement experience of CDM coordinators varies from facility to facility. HIM professionals may help the CDM team understand the rules of using a **Healthcare Common Procedure Coding System (HCPCS) code**, understand new coding guidelines released for a **Current Procedural Terminology (CPT)** code, understand how new Centers for Medicare and Medicaid Services (CMS) regulations affect the CDM, and communicate coding rules and regulations to various clinical or ancillary department managers. The **Healthcare Common Procedure Coding System (HCPCS)** is a two-tiered system of procedural codes used primarily for ambulatory care and physician services. A HCPCS code is a code that is part of the Healthcare Common Procedure Coding System. CPT is used throughout the US to report diagnostic and surgical services and procedures.

Additionally, it is valuable for the HIM department and CDM team to have a good working relationship. By exploring each professional's roles and responsibilities, they may realize they have more in common than they thought. When these two units work together, they can significantly affect key performance indicators established for the revenue cycle, thereby improving the efficiency of providing quality service for all patients. Management of the CDM is crucial to the efficiency of the revenue cycle. This topic is discussed later in this chapter.

Charge Description Master and the Revenue Cycle

In addition to producing claims, CDM data can be used for utilization management. Each time a unit of service is included on a claim, the CDM item number is also recorded. Thus, at any given time, the number of services performed or the number of units of rendered services can be calculated. This is extremely helpful for utilization management. For example, the radiology department may want to track how many chest x-rays it performs per month. Further, the department manager wants to confirm that every chest x-ray procedure was billed. The department will most likely have internal records of the number of x-rays performed by month, but comparing that volume with the units of service billed according to the CDM will allow the radiology department to identify whether there is a charge capture issue.

Like utilization management, the resource consumption level can be monitored in a consistent and reliable manner with the help of the CDM. The CDM, by using standardized code sets, allows a facility to track the types of services utilized by a specific patient population. For example, the cardiac catheterization unit wants to know what drugs were administered to patients who underwent catheterizations in May. By using the charge code for cardiac catheterization procedures, the department can pull billing details from the facility's data warehouse. The department can then analyze the data to determine which types of resources patients most often consume. The department may be particularly interested in recovery room time. Because recovery room time is reported on claims, the service has a unique charge code. Therefore, the analysis would be able to determine the average length of time that patients spend in the recovery room post-procedure. This is important not only for cost determination, but also for staffing and patient scheduling considerations. Using CDM data elements, a data analyst can perform this review very easily. Without a CDM, a data abstraction professional would need to review medical records to find the data, which can be very time consuming.

The required data elements reported on the claim represent the charge. This can be confusing because there are two meanings of **charge** in healthcare. The first is the charge data on the claim that are used to report services and supplies to third-party payers. The second is the charge or price for the service or supplies. The price is one required data element in the charge. In a process known as **hard coding**, a unique identifier triggers a charge from the CDM to be posted to the patient's account. Noncomplex services that do not require the expertise of a coding professional may be reported via hard coding. Additionally, repetitive services, such as radiology and laboratory procedures, are often hard coded.

The CDM is a vital component of the revenue cycle. The accuracy of the CDM data elements is crucial to ensure claims are error-free and complete. Thus, governance of the CDM data elements is a year-round endeavor requiring a multidisciplinary team. The next sections will explore CDM structure and CDM maintenance.

CDM Structure

Although each CDM is unique, standard data elements are included in a CDM. HIM professionals should be familiar with each of the CDM data elements and the elements' importance to the claim production process. A CDM **line item** is a single line of a CDM that includes all the required data elements. Table 10.1 displays sample line items from a CDM.

The first line item in table 10.1 is for the supply of Dermagraft, which is used in a synthetic skin grafting procedure. The line item contains seven data elements in this example. Some of the data elements are hospital-specific and used internally for management purposes. Other data elements, such as revenue codes, are used by all facilities and included on the claim form. Review the active line item for venipuncture in table 10.1 and examine how the venipuncture service is reported on a claim form. Figure 10.3 displays the CDM data elements on an excerpt from a UB-04 claim form.

Compare data elements included in the CDM to data elements required for claim submission. Note that only the revenue code, description, HCPCS code, and charge data elements from the CDM populate the UB-04 claim

Table 10.1. **Sample CDM**

Department Code	Charge Code*	Charge Description	Revenue Code	HCPCS Code**	Charge***	Charge Status Indicator
700	7008989	Dermagraft (Synth skin graft)	0252	Q4106	$1,525.00	Active
700	7005202	XR shoulder, complete	0320	73030	$350.00	Active
700	7005203	Regular OR—1st hour	0360		$4,687.00	Active
700	7005205	Regular OR—½ hour	0360		$1,682.00	Active
715	7157059	Open heart—1st hour	0360		$5,589.00	Active
715	7157060	Open heart—½ hour	0360		$2,782.00	Active
465	7605161	P.T. Eval	0424	97001	$295.00	Active
800	8004557	ED visit level 3	0450	99283	$586.00	Active
822	8224210	Albumin 5% saline	0250	P9045	$265.00	Active
367	3675839	Speech screening	0440	V5362	$298.00	Active
367	3675840	Language screening	0440	V5363	$298.00	Active
367	3675841	Dysphagia screening	0440	V5364	$298.00	Active
200	2578961	Venipuncture	0300	G0001	$18.00	Inactive
200	2578989	Venipuncture	0300	36415	$18.00	Active
110	1478951	MRI upper extremity without dye	0610	73218	$817.00	Active
110	1478952	MRI upper extremity with dye	0610	73219	$857.00	Active
110	1478953	MRI upper extremity without and with dye	0610	73220	$897.00	Active

* Also called item number, charge number, item code, service code, and service number.
** When blank, Healthcare Common Procedure Coding System (HCPCS) code is determined via coding in health information management (HIM) department for certain revenue codes.
*** Charge is fictitious and should not be used for rate setting.

form. The remaining data elements, such as charge code, are used for internal controls, operations, and analyses. Next, examine the data elements on the claim form that are not in the CDM. These data elements, such as service date and service units, are unique to the encounter and may be different for each patient. In the sections that follow, each data element of the CDM is discussed in detail.

Charge Code

The **charge code**, also known as the service code, item code, charge description number, or charge identifier, is a hospital-specific internally assigned code used to identify a supply or service. The code is typically numeric but could also be alphanumeric. Charge codes are assigned or distributed by a designated person, typically in the IT

Figure 10.3.   Sample UB-04 claim form

42 REV CD	43 DESCRIPTION	44 HCPCS/RATES	45 SERV. DATE	46 SERV. UNITS	47 TOTAL CHARGES		48 NON-COVERED CHARGES		49
0300	VENIPUNCTURE	36415	7/12/20	1	18	00			
0300	METABOLIC PANEL BASIC (CHEM 7)	80048	7/12/20	1	264	00			
0301	MAGNESIUM	83735	7/12/20	1	82	00			
0301	TROPONINI	84484	7/12/20	1	221	00			
0301	CBC	85025	7/12/20	1	82	00			
0320	XR SHOULDER COMPLETE	73030	7/12/20	1	350	00			
0424	P.T. EVAL	97001	7/12/20	1	295	00			
0450	ED STRAPPING SHOULDER	29240	7/12/20	1	640	00			
0450	ED VISIT LEVEL 3	99283	7/12/20	1	586	00			
0636	MORPHINE SULFATE 10 MG	J2270	7/12/20	2	308	00			
0636	LACTATED RINGERS 1000CC	J7120	7/12/20	1	75	00			

Source: Adapted from CDC n.d.

department or the CDM unit. The methodology for assignment depends on the facility. Similar to typical health record number schemes, the charge code number may be distributed in a sequential numeric order, or a facility may reserve numerical sections by ancillary service. For example, charge code number set 100000 to 199999 is reserved for radiology.

Regardless of the distribution methodology, each charge code number must be unique, and the CDM unit must ensure there are not duplicate charge codes in the CDM. When multiple identical charge codes are present in a CDM, the facility may inadvertently submit billing data elements for the wrong service or procedure on the claim. Therefore, the CDM coordinator should schedule and complete duplicate charge code audits throughout the year.

Department Code

A **department code** is a hospital-specific number that is assigned to each clinical or ancillary department that provides services to patients. Alternative terminology for this data element may be *general ledger number*. The department code is used to identify the area within the healthcare facility that delivers the service or supply. Department codes usually correspond with an ancillary or clinical service, such as speech therapy, or with a physical area, such as the emergency department.

Revenue Code

A **revenue code** is a four-digit numeric code required for billing on the UB-04 claim form or the 837I. Revenue codes are maintained by the National Uniform Billing Committee and, therefore, are standard in the US, with the same code set used by all facilities. Revenue code assignment is usually driven by the ancillary department or location where the service is performed. Revenue code reporting requirements for Medicare are detailed in the *Medicare Claims Processing Manual*, chapter 25, section 75.4 (CMS 2021). The *Medicare Claims Processing Manual* is an online publication that offers guidance for producing claims for all healthcare settings. At each facility, the revenue codes reported on claims are used in the end-of-year cost reporting process to aggregate charge and cost data.

Although the revenue code list is standardized, the combination of HCPCS code and revenue code can be somewhat facility specific. Medicare and other third-party payers issue transmittals and bulletins that provide instruction for revenue and HCPCS code combinations. Additionally, the Medicare Code Editor (MCE) and the Outpatient Code Editor (OCE) used by the Medicare administrative contractors (MACs) contain revenue code and HCPCS code edits to ensure the appropriate combinations are reported on claims.

In addition to identifying the service area or type of service performed, revenue codes are used by third-party payers to identify payment methodologies in their contracts. Therefore, the revenue code assignment in the CDM must be reviewed annually by the CDM analyst and hospital contract management team. For example, consider the following contract language for three payers at a facility. Payer one indicates in the contract that MRI services identified by revenue code 0610 will be reimbursed at 60 percent of the billed charges. The second payer, Medicare, specifies that the most specific revenue code should be used for MRI services and that facilities should report the applicable revenue code in range 0610 to 0614. The third payer specifies that MRI services will be reimbursed based on the HCPCS code regardless of the revenue code reported. CDM analysts must work closely with hospital contract managers to ensure the CDM meets the reporting needs for all three of these payers, not just major payers like Medicare.

HCPCS codes are the current code set utilized to report individual services, procedures, and supplies rendered to patients. The HCPCS code set is discussed in detail later in this chapter. HCPCS codes were established by HIPAA as the designated code set for use on electronic transactions by all healthcare facilities and insurers for the services, procedures, and supplies rendered in outpatient settings. Thus, the use of HCPCS codes, when available, is mandatory. However, it is important to remember that HCPCS codes are not available for all services and supplies provided to patients. For example, nursing services, patient care associate services, case management services, and some medications do not have HCPCS codes. Therefore, this data element will be blank for some line items.

Charge Description

Charge description is an explanatory phrase that is assigned to describe a procedure, service, or supply. The charge description is based on the official HCPCS description when applicable, but the field is often limited by the character length allowed by the EHR or financial system and cannot always accommodate the official description. Therefore, hospitals develop their own descriptions for many line items in the CDM.

The American Medical Association (AMA) and CMS provide an official long description for each HCPCS code. Additionally, a short description is provided for use in space-limited fields within hospital systems. The CDM team must decide whether the short description of the code should be used as the hospital description or whether a modified description would be better for the facility. Likewise, a list of commonly used abbreviations should be maintained to provide consistency through the CDM. The dilemma is that most practitioners are not familiar with the official HCPCS code description; rather, they use working lay titles for the procedures and services they perform or provide. Therefore, using the official short descriptions in the CDM may be confusing for service providers. Conversely, healthcare consumers may better understand the official short or long description than the lay term used by practitioners. As hospitals work to improve customer service with their patients, they strive to produce a patient bill that the patient can easily comprehend. To illustrate this point, table 10.2 compares a few lay descriptions to some official short descriptions.

In examples A and B, it is not likely that the average patient would be able to identify the service they received from the charge description. If someone is not familiar with coding, they will not likely be able to identify which service "SLP treatment" represents. It is more likely that only ancillary therapists would understand the hospital lay description for these therapy services. Likewise, in examples C and D, perhaps only radiology technicians, radiologists, physicians, and coders might understand the hospital lay descriptions for these services. Again, it is unlikely that the average patient would be able to connect "SP arterio renal bilateral" to the catheterization that they received.

Table 10.2.   Sample charge descriptions (lay descriptions) versus short descriptions

Example	Charge Description	Code	Short Description
A	SLP treatment	92507	Speech/hearing therapy
B	CPM setup	97001	PT evaluation
C	Treatment aids—interim	77333	Radiation treatment aid(s); intermediate
D	SP arterio renal bilateral	36246	Place catheter in artery; initial second order

There are no hard and fast rules regarding the charge description that must be used in the CDM. Each facility must determine which method works best. The Healthcare Financial Management Association (HFMA) has published extensively on patient-friendly billing. HFMA launched the Patient Friendly Billing Project to encourage facilities to improve billing for patients (HFMA n.d.). The philosophy of the project is based on the following ideals:

- The needs of patients and family members should be paramount when designing administrative processes and communications.

- Information gathering should be coordinated with other providers and insurers, and this collection process should be done efficiently, privately, and with as little duplication as possible.

- When possible, communication of financial information should not occur during the medical encounter.

- The average reader should easily understand the language and format of financial communications.

- Continuous improvement of the billing process should be made by implementing better practices and incorporating feedback from patients and consumers. (HFMA n.d.)

Though many revenue cycle areas are impacted by this project, the patient's ability to understand their healthcare bill should drive the charge description development.

Charge

Recall that the charge, or price, is the dollar amount that the hospital requests for payment when providing the item or service to the patient. This term can be confusing. Healthcare professionals use the term *charge* as a verb to refer to the act of collecting the data elements for all services and supplies. They also use the term to mean price. The CDM team does not typically set the price. A team within finance analyzes and updates the charge structure and charges on a regular basis. However, CDM analysts may identify charge oddities, and these issues should be forwarded to the revenue cycle team for investigation.

Modifier

A **modifier** is a two-digit alphabetic, alphanumeric, or numeric code used by providers and facilities to identify or flag a service that has been modified in some way or to provide more specific information about the procedure or service. There are two sources of modifiers. The first source of modifiers includes those that are part of the CPT code set. The second source of modifiers includes those that are part of the HCPCS Level II code set.

Because the use of a modifier can alter the meaning of the code, it is important that modifiers only be applied to HCPCS codes when supported by documentation in the medical record. Thus, inclusion of modifiers in the CDM is rare, but some facilities do use this practice. CDM teams should pay close attention to modifier reporting guidelines if they choose to include a modifier in the CDM. CDM units should consider all compliance implications that could arise because, when included as a line item data element, the modifier is reported with the associated HCPCS code every time the charge code is activated.

Charge Status Indicator

A **charge status indicator** is an identifier used to indicate whether a CDM line item is active or inactive. Hospitals may or may not maintain charge status in the CDM. Most facilities choose not to delete line items from their CDM to preserve historic practices. Instead, they use a charge status indicator. This allows the facility to maintain the integrity of line items that have been used in the past and that may require review at later dates by Medicare and other third-party payers. It is also a way to identify whether new CDM line items are needed. In the CDM line-item addition process, the requested line item can be compared to inactive line items. If there is a match, the appropriate discussions can take place about why the line item was moved to inactive status and to determine whether the new line item is necessary.

Payer Identifier

Payer identifier codes are used to differentiate payers that may have specific or special billing protocol in the payer-hospital contract. For example, CMS requires the use of HCPCS code G0463 for a new office visit, while most commercial payers require CPT codes in the range 99202 to 99205. It is important for the CDM team to review the payer identifier assignment on a regular basis. Each time a payer contract is revised, the CDM team must work with the contract management unit to determine whether changes in payer identifier assignment are warranted.

For example, a facility's largest payer, Super Payer, is adopting the CMS outpatient prospective payment system (OPPS) methodology. Previously, Super Payer paid a percent of billed charges and did not require facilities to use HCPCS Level II codes. However, with the movement to OPPS, they will now require HCPCS Level II codes, and Super Payer is adopting the same reporting requirements as Medicare. The payer identifier assignment for Super Payer may need to be revisited before the switch in their methodology, as displayed in table 10.3.

Charge Description Master Maintenance

CDM maintenance is an ongoing process at healthcare facilities, physician offices, hospitals, imaging centers, and freestanding laboratory facilities. CDM maintenance is an important compliance task used to ensure revenue integrity. Numerous events throughout the year provide cause for CDM maintenance. HCPCS codes are updated regularly throughout the year, as are billing and coding guidance documents. Likewise, payer contracts are usually negotiated based on the facility's fiscal year. Understanding the hospital's financial calendar is an important part of planning for ongoing CDM maintenance.

Each year, the CDM coordinator should ensure the proper resources are allocated for CDM maintenance. Updated code books, as well as national, uniform billing data set information, are required. Additionally, payer instructions such as the *Medicare Claims Processing Manual* should be available so that crucial instructions can be located easily and reviewed. Any publications specific to the state in which the facility operates should be present as well (Dietz 2005, 3). Many payer resources, such as the *Medicare Claims Processing Manual*, are available online. A CDM team may consider having a shared location to house the links to these documents to ensure all team members are able to access the necessary documents without having to spend time searching online.

Charge Description Master Maintenance Process

Although facilities may use different management structures, the CDM unit or team, CDM committee, or revenue cycle team will need to oversee the CDM maintenance process. Oversight should not be a single individual's

Table 10.3.   Example of effect on payer identifier by payer reimbursement methodology change

Super Payer—Reimbursement Methodology Is Percent of Billed Charges						
Charge Code	Department Number	Revenue Code	HCPCS Code	HCPCS Code CMS	Description	Charge*
12345	301	0481	92928	C9600	Coronary stent placement, drug-eluting stent—Medicare	$12,375.00

Super Payer—Reimbursement Methodology Is OPPS						
Charge Code	Department Number	Revenue Code	HCPCS Code	HCPCS Code CMS and Super Payer	Description	Charge*
12345	301	0481	92928	C9600	Coronary stent placement, drug-eluting stent—Medicare	$12,375.00

*Charge is fictitious and should not be used for rate setting.

responsibility because diverse perspectives and expertise are required to create a comprehensive plan. One of the team's major responsibilities is developing policies and procedures for the CDM maintenance process. While doing so, they should consider the following questions:

- Do policies cover how coding and billing regulations are communicated within the organization?
- Do policies address resources and instructions for code updates?
- Do policies require coders and billers to document any advice received from the MAC?
- Are CDM risk areas addressed in policies and procedures?
- Do policies define how consultants may be used in CDM maintenance?

After the policies and procedures are put into place, the team is ready to start building their maintenance plan.

CDM maintenance is incredibly detailed and must be approached methodically. Thus, the maintenance plan should consist of several organized and structured processes. CDM coordinators should approach CDM maintenance with a project management plan. A CDM maintenance plan will allow all individuals and departments included in the processes to understand how their component(s) fit into the larger maintenance plan. Likewise, each participant will understand their duties and be fully aware of the expected timeline for completion. Not only does this help individuals stay on task, but it can greatly benefit new employees who may not be familiar with the facility's internal process.

Working with Ancillary and Clinical Areas

Ancillary and other clinical areas play a large role in CDM maintenance. Their clinical expertise combined with the coding knowledge of the CDM coordinator or HIM representative will allow a facility to have a current, accurate, and complete CDM. It is important to remember that the primary focus of clinical and ancillary areas is patient care, so the CDM coordinator must respectfully engage the departments in the CDM maintenance process.

Having a good working relationship with clinical and ancillary areas is important for the maintenance process. Who better to explain services, service components, and service delivery techniques than health professionals themselves? Understanding the service is the key to assigning the appropriate HCPCS code for the line item. For example, interventional radiology is an incredibly challenging service area for many coders and CDM professionals. This service area requires code selection from both the surgical and radiology sections of the code book. Understanding which codes are used together for which procedures is crucial. Therefore, having a clinician from the interventional radiology department explain which procedures are performed by the facility and how the components work together is paramount. This type of valuable interaction will provide the clinical insight needed to ensure these complex cases are accurately and completely reported by the facility.

As important as it is for clinical and ancillary areas to share their expertise with the CDM coordinator, it is equally important for the CDM team to explain the compliance or billing implications of poor CDM maintenance with the clinical areas. It is much easier to get buy-in from healthcare professionals when they understand the reasoning behind a set process or protocol. Providing an example with implications is an effective way to help ancillary and clinical professionals understand why proper code selection is vital in the CDM maintenance process. Example 10.1 provides an example of a CDM charge capture issue.

Example 10.1

A CDM charge analyst is reviewing the line items for the neurology clinic. The analyst identifies three charge codes with the same description: autonomic nerve function test. The clinical professionals may understand the difference between tests one, two, and three even though the description is the same. However, the charge capture staff may not. Therefore, the charge analyst examines the issue in detail. Review of the utilization report reveals that the charge code listed first is reported 98 percent of the time. The neurology clinic manager

(continued)

Example 10.1 *(continued)*

states that the utilization pattern does not match their internal procedure statistics. Therefore, a sample of medical records is audited to determine which service was performed. The results of the audit show that the wrong charge code was activated 65 percent of the time. Because the wrong charge code was activated, the wrong CPT code (95921 rather than 95922 or 95923) was reported for several encounters. Because of the charge capture error, the facility was overpaid by Medicare for several claims and must now resubmit the claims with the corrected CPT code and pay back the overpayment amount. The CDM team must work with the neurology clinic manager to revise the charge descriptions so they better differentiate the three tests.

Example 10.1 illustrates how important it is for clinical areas to understand CDM functionality. Appreciating the complexities of each other's roles and responsibilities will strengthen the relationship between the CDM team and the clinical and ancillary areas.

CDM Maintenance Process Activities

The CDM team will engage in numerous maintenance activities throughout the year. To be able to understand and effectively communicate the intent of the maintenance activities, the CDM team should establish a scope for each review. By defining the scope, each participant will understand the intent and extent of the review. The CDM coordinator will be able to communicate what is included and what is not included in each review activity to the finance team and the revenue cycle team.

Although each facility is different, the following technical activities should be included in the CDM maintenance plan for each review:

- Review of current statistics
- HCPCS code review
- Revenue code review
- Modifier review (Dietz 2005, 3)

Each of these line-item components should be addressed in the review. However, it is not enough to just review each component individually to ensure it is a valid data element. Rather, the whole line item should be reviewed to ensure the components fit together properly. This is where CDM maintenance can become very complex. The reviewer must ensure the line-item components meet the requirements for each payer as well as meet the requirements established under compliance guidance.

There is much to consider, research, and verify during the CDM maintenance process, so having a thorough review plan is crucial. Mapping out each task in the plan will prompt the reviewer to complete all planned activities. Likewise, it is during this process that the CDM analysts must adhere to review policies and procedures.

The responsibility of charge setting varies from hospital to hospital. Most often, this activity is the finance department's responsibility, so the CDM team may or may not perform charge review. However, the CDM team can assist the finance department by identifying charges that appear to be outside normal limits. For example, the CDM team could identify all line items that are missing a charge. Likewise, it could identify line items that have a charge lower than the Medicare reimbursement rate. The CDM team must regularly complete ongoing maintenance activities. Issues will always arise and must be addressed immediately. However, the majority of maintenance can be scheduled, so CDM team staffing needs for these activities can be projected.

Code and Payment System Updates

The CPT Editorial Research and Development Department supports the modification process for the CPT code set. The CPT Editorial Panel meets three times per year to consider proposals for changes to CPT (AMA n.d.). The CPT Advisory Committee of the AMA, which comprises representatives of more than 90 medical specialty societies and other healthcare professional organizations, supports the editorial panel. To stay current with new technologies and pioneering procedures, CPT is revised each year, with changes effective January 1 of the following year.

The updated code set is released before January 1, so the CDM maintenance plan should include steps for the acquisition of the new code set as well as adequate time for additions, deletions, and modifications to be reviewed and incorporated into the CDM. This makes December a very busy time of year for the CDM team. The CDM coordinator should give special attention to time-off requests for the CDM team members to ensure line items will be ready for use by January 1. Additionally, the CDM coordinator needs to schedule the annual maintenance with IT and other revenue cycle team representatives. Not only do the CDM line items need to be up to date, but the team must ensure adequate time is provided for IT to update systems and to ensure that interfaces between the EHR, CDM, and finance system remain intact. If a paper-based charge capture process is used, the ancillary or clinical units must have adequate time to ensure their documents are up to date and staff is properly educated on the changes.

Permanent HCPCS Level II codes are maintained by the CMS HCPCS Workgroup. Permanent national codes are updated annually on January 1. Temporary codes can be added, changed, or deleted quarterly. Like the CPT code updates, the HCPCS Level II code updates must be planned for as well. But in addition to the yearly updates, CDM coordinators must plan for quarterly updates to the temporary HCPCS Level II codes. HCPCS Level II code updates require coordination with a variety of areas in the healthcare facility. The code set contains not only procedure or service codes, but also drug codes, supply codes, durable medical equipment codes, and implantable device codes. The CDM team must work closely with materials management and the pharmacy department to ensure the CDM line items properly represent the drugs, biologicals, and devices used by the facility.

New drug, device, and supply codes should be closely reviewed during the HCPCS Level II update. Just because the HCPCS Level II code is new does not mean the drug, device, or supply it represents is new to the marketplace. For example, a drug may be manufactured and administered for several years before it is assigned a HCPCS Level II code. It is important to ensure a line item is updated with the HCPCS Level II code rather than a new line item being added.

CMS updates its prospective payment systems (PPSs) on a regular schedule throughout the year. For example, the Medicare hospital acute inpatient payment system is updated on the federal fiscal year, with an effective date of October 1. The Medicare hospital outpatient payment system is updated on the calendar year, with an effective date of January 1. Depending on the type of facility or facilities included under the healthcare entity, the CDM coordinator will need to plan for the review of payment system rules and the incorporation of rule changes into the CDM. CMS's proposed and final rules are posted on the CMS website.

Contract Updates

Throughout a payer contract effective period, the payer may send out policy alerts. Policy alerts contain billing and coding requirements specific to that payer. It is important that the payer contract unit at the facility provide a copy or summary of the policy alerts to the revenue cycle team or CDM unit. The policy alert may not only require modification to the CDM, but it may also warrant changes to charge capture, as well as education for clinical or ancillary areas.

Although hospitals and other healthcare facilities may prefer payer contracts to align with their fiscal year, there may be payers whose set effective period differs from the facility's fiscal year. Thus, a schedule of payer contract updates should be considered in the CDM maintenance plan. The CDM coordinator and payer contract unit must work together to ensure the CDM reflects billing and coding protocol outlined in the payer contracts.

Ongoing CDM Maintenance

Even with policies, procedures, and maintenance plans in place, issues will always arise that need immediate attention. When issues surface, the CDM coordinator must be ready to execute a CDM review to help identify the root cause and address it quickly. Reimbursement for services is at stake and the internal cost of claim correction and resubmission can be significant.

Table 10.4.   CDM maintenance issues

Issue	Possible Result	Risk Area
Undercharging for services	Underpayment	Revenue loss
Overcharging for services	Overpayment	Compliance
Incorrect HCPCS or diagnosis code	Claims rejection/denial	Revenue loss
Incorrect revenue code	Claims rejection/denial	Revenue loss

Not only is CDM maintenance very detail-oriented and complicated, it is also time consuming. To assist facilities with CDM maintenance, many companies provide CDM maintenance software packages. Although each maintenance program will have unique and proprietary features, most provide software that will identify revenue codes, HCPCS codes, and compliance issues for the facility. For example, the program will identify all codes in the client CDM that have been deleted according to the CPT annual update and will provide the facility with replacement choices.

Some of the maintenance programs are installed at the facility and some are provided online. It is important to remember that many of these packages are based on Medicare guidelines, though some also provide state-level Medicaid regulations. Individual payer regulations are typically not included in these packages, so specific coding and billing guidance by private payers must be considered and monitored by the facility. Failure to effectively maintain the CDM puts a facility at risk for compliance violations and the loss of reimbursement, as outlined in table 10.4.

Because many reimbursement methodologies depend on the accuracy of claim data elements, it is vital that the correct information is reported to third-party payers. This key information is maintained in the CDM; therefore, it is critical that the CDM be precise.

Check Your Understanding 10.1

1. List an advantage of CPOE over paper charge capture.

2. Describe one way barcode scanning enhances the charge capture process.

3. The main purpose of the CDM is to produce claims. Describe an alternative use of the CDM or CDM data.

4. List the basic data elements of a CDM, identifying which data elements are hospital-specific and which are nationally recognized.

5. Explain the importance of ensuring unique charge codes in the CDM.

Code Sets for Diagnosis, Procedure, and Supply Reporting

A key component of claim production is communicating the clinical reason for treatment and the procedures that were performed for that condition. Facilities use diagnosis and procedure code sets to communicate this information. Diagnosis codes are used to establish medical necessity and record complication and comorbid conditions. Procedure codes are used to record the treatments, services, and supplies provided to the beneficiary. Therefore, a baseline knowledge of the approved code sets and their functionalities is essential for HIM and other healthcare professionals. HIPAA designated the code sets to use when reporting healthcare services to public and private insurers. The HIPAA-compliant code sets are listed in table 10.5.

Table 10.5.   HIPAA-designated code sets

| Provider | Inpatient | | Outpatient | |
	Diagnosis	Procedure	Diagnosis	Procedure
Physician	ICD-10-CM	CPT	ICD-10-CM	HCPCS (CPT and HCPCS Level II)
Facility	ICD-10-CM	ICD-10-PCS	ICD-10-CM	HCPCS (CPT and HCPCS Level II)

The *International Classification of Diseases*

The *International Classification of Diseases* (ICD) coding and **classification system** is used throughout the world for mortality reporting. A classification system is a system for grouping similar diseases and procedures and organizing related information for easy retrieval. The ICD classification system assigns alphanumeric codes to represent specific diseases. The ICD is maintained by the **World Health Organization (WHO)** and is updated to a new version (revision) approximately every 10 years. The WHO directs and coordinates international health within the United Nations' system. The WHO manages the ICD, and countries throughout the world use this classification system to collect morbidity and mortality information.

ICD-11

The WHO has released the eleventh revision of ICD, which is referred to as ICD-11. As of 2023, 64 states and countries are in various stages of implementing ICD-11. Unlike previous versions of ICD, ICD-11 is ready for use in electronic environments. ICD-11 is fully electronic and provides an index-based search algorithm that can interpret more than 1.6 million terms (WHO n.d.). The WHO provides free container software for ICD-11 to support easy installation and online or offline use. The WHO believes the use of this software will result in less user training (WHO n.d.).

ICD-11 allows for more precise and detailed coding than ICD-10. Examples of these coding improvements include the following:

* Codes for antimicrobial resistance
* Codes for full documentation of patient safety
* Details for cancer registration
* Specific codes for the clinical stages of HIV
* Up-to-date codes for the complications of diabetes
* Codes for skin cancers basalioma, and melanoma subtypes
* Classification of heart valve diseases and pulmonary hypertension that match current diagnostic and treatment practices (WHO n.d.)

Additionally, there are new core chapters for "Diseases of the Immune System," "Sleep-Wake Disorders," and "Conditions Related to Sexual Health." Overall, the clinical changes in ICD-11 align the classification with the most current information about disease treatment and prevention (WHO n.d.). ICD has increased transparency for changes and modifications to ICD-11 through a proposal platform. Anyone can suggest code changes or modifications to ICD-11, which can be viewed and discussed online.

ICD-11 is free for use in all countries, and the WHO provides user guides, tools, and training materials to help countries with implementation. In the US, the Centers for Disease Control and Prevention began using ICD-11 in 2022 for acute-illness and mortality reporting.

ICD-10-CM and ICD-10-PCS

Although the US has adopted ICD-11 in limited circumstances, the predominant classification system remains the *International Classification of Diseases, Tenth Revision, Clinical Modification* (**ICD-10-CM**) to report diagnoses and the *International Classification of Diseases, Tenth Revision, Procedure Coding System* (**ICD-10-PCS**) to report inpatient procedures (table 10.5). ICD-10-CM and ICD-10-PCS were implemented on October 1, 2015. These systems, referred to by many as ICD-10-CM/PCS, communicate diagnoses and inpatient procedures for public and private reimbursement systems.

The US clinical modification, ICD-10-CM, was developed by the **National Center for Health Statistics (NCHS)**. Although the international version of ICD focuses on acute illnesses and mortality, ICD-10-CM includes morbidity or chronic conditions. ICD-10-PCS was developed by CMS to provide a classification system for reporting inpatient procedures in the US. Several features in ICD-10-CM allow for a greater level of specificity and clinical detail than the previous versions of ICD, such as laterality, additional combination codes, and expanded code categories (Casto 2016, 1). There are many benefits associated with ICD-10-CM and ICD-10-PCS that allow for a precise capture of healthcare data:

- Improved ability to measure healthcare service, including quality and safety data

- Augmented sensitivity when refining grouping and reimbursement methodologies

- Expanded ability to conduct public health surveillance

- Decreased need to include supporting documentation with claims

- Strengthened ability to distinguish advances in medicine and medical technology

- Enhanced detail on socioeconomic conditions, family relationships, ambulatory care conditions, conditions related to lifestyle, and the results of screening tests

- Increased use of administrative data to evaluate medical processes and outcomes, to conduct biosurveillance, and to support value-based purchasing initiatives (AHA n.d.)

Providers use the ICD-10-CM and ICD-10-PCS classification system to determine payment categories for various PPSs, including the following:

- Hospital inpatient: Medicare severity diagnosis-related groups (MS-DRGs)

- Hospital rehabilitation: case-mix groups (CMGs)

- Long-term care: long-term care Medicare severity diagnosis-related groups (LTC-MS-DRGs)

- Home health: home health resource groups (HHRGs)

In the sections that follow, we will discuss the structure, maintenance, and reporting guidelines for ICD-10-CM and ICD-10-PCS.

Structure of ICD-10-CM

ICD-10-CM contains two sections: the Alphabetic Index and the Tabular List of Disease and Injuries. The Alphabetic Index includes the indices and tables that are used during the code selection process. The Tabular List of Diseases and Injuries provides 21 chapters that list all possible codes for each body system. Figure 10.4 provides the table of contents from AHIMA's 2023 *ICD-10-CM Code Book*.

Figure 10.4.   ICD-10-CM 2023 table of contents

Contents

Source: © AHIMA.

Figure 10.5.   ICD-10-CM diagnoses code structure

S10.11XA	
S10	Superficial injury of neck
S10.1	Other and unspecified superficial injuries of throat
S10.11	Abrasion of throat
S10.11XA	Abrasion of throat, initial encounter

ICD-10-CM diagnosis codes vary in length from three to seven characters; codes of four or more characters have a decimal point placed after the third character. The first three characters are a category code. The fourth and fifth characters are subcategory codes that provide the specificity necessary to accurately describe a patient's clinical condition. Some codes have a seventh character to further describe the circumstances of the condition. If a code requires a seventh character and is not six characters in length, a placeholder X must be used to fill in the empty sixth character slot, as shown in figure 10.5.

Structure of ICD-10-PCS

ICD-10-PCS contains four sections: Index, Sections, Code Listings, and Appendices, as shown in the 2023 ICD-10-PCS table of contents (figure 10.6). The sections of ICD-10-PCS consist of the following:

- Medical and Surgical (001–0YW)

- Obstetrics (102–10Y)

- Placement (2W0–2Y5)

- Administration (302–3E1)

- Measurement and Monitoring (4A0–4B0)

- Extracorporeal or Systemic Assistance and Performance (5A0–5A2)

- Extracorporeal or Systemic Therapies (6A0–6AB)

- Osteopathic (7W0)

- Other Procedures Section (8C0–8E0)

- Chiropractic (9WB)

- Imaging (B00–BY4)

- Nuclear Medicine (C01–CW7)

- Radiation Therapy (D00–DWY)

- Physical Rehabilitation and Diagnostic Audiology (F00–F15)

- Mental Health (GZ1–GZJ)

- Substance Abuse Treatment (HZ2–HZ9)

- New Technology (X2A–XY0)

Within each section are the tables that are used to construct the procedure code.

ICD-10-PCS has a logical, consistent code structure. Coding professionals use the Index to locate the appropriate table for code selection, using the procedure's root operation as the main term. The first three characters of the code identify the table to be used for code assignment. After the table is identified, codes must be constructed by choosing accurate values to complete the seven-character code. The spaces of the code are called *characters* and are filled with individual letters and numbers called *values* (figure 10.7).

Using the example in figure 10.7, the procedure is a mitral valve biopsy. In ICD-10-PCS, the root operation for biopsy is Excision (partial removal). Using the Index, the coding professional would locate the main term *Excision* and subterm *Valve* to see that the table to be used to construct the code is Table 02B in the Tables section of ICD-10-PCS. The coding professional would review the value choices for the remaining four characters in Table 02B and make the final determination based on the medical record documentation in the health record. Because this is a biopsy procedure, the coding professional would choose the seventh character of X indicating that the procedure was diagnostic in nature.

Figure 10.6.   ICD-10-PCS 2023 table of contents

Contents

Source: © AHIMA.

Figure 10.7.   Sample PCS code structure, 02BG0ZX Excision of mitral valve, open approach, diagnostic

Character 1	Character 2	Character 3	Character 4	Character 5	Character 6	Character 7
Section	Body System	Operation	Body Part	Approach	Device	Qualifier
0	2	B	G	0	Z	X
Medical and Surgical	Heart and Great Vessels	Excision	Mitral Valve	Open	No Device	Diagnostic

Maintenance of ICD-10-CM and ICD-10-PCS

The **ICD-10-CM/PCS Coordination and Maintenance Committee**, composed of NCHS and CMS, is responsible for maintaining the US clinical modification version of the code set. NCHS makes determinations regarding diagnosis issues, whereas CMS maintains the procedures. Advisory in nature, the committee was created in 1985 to discuss possible updates and revisions to the US clinical modification of ICD. The director of NCHS and the administrator of CMS make the final determinations.

The committee holds public meetings every year in spring and fall, and suggestions for new codes, modifications, and deletions are submitted by members of both public and private sectors. Proposals for code changes are submitted before the semiannual meetings and include a description of the diagnosis or procedure and the rationale for the requested modification. Supporting references, literature, statistics, and cost information may also be submitted. Requests must follow industry-accepted ICD-10-CM and ICD-10-PCS coding conventions. Each year after the fall meeting, the committee determines code modifications to become effective October 1 of the following year. In addition, CMS has the option to add more new codes to the annual update after the spring meeting. This supplemental opportunity was added to address the healthcare community's concerns about limitations of code maintenance. Meeting materials and proposals for diagnosis issues are located on the NCHS portion of the Centers for Disease Control and Prevention website. Meeting materials and proposals for procedure issues are located on the CMS website.

ICD-10-CM and ICD-10-PCS Coding Guidelines

Because ICD-10-CM and ICD-10-PCS codes serve as the communication vehicle between providers and insurers, it is always crucial to follow ICD-10-CM and ICD-10-PCS guidelines. Establishing medical necessity and ensuring accurate reimbursement depends on timely, accurate, and complete coding of services and procedures. The ICD-10-CM Official Coding Guidelines for Coding and Reporting are available for download from the NCHS and CMS websites. The ICD-10-PCS Official Coding Guidelines for Coding and Reporting are available for download from the CMS website. Additionally, the Cooperating Parties—NCHS, CMS, American Hospital Association (AHA), and AHIMA—and the Editorial Advisory Board are responsible for publishing additional coding guidance for ICD-10-CM and ICD-10-PCS. This additional coding guidance is published in the ***AHA Coding Clinic for ICD-10-CM and ICD-10-PCS***, the only official quarterly newsletter for ICD-10-CM and ICD-10-PCS coding guidance and advice. *Coding Clinic* is published quarterly and includes the following information:

- Official coding advice and coding guidelines
- Correct code assignments for new technologies and newly identified diseases
- Articles and topics that offer practical information and improve data quality
- Conduit for disseminating coding changes and corrections to hospitals and other parties
- "Ask the Editor" section that uses practical examples to address questions (AHA n.d.)

Coding Clinic should be a component of all coding education and compliance programs for healthcare provider and facility coding units.

Healthcare Common Procedure Coding System

As mentioned earlier in this chapter, HCPCS is a two-tiered system of procedural codes used primarily for ambulatory care and physician services. The first tier is CPT (HCPCS Level I) and the second tier is HCPCS Level II. The structure, maintenance, and guidelines for each tier are discussed in the next section. HCPCS codes are frequently included in the CDM for convenience and to facilitate communication between providers and payers about services and supplies.

Current Procedural Terminology (HCPCS Level I)

CPT is a coding system that is used to report diagnostic and surgical services and procedures that are provided to patients. Created and first published by the AMA in 1966, CPT was designed to be a means of effective and dependable communication among physicians, patients, and third-party payers (Palkie 2020, 152). The terminology provides a uniform coding scheme that accurately describes medical, surgical, and diagnostic services. The CPT coding system is used by physicians to report services and procedures performed in the hospital inpatient and outpatient setting and by facilities for outpatient services and procedures (table 10.5). CPT has several uses:

- Communication vehicle for public and private reimbursement systems
- Development of guidelines for medical care review
- Basis for local, regional, and national use comparisons
- Medical education and research

The code set was adopted into HCPCS in 1985 and became the HCPCS Level I code set for Medicare reporting, so CPT is referred to as HCPCS Level I as well as CPT in the coding and reimbursement communities. The structure, maintenance, and guidelines for CPT follow.

Structure of CPT

The code set is divided into six main sections, known as Category I codes, plus two types of supplementary codes (Category II and Category III codes), and modifiers.

Category I CPT codes consist of the following six sections:

- Evaluation and Management (99201–99499)
- Anesthesia (00100–01999)
- Surgery (10004–68899)
- Radiology (70010–79999)
- Pathology and Laboratory (80047–89398, 0001U–0138U)
- Medicine (90399–99607)

The Surgery section is further divided as follows:

Integumentary System	10004 to 19499
Musculoskeletal System	20005 to 29999
Respiratory System	30000 to 32999
Cardiovascular System	33010 to 39599
Digestive System	40490 to 49999
Urinary System	50010 to 53899
Male Genital System	54000 to 55980
Female Genital System	56405 to 58999
Maternity Care and Delivery	59000 to 59899
Endocrine System	60000 to 60699
Nervous System	61000 to 64999
Eye and Ocular Adnexa	65091 to 68899
Auditory System	69000 to 69979
Operating Microscope	69990

Table 10.6 contains sample CPT codes. Each code is five characters in length. The code descriptions reflect language used by physicians and clinicians. Each of the three code categories in the CPT coding system serves a different and unique purpose.

Category I CPT codes describe a procedure or service that is consistent with contemporary medical practice and that is performed by many physicians in clinical practice in multiple locations (Beebe 2003, 84). The US Food and Drug Administration (FDA) must approve the specific use of devices and drugs for all services in this category. Category I codes are represented by a five-character numeric code.

Within Category I codes, there are unlisted codes. Unlisted codes are used to report services and procedures that are not represented by an existing code. Typically, unlisted codes are used for new or innovative procedures that have not been added to the CPT coding system. When an unlisted code is reported, supporting documentation should be submitted to the third-party payer to establish correct coding and medical necessity for that service.

Category II CPT codes were created to facilitate data collection for certain services and test results that contribute to positive health outcomes and high-quality patient care (Beebe 2003, 84). Category II is a set of optional tracking codes for performance measurement. The services included in this category are often part of the Evaluation and Management service or other component part of a service. Category II codes have been implemented to help medical practices and facilities reduce operational costs by replacing time-consuming medical record documentation reviews and surveys with this streamlined code tracking system (Beebe 2003, 84). Use of Category II codes is optional, and they cannot be used as substitutes for Category I codes. Category II codes are represented by a five-character alphanumeric code with the character *F* in the last position—for example, 1234F.

Category III CPT codes represent emerging technologies. This category of codes was created to help facilitate data collection and assessment of new services and procedures (Beebe 2003, 85). To qualify for inclusion in this category, a service or procedure must have relevance for research, either ongoing or planned. Like Category II codes, Category III codes are represented by an alphanumeric five-character code, but Category III codes have the character *T* in the last field—for example, 1234T.

Table 10.6.   Sample CPT codes

Code	Code Description
13100	Repair, complex, trunk; 1.1 cm to 2.5 cm
26580	Repair cleft hand
33910	Pulmonary artery embolectomy; with cardiopulmonary bypass
44640	Closure of intestinal cutaneous fistula
45399	Unlisted procedure, colon
50945	Laparoscopy, surgical; ureterolithotomy
62270	Spinal puncture, lumbar, diagnostic
71045	Radiologic examination, chest; single view
85004	Blood count: automated differential WBC count
93005	Electrocardiogram, routine ECG with at least 12 leads; tracing only, without interpretation and report

Source: AMA 2021.

In addition to the three categories of codes, CPT contains modifiers for use by physicians and other healthcare providers. A physician or facility uses a modifier to flag a service provided to a patient that has been altered by some special circumstance but for which the basic code description itself has not changed. The following are common reasons to use a modifier:

- A service or procedure has been increased or reduced.
- Only part of a service was performed.
- A bilateral procedure was performed.
- A service or procedure was performed more than once.
- Unusual events occurred during a procedure or service. (AMA 2021, xvii)

Health record documentation must support the use of a modifier because the modifier may change the reimbursement for the service or procedure. Appendix A of CPT provides guidelines for the correct use of modifiers. For example, modifier 91 is used to indicate that a clinical laboratory test was repeated. Rules governing the usage of this modifier specify that it may not be used when an equipment or testing failure has occurred, but rather only when the test has been reordered to determine whether a change in the result has occurred. Accordingly, using modifier 91 relays to the third-party payer that the duplicate code reported was not accidental or fraudulent but instead was correct, and that the physician ordered the test twice based on medically necessary foundations. However, failure to have supporting documentation in the medical record that establishes medical necessity can result in claim denials and fraud or abuse penalties.

Maintenance of CPT

The CPT Editorial Research and Development Department supports the modification process for the code set. A 16-member CPT Editorial Panel meets four times yearly to consider proposed changes to CPT. The Editorial Panel is supported by a CPT Advisory Committee comprised of representatives from more than 90 medical specialty societies and other healthcare professional organizations.

Requesting a Code Modification for CPT

CPT coding modifications are submitted to the CPT Editorial Research and Development Department at the AMA. The Coding Change Request Form, which is found on the AMA website, must be used and submitted along with supporting documentation and clinical vignettes. A coding modification may be requested for all three categories of codes. After the Coding Change Request Form is received, it is reviewed for completeness by the AMA staff. If the form is complete, Coding Change Request Forms for Category I and Category III codes are forwarded to the CPT Advisory Committee for a detailed review.

Coding Change Request Forms for Category II *CPT codes* are sent to the Performance Measurement Advisory Group for review. These requests must receive a two-thirds majority opinion from the advisory group before they are passed on to the CPT Advisory Committee. The AMA established the Performance Measurement Advisory Group to help create and maintain the performance measurement codes (Beebe 2003, 84). The group consists of representatives from various organizations, AMA's CPT and clinical quality improvement staffs, the CPT Editorial Panel, health services researchers, and other knowledgeable experts.

After review by the CPT Advisory Committee, those requests that warrant final review are submitted to the CPT Editorial Panel responsible for final decisions on all coding modifications (AMA n.d.). A calendar for code submission deadlines and regular meetings for the CPT Advisory Committee and the CPT Editorial Panel is posted on the AMA website.

CPT Coding Guidelines

The AMA provides several resources regarding the appropriate use of CPT. The official monthly newsletter for CPT coding issues and guidance is *CPT Assistant* (AMA 1989–2023). *CPT Assistant* contains the following helpful features:

- Coding communication that provides up-to-date information on codes and trends
- Clinical vignettes that offer insight into confusing coding and modifier usage scenarios
- Coding consultation that covers the most frequently asked questions

All coding education and compliance programs should include the use of *CPT Assistant*.

HCPCS Level II

HCPCS was developed by CMS in the 1980s to report services, supplies, and procedures not represented in the CPT (HCPCS Level I) code set but submitted for reimbursement (CMS 2023). The descriptions identify items or services rather than specific brand names and do not endorse any manufacturer. Specifically, the code set includes the following:

- Medical and surgical supplies
- Enteral and parenteral therapy
- Detailed procedures required for OPPS
- Dental procedures
- Durable medical equipment
- Temporary codes for procedures and professional services
- Behavioral health and substance use treatment services
- Drugs, biologicals, and chemotherapy drugs
- Orthotics and prosthetics
- Laboratory services
- Temporary codes assigned by CMS
- Diagnostic radiology
- Temporary national codes established by private payers
- Vision services

This alphanumeric code set is a standardized coding system that provides an established environment for claims submission and processing. Both private and public health insurers manage the system. The existence of a particular code does not guarantee or indicate coverage or reimbursement by Medicare, Medicaid, or other third-party payers. A sample of HCPCS Level II codes are included in table 10.7. There are several types of codes included in HCPCS Level II, including national and dental codes.

All public and private health insurers use HCPCS Level II national codes. National codes are alphanumeric, with five characters, including an alpha character in the first position—for example, A2345. The alpha character designates the category to which the code is classified. The national codes are maintained by CMS.

Within the national codes are "miscellaneous/not otherwise classified" codes. These codes enable suppliers and healthcare providers to report items or services that have not been incorporated into the coding system but that nonetheless have been approved for marketing by the FDA (CMS 2022). Miscellaneous codes are manually reviewed and must be submitted with accompanying pricing and documentation of medical necessity.

Table 10.7.   **Sample HCPCS Level II codes**

Code	Description
A4215	Needle, sterile, any size, each
B4081	Nasogastric tubing with stylet
C8903	Magnetic resonance imaging with contrast, breast; unilateral
E0966	Manual wheelchair accessory, headrest extension, each
G0378	Hospital observation service, per hour
J1644	Injection, heparin sodium, per 1000 units
L8679	Implantable neurostimulator, pulse generator, any type
Q9958	High osmolar contrast material, up to 149 mg/ml iodine concentration, per ml
S9131	Physical therapy; in the home, per diem

Source: CMS 2023.

The Code on Dental Procedures and Nomenclature (CDT Code), commonly known as dental codes, constitutes a separate category of HCPCS Level II codes. The codes are copyrighted and maintained by the American Dental Association (ADA). Dental codes are easily identified because they begin with the letter *D*.

Like CPT, HCPCS Level II allows for modifiers. HCPCS Level II modifiers are two-character alpha or alphanumeric codes. A modifier is designed to give Medicare and other third-party payers additional information needed to process a claim. Many HCPCS Level II modifiers indicate body areas that allow for specific information to be provided to third-party payers. Table 10.8 provides examples of HCPCS Level II modifiers.

Maintenance of HCPCS Level II Coding System

HCPCS Level II codes are maintained and distributed by CMS. Temporary codes can be added, changed, or deleted on a quarterly basis. Additionally, CMS decides when a temporary code should transition to a permanent code. However, there is no time limit for an item, supply, or service remaining a temporary code.

Requesting a Code Modification for HCPCS Level II

There are three types of coding modifications to HCPCS Level II codes that users can request: a code may be added to the code set, the language used to describe an existing code may be changed, and an existing code may be deleted. The HCPCS Level II coding review process is a continual process with the submission deadline posted annually on the CMS website.

Table 10.8.   **HCPCS Level II modifier examples**

	HCPCS Level II Modifiers
LT	Left side
RT	Right side
E1	Upper left, eyelid
F1	Left hand, second digit

Source: CMS 2023.

Requests for code changes may be submitted anytime during the year. The proper request format can be found on the CMS website. Requests for coding modifications are submitted to the National Level II HCPCS Coding Program at CMS. After a request is submitted, the CMS HCPCS Workgroup reviews it at one of its regular monthly meetings. After considering the request, CMS will make a recommendation that usually falls into one of the following categories:

- Add a code
- Use an existing code that describes the item or service
- Use an existing code for miscellaneous items or services
- Revise an existing code
- Delete an existing code

CMS is responsible for approving all coding modifications. After the decision is made regarding a request, CMS will send a decision letter to the requester. If the requester is unsatisfied with the decision, a new request with new supporting information may be submitted for reconsideration and evaluation (CMS 2023).

HCPCS Level II Coding Guidelines

AHA Coding Clinic for HCPCS is a resource newsletter that provides coding advice for the users of HCPCS Level II. This quarterly newsletter was first introduced in March 2001 and is published by the AHA's Central Office on HCPCS. The newsletter includes an "Ask the Editor" section providing actual examples, correct code assignment for new technologies, articles, and a bulletin of coding changes and corrections. Although this is not official coding guidance, it is expert. Unlike ICD-10-CM, ICD-10-PCS, and CPT, there are no official coding guidelines for HCPCS Level II other than coverage determinations issued by CMS and its MAC. It is important to keep in mind that coding does not dictate coverage of medical services or reimbursement policies.

Check Your Understanding 10.2

1. The code sets to be used for reporting healthcare services by public and private insurers were designated by what legislation?

2. Dr. Shah is a urologist that performs surgery at Community Hospital. He performs approximately 12 inpatient surgeries per month. His office staff generates claims for his surgeries. What procedure code set should his staff use to report inpatient surgeries on the provider (physician) claim?

3. What organization maintains the ICD-10-CM and ICD-10-PCS code sets?

4. What organization maintains the CPT code set?

5. Which code set includes detailed codes for chemotherapy drugs?

The Coding Process

When care is provided at a facility-based service area, two claims for reimbursement are submitted to the payer. One claim is submitted for services and supplies provided by the facility. These charges detail the volume and intensity of resources used to treat the patient. The charges are submitted on the UB-04 or 837I claim format for facilities. Claim formats are discussed in more detail in chapter 11, "Revenue Cycle Back-End Processes—Claims Production and Revenue Collection," when the claims generation process is explored. The second claim submitted to the payer is for the physician or other health professional services. This claim represents the complexity of the physician work provided during the encounter. Examples of physician work include performing an evaluation, providing a consultation, or performing a surgery. These charges are submitted on the CMS-1500 or 837P claim format for physicians and other health professionals. In the following section, we will discuss the coding process for each claim type.

Facility Coding

Facility coding is the process of determining the diagnosis and procedure codes that should be submitted on the facility claim (UB-04/837I). The facility claim requests reimbursement for the hospital or facility, not for the physician. Inpatient admissions and moderate-to-complex ambulatory surgery encounters require coding professionals to assign diagnoses and operating room procedures. Coding professionals read and closely examine the physician documentation to determine the correct diagnosis and procedure codes. This process is often referred to as **soft coding**. During soft coding, diagnoses and procedures are identified, coded, and then abstracted into the HIM coding system by a coding professional. This system works within the EHR to include the codes on the claim form prior to submission to the payer. It is important to remember that numerous services and procedures are hard coded via the CDM and not soft coded. For example, services like chest x-rays and laboratory tests are hard coded. A coding professional does not assign CPT procedure codes for these services. Hard-coded services and soft-coded diagnoses and procedures are included on the claim form to complete the facility coding process.

Facility coding professionals are trained in ICD-10-CM diagnosis coding, ICD-10-PCS inpatient procedure coding, and HCPCS coding, which is used for outpatient encounters. Facility coding professionals are experts in coding and billing guidance related to facility-based payment systems such as MS-DRGs and APCs, discussed in chapter 5, "Medicare Hospital Acute Inpatient Payment System," and chapter 7, "Medicare Hospital Outpatient Payment System," respectively. Most coding units have designated inpatient coding professionals and outpatient coding professionals. This allows the coding professionals to specialize in the code sets, conditions, and procedures that are most often encountered in their assigned role. This approach can improve quality and productivity because the coding professionals become experts in their clinical domains. However, one drawback is that the coding professionals may lose some of their skill in coding other clinical areas or with other code sets, such as HCPCS. Example 10.2 illustrates the facility coding process.

Example 10.2

At a large metropolitan hospital, the coding team would consist of an inpatient coding team and an outpatient coding team. The inpatient coding team would have coding professionals that excel in ICD-10-CM and ICD-10-PCS coding. The team may even be divided by clinical areas. For example, there may be one or more coding professionals designated to code complex cardiovascular procedures, such as heart transplants, implantation of heart assist systems, and coronary artery bypass procedures. Additionally, the team may have a coding professional designated to code deliveries and births. While an uncomplicated birth may be routine and familiar to most coders, complex pregnancies and births are difficult to code and may require a coding professional with extensive experience.

Professional Coding

Like facility coding, diagnosis and procedure codes are required for the professional claim (CMS-1500/837P). Professional coding is performed by coding professionals that specialize in HCPCS coding. As discussed earlier, HCPCS coding consists of CPT coding and HCPCS Level II coding. Remember that physicians and other clinicians report HCPCS codes for the services and procedures they perform regardless of the setting. They do not report ICD-10-PCS codes on professional bills.

Professional coders must be well versed in diagnosis coding. Although professional reimbursement rates are not dependent on diagnosis codes, as illustrated in the resource-based relative value scale (RBRVS) section of this text, the diagnosis code(s) are required to determine medical necessity. When completing the professional claim, coding professionals must link the diagnosis code(s) to the associated HCPCS code in order to establish medical necessity. This linking is unique to professional coding. It is also a critical step to receive reimbursement.

Single Path Coding

Traditionally, facility coding and professional coding have been separate functions. In most facilities, these functions have different reporting units and managers and may even use different platforms to capture diagnosis and procedure codes. However, there is a growing trend to explore single path coding. **Single path coding** is a process where one coding professional assigns the codes required for both facility and professional claims during the same coding session. Single path coding streamlines the coding processes because it eliminates two different coding teams looking at the same documentation. Instead, one team views the medical documentation one time to complete coding for both the facility and the professional claims. Some benefits of single path coding include the following:

- Eliminate duplicate processes
- Optimize productivity
- Enhance coding accuracy
- Reduce or eliminate variances between professional and facility outpatient HCPCS codes (Goar 2018, 22)

Single path coding is especially effective in the outpatient setting, where the procedure coding set, HCPCS, is the same for facility and professional claims. This new approach also lends itself to improving coding performance for risk adjusted coding and hierarchical condition category (HCC) coding. While risk adjusted coding models, such as the HCC model implemented by Medicare, are prevalent in the professional reimbursement methodologies, they are migrating toward facility value-based purchasing programs.

Single path coding is more challenging for the inpatient setting, where the coding professional must be well versed in ICD-10-PCS and HCPCS coding. To this point, expanding the coding professional's proficiency in multiple code sets is key. Coding managers should perform a gap analysis to determine which coding professionals need to improve skills in specific code sets.

Most departments moving toward single path coding are using a staged approach (Goar 2018, 22). Facilities may choose to start in one ancillary area, such as radiology. Once success is gained and the process refined, facilities may choose to move on to clinic areas such as pain management, and then finally on to same-day surgery. Since success depends on a good single path coding platform, cohesive teamwork, and well-cross-trained coding professionals, implementation throughout all coding processes could take a significant amount of time and resources. However, if gains in quality, productivity, and cost reduction are achieved, single path coding could improve the facility's revenue integrity position.

Patient Connection

Nick is an analyst at Memorial Hospital. He is reviewing charge capture data for knee arthroplasty surgeries. He is focusing on admissions where the length of stay (LOS) was greater than the Medicare average LOS. He is examining the admission for patient Malakai. The surgeon for the case is Dr. Shah. Nick has created the following table for this admission based on his medical record review.

Patient Care Day	Charge Type	Documented in Health Record	Reported on Claim	Missed Charge
1	Operating room	√	√	
	Anesthesia	√	√	
	Pharmacy (pre- and postop meds)	√	√	
	Supply (implants used during surgery)	√	√	
	Recovery room	√		√
	Room rate	√	√	

(continued)

Patient Care Day	Charge Type	Documented in Health Record	Reported on Claim	Missed Charge
2	Laboratory tests	√	√	
	Pharmacy (pain medication)	√	√	
	Supply (pressure stockings)	√	√	
	Physical therapy	√	√	
	Respiratory therapy			√
	Room rate		√	
3	Pharmacy (pain medication and laxative)	√	√	
	Physical therapy	√	√	
	Respiratory therapy	√		√
	Room rate	√	√	
4	Physical therapy	√	√	
	Occupational therapy	√	√	
	Respiratory therapy	√	√	√
	Room rate	√		
5	Laboratory test – culture	√		√
	Pharmacy (IV antibiotic)	√	√	
	Physical therapy	√	√	
	Occupational therapy	√	√	
	Respiratory therapy	√		√
	Room rate	√	√	
6	No charges (discharged in morning)	√		

Through analysis, Nick identified that several charges were missed during the charge capture process for this admission. Patient Malakai was moved to the recovery room after surgery, but the charge was not captured through the CPOE. Malakai was given respiratory therapy on days 2, 3, 4, and 5, but none of these charges were captured. Lastly, Malakai had a wound culture on day 5 that identified a surgical wound infection. This charge was not captured in the CPOE.

After reviewing over 50 patient records, Nick found several similar missed charges. His summary recommends the following next steps:

- Meet with the director of respiratory therapy to determine the root cause of the missed charges for the ancillary services
- Meet with the laboratory director to perform root cause analysis for missed culture charges
- Meet with the recovery room nurse manager to identify possible causes for missed charges in this area

Through this analysis, Nick identified $72,500 in missed charges, which translated to $20,375 in missed reimbursement.

Chapter 10 Review Quiz

1. How does CPOE reduce errors and improve patient safety?

2. Describe the barcoding process.

3. Identify and discuss a risk area that is of concern when the CDM is not properly maintained.

4. Why is the charge description construction an important CDM task?

5. How does CDM maintenance support the revenue integrity principle of compliance adherence and legitimate reimbursement?

6. Match each coding system on the left with its description of uses on the right.

   ICD-10-CM and ICD-10-PCS   ____   a. Medical and surgical supplies

   HCPCS Level II   ____   b. Physician inpatient or outpatient procedures

   CPT   ____   c. Diagnoses and inpatient procedures

7. Describe the difference between WHO versions of ICD and US versions of ICD (clinical modification).

8. Match the governing bodies on the left with their associated code sets on the right.

   CMS   ____   a. ICD-10-PCS

   NCHS   ____   b. CPT

   AMA   ____   c. ICD-10-CM

9. Describe the differences between hard and soft coding.

10. How does single path coding support the revenue integrity principle of obtaining operational efficiency?

References

AHA (American Hospital Association). n.d. "AHA Coding Clinic Advisor." Accessed February 24, 2023. https://www.codingclinicadvisor.com/about-icd-10-coding.

AMA (American Medical Association). 2021. *Current Procedural Terminology 2022*. Chicago: AMA.

AMA (American Medical Association). 1989 to 2023. *CPT Assistant*. Chicago: AMA.

AMA (American Medical Association). n.d. "The CPT Code Process." Accessed February 24, 2023. https://www.ama-assn.org/about/cpt-editorial-panel/cpt-code-process.

Beebe, M. 2003. CPT Category III codes cover new, emerging technologies: New codes developed to address issues in light of HIPAA. *Journal of AHIMA* 74(9):84–85.

Casto, A. 2016. *ICD-10-CM Code Book 2016*. Chicago: AHIMA.

Casto, A. 2011. "The Charge Description Master." Chapter 7 in *Effective Management of Coding Services*, 3rd ed., edited by L. A. Schraffenberger and L. Kuehn. Chicago: AHIMA.

CDC (Centers for Disease Control and Prevention). n.d. "UB-40-P." Accessed February 24, 2023. https://www.cdc.gov/wtc/pdfs/policies/ub-40-P.pdf.

CMS (Centers for Medicare and Medicaid Services). 2023. "HCPCS-General Information." https://www.cms .gov/Medicare/Coding/MedHCPCSGenInfo.

CMS (Centers for Medicare and Medicaid Services). 2022. Healthcare Common Procedure Coding System (HCPCS) Level II Coding Procedures. https://www.cms.gov/Medicare/Coding/MedHCPCSGenInfo/ Downloads/2018-11-30-HCPCS-Level2-Coding-Procedure.pdf.

CMS (Centers for Medicare and Medicaid Services). 2021. "Completing and Processing the Form." Chapter 25 in *Medicare Claims Processing Manual*. https://www.cms.gov/Regulations-and-Guidance/Guidance/Manuals /Downloads/clm104c25.pdf.

Dietz, M. S. 2005. Ensure equitable reimbursement through an accurate charge description master. *Proceedings from AHIMA's 77th National Convention and Exhibit*. Chicago: AHIMA.

Goar, E. S. 2018. A singular effort. *For the Record* 30(1):22. https://www.fortherecordmag.com/archives /0118p22.shtml.

HealthIT.gov. n.d. "What Is a Computerized Provider Order Entry?" Accessed February 24, 2023. https://www .healthit.gov/faq/what-computerized-provider-order-entry.

HFMA (Healthcare Financial Management Association). n.d. "Patient Friendly Billing Project." Accessed February 24, 2023. https://www.hfma.org/guidance/patient-friendly-billing-project/.

Palkie, B. 2020. "Clinical Classifications, Vocabularies, Terminologies, and Standards." Chapter 5 in *Health Information Management: Concepts, Principles, and Practice*, 6th ed., edited by P. Oachs and A. Watters. Chicago: AHIMA.

WHO (World Health Organization). n.d. "ICD-11 Fact Sheet." Accessed February 24, 2023. https://icd.who.int/en /docs/icd11factsheet_en.pdf.

Chapter 11
Revenue Cycle Back-End Processes— Claims Production and Revenue Collection

Learning Objectives

❖ Describe claims production

❖ Identify HIPAA electronic transactions and designated code sets

❖ Describe accrual accounting

❖ Explain data elements included in an explanation of benefits document

❖ Describe claims reconciliation

Key Terms

Accounts receivable (AR)
Accrual accounting
Adjudication
Cash accounting
Contractual allowance

Days in accounts receivable
Explanation of benefits (EOB)
Medicare summary notice (MSN)
Remittance advice (RA)
Scrubbers

In this chapter, the final component of the revenue cycle is explored. The back-end processes involve preparing the claim for submission to the payer and ensuring that expected reimbursement is collected. Figure 11.1 shows a refresher of the revenue cycle components and highlights the processes for the back end of the revenue cycle.

There are several back-end processes, as shown in figure 11.1, and all of them support the collection of the correct reimbursement for the services provided during patient treatment. Patient financial services is typically the department responsible for these processes. In the next section, the claims production process is discussed in detail.

Claims Production

After charge capture is complete, the facility or provider prepares the claim for submission to the third-party payer. The first step is to review the claims data for accuracy and completeness. Many facilities have internal auditing systems, known as **scrubbers**. The auditing system runs each claim through a set of edits specifically designed for the patient's third-party payer. The auditing system identifies data that have failed edits and flags the claim for correction. Examples of errors that cause claim rejections or denials if not caught by the scrubber are as follows:

- Incompatible dates of service

- Nonspecific or inaccurate diagnosis and procedure codes

- Lack of medical necessity

- Inaccurate revenue code assignment

Figure 11.1.   Components of the revenue cycle

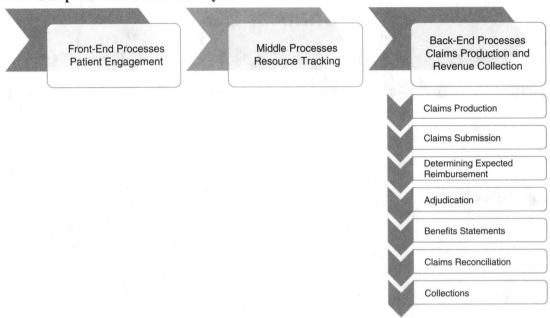

The auditing process prevents facilities from sending incomplete or inaccurate claims to the payer. Facilities that do not have a scrubber may perform a hand audit of a sample of claims. Health information management (HIM) and reimbursement specialists review claims in conjunction with medical record documentation to determine whether all services, diagnoses, and procedures were accurately reported. If errors are found, they can be corrected before claim submission.

More than just data elements identified during charge capture are included on the claim. Beneficiary information collected during scheduling, precertification, and registration is included on the claim. Information about the healthcare facility and providers is also included on the claim. Table 11.1 provides a listing of essential data for healthcare insurance claims.

Claims Submission

After being reviewed and corrected, the claim can be submitted to the third-party payer for payment. The Health Insurance Portability and Accountability Act of 1996 (HIPAA) added a new part to the Social Security Act, titled Administrative Simplification. The purpose of this section is to improve the efficiency and effectiveness of the healthcare delivery system. Through this section, Medicare has established standards and requirements for the electronic exchange of certain health information (HHS 2003, 8381). The final rule on Standards for Electronic Transactions and Code Sets, also known as the Transactions Rule, identified eight electronic transactions (table 11.2) and six code sets (table 11.3). This rule ensures all providers, third-party payers, claims clearinghouses, and so forth use the same sets of codes to communicate coded health information, ensuring standardization for systems and applications across the healthcare continuum. Not only does this support standardization, but it also supports administrative simplification. Providers now maintain a select number of code sets at their current version, rather than maintaining different versions (current and old) of many code sets based on payer specification.

Healthcare claims, healthcare payment and remittance advice (RA), and coordination of benefits are included in the electronic transactions. RA and coordination of benefits are documents regarding the claim processing outcome and are discussed later in this chapter. Since October 16, 2003, all healthcare facilities have been required to electronically submit and receive healthcare claims, RA, and coordination of benefits. Thus, today, most facilities submit claims via the 837I electronic format, which replaces the paper UB-04/CMS-1450 billing form. Physicians and other applicable professionals submit claims via the 837P electronic format, which takes the place of the paper

Table 11.1.   Essential data for healthcare insurance claims

Data Element	Description
Patient or client name	Patient or client's name. Patients and clients should strive to list their names consistently across sites of care and insurance policies (do not mix nicknames and given names or surnames).
Patient or client's health record number	Health record number that the provider uses to identify the patient or client's record across time.
Patient or client's account number	Identifier of specific episode-of-care, date of service, or hospitalization.
Patient or client's demographic data	Date of birth, sex, marital status, address, telephone number, relationship to subscriber, and circumstances of condition (such as related to automobile accident).
Subscriber (member, policyholder, certificate holder, or insured) name	Purchaser of the healthcare insurance or the member of group for which an employer or association has purchased insurance.
Subscriber's demographic data	Address and telephone number.
Subscriber (member) number (identifier)	Unique code used to identify the subscriber's policy.
Group or plan number (identifier)	Unique code used to identify a set of benefits of one group or type of plan.
Prior approval number (precertification or preauthorization number, if applicable)	Number indicating that the healthcare insurance company has been notified and has approved healthcare services prior to their receipt.
Provider name	Name of the hospital, physician, or other entity that rendered healthcare services.
National provider identifier (NPI)	Unique 10-digit code for healthcare providers (required by the Health Insurance Portability and Accountability Act of 1996).
Provider's address and telephone number	Address and telephone number of entity that rendered healthcare services and that will be reimbursed by the claim.
Date(s) of service	Date when the healthcare service was rendered.
Diagnosis code	*International Classification of Diseases* code representing the disease, condition, or status of the patient or client.
Procedure code	*International Classification of Diseases* code, Current Procedural Terminology code, or Healthcare Common Procedure Coding System code representing the procedure or service.
Revenue code	Four-digit code identifying specific accommodation, ancillary service, or billing calculation related to the services on the bill. Indicates where the service was performed and summarizes other services and supplies used for treatment.

(continued)

Table 11.1. *(continued)*

Data Element	Description
Itemized charges for services	Detailed list of each service and its cost.
Number of services (or duration of time)	Details related to number of services or length of time service was rendered.
Secondary or other healthcare insurance information	Another entity that may be responsible to reimburse the provider for the healthcare services rendered (such as automobile insurance or workers' compensation).

Table 11.2.   HIPAA electronic transactions

Healthcare claims or equivalent encounter information
Eligibility for a health plan
Referral certification and authorization
Healthcare claim status
Enrollment and disenrollment in a health plan
Healthcare payment and remittance advice
Health plan premium payments
Coordination of benefits

Source: CMS 2022a.

Table 11.3.   HIPAA code sets

International Classification of Diseases, Tenth Revision, Clinical Modification (CM) and *Procedure Coding System (PCS)*
National Drug Codes (NDCs)
Code on Dental Procedures and Nomenclature (CDT)
Healthcare Common Procedure Coding System (HCPCS)
Current Procedural Terminology (CPT), 4th ed.

Source: CMS 2022b.

CMS-1500 billing form. Some facilities continue to use paper forms for certain third-party payers. For example, a facility may use a paper form for a state employee's workers' compensation payer. Additionally, when a visual display of a claim is provided for education, auditing, or analysis, it typically follows the paper format.

Determining Expected Reimbursement

After the submission of a clean claim, the provider uses the data from the claim and the contract terms for the insurance company to calculate the expected payment. The expected reimbursement is calculated for two primary reasons. First, the provider will add the expected payment to their amount of **accounts receivable (AR)**. AR are amounts owed to a facility by patients or insurance companies who received services but whose payments will be made at a later date. The second reason for calculating the expected reimbursement for each claim is to ensure that the third-party payer is paying the correct amount and that the amount to be collected from the patient is billed in a timely fashion.

Hospitals and most other healthcare providers use the accrual method of accounting. The details of accounting methods are beyond the scope of this text, but the general concept of cash versus **accrual accounting** is important to understand as it pertains to the revenue cycle. When using the accrual method of accounting, an AR amount is recorded when services are provided to a patient (White 2018, 23). This is essentially a placeholder used to account for the fact that the effort to provide the services was expensed, but the payment is expected later. Accruals or AR allow the provider to apply a concept called "the matching principle" by accounting for the expense to provide the services and the reimbursement earned in the same period. **Cash accounting** is the other method of accounting. In cash accounting, all amounts are recorded when the cash or funds are exchanged (White 2018, 22–23). This is not the preferred accounting method to use for healthcare because there is often a significant delay between the date that services are provided and when the payment is received.

After the claim is submitted to a third-party payer for reimbursement, time is allowed for the payer to remit a payment. Typical performance statistics maintained by the AR department include days in AR and aging of accounts. **Days in accounts receivable** is calculated by dividing the ending AR balance for a given period by the average revenue per day. An example of calculating days in accounts receivable is provided in example 11.1.

Example 11.1

If the average expected revenue per day for a hospital is $250,000, and it has $10,000,000 in AR at the end of the month, then the number of days in AR is 10,000,000/250,000 = 40 DAR or days in AR.

Facilities typically set performance goals for this standard. Aging of accounts is maintained in 30-day increments (0 to 30 days, 31 to 60 days, and so forth). Facilities monitor the number of accounts and the total dollar value in each increment. The older the account or the longer the account remains unpaid, the less likely the facility will receive reimbursement for the encounter.

Adjudication

Once the claims are submitted to the third-party payer, the payer adjudicates the claims. **Adjudication** is the determination of the reimbursement amount based on the beneficiary's insurance plan benefits. When clean claims are submitted, electronic adjudication can occur. Four outcomes may occur from adjudication: payment, suspend, reject, or deny. If the outcome is "payment," then the reimbursement for the claim is paid without review or further processing.

If the outcome is "suspend," a claims examiner or claims analyst must review the claim. Claims may be suspended if they have claim attachments. In the adjudication of a claim, a claim attachment documents supplemental information that assists claims examiners in understanding specific services received by an individual and in determining payment. Examples of claim attachments include proof of prior authorization or documentation supporting medical necessity.

A "reject" outcome can occur at the claim level or the line-item level. For the UB-04 claim form, the line-item-level detail is entered into form locators 42 to 48 lines. Figure 11.2 displays the line-item-level section for a sample claim.

The payer may reject single or multiple line items on the claim but approve payment for the remaining lines. For most payers, a rejection indicates that the provider may correct the erroneous data element and submit the claim for readjudication. An example would be a missing or incorrect modifier, incorrect date of service, or missing HCPCS code.

A "denial" outcome may also be a claim denial or line-item denial. For most payers, a denial indicates that the provider must go through the appeals process if they disagree with the adjudication decision. Figure 11.3 illustrates the adjudication process.

Figure 11.2.   Line-item-level section for a sample claim

42 REV CD	43 DESCRIPTION	44 HCPCS/RATES	45 SERV. DATE	46 SERV. UNITS	47 TOTAL CHARGES		48 NON-COVERED CHARGES	49
0300	VENIPUNCTURE	36415	7/12/20	1	18	00		
0300	METABOLIC PANEL BASIC (CHEM 7)	80048	7/12/20	1	264	00		
0301	MAGNESIUM	83735	7/12/20	1	82	00		
0301	TROPONINI	84484	7/12/20	1	221	00		
0301	CBC	85025	7/12/20	1	82	00		
0320	XR SHOULDER COMPLETE	73030	7/12/20	1	350	00		
0424	P.T. EVAL	97001	7/12/20	1	295	00		
0450	ED STRAPPING SHOULDER	29240	7/12/20	1	640	00		
0450	ED VISIT LEVEL 3	99283	7/12/20	1	586	00		
0636	MORPHINE SULFATE 10 MG	J2270	7/12/20	2	308	00		
0636	LACTATED RINGERS 1000CC	J7120	7/12/20	1	75	00		

Source: Adapted from CDC n.d.

Figure 11.3.   Adjudication process

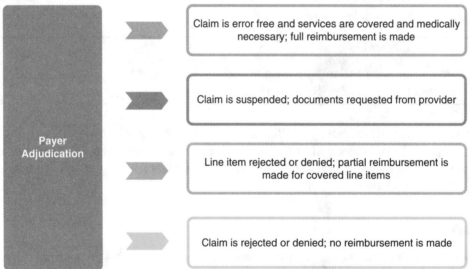

Medicare claims for Part A services and hospital-based Medicare Part B services are submitted to a designated A/B Medicare administrative contractor (MAC). MACs contract with Medicare to process claims for a specific region (CMS 2023a). The MAC adjudicates claims and administers reimbursement to providers for covered services on behalf of Medicare. MACs also conduct improper payment reviews. This MAC function is discussed further in chapter 13, "Revenue Compliance." Figure 11.4 shows the A/B MAC jurisdictions. After adjudication, third-party payers and MACs create benefits statements, as discussed in the next section.

Check Your Understanding 11.1

1. Why are auditing systems used during the claims production process?

2. Define accounts receivable.

3. What are the four outcomes of adjudication?

4. Which adjudication outcome requires the provider to appeal if they disagree with the insurance company's claim determination?

5. What is the government name for companies that process healthcare claims on behalf of Medicare?

Figure 11.4.   A/B MAC jurisdictions

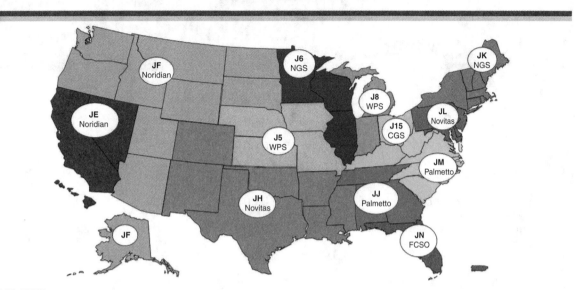

Source: CMS 2023b.

Benefits Statements

In addition to processing the claim for payment, third-party payers prepare an **explanation of benefits (EOB)** that is delivered to the patient. The EOB is a statement that describes services delivered, charges covered, reimbursement made, and benefit limits and denials. Specifically, for Medicare patients, MACs prepare **Medicare summary notices (MSNs)**. The MSN details amounts billed by the provider, amounts approved by Medicare, how much Medicare reimbursed the provider, and what the patient must pay the provider by way of deductible and copayments (CMS 2023c). Appendix F at the back of this text provides a sample MSN. EOBs and MSNs are part of the Transactions Rule and are sent to the patient via postal mail. Figure 11.5 is an example of an EOB.

EOB details can be challenging for beneficiaries to understand. The first set of data elements to discuss is charge, allowable charge, and contractual allowance. The charge is the actual charge the provider submitted to the insurance company for the healthcare service. As discussed earlier in the text, it is the price of the service or supply. The allowable charge is the amount that the payer has agreed to reimburse for the service provided to the beneficiary. The provider has agreed to accept the payment of the allowable charge as payment in full. The allowable charge is determined during the contract negotiation between the payer and the provider. The allowable charge is divided into two portions: the benefit payment for which the payer is responsible and the cost-sharing amount for which the beneficiary is responsible. The **contractual allowance** is the difference between the charge and the allowable charge. The contractual allowance is really an adjustment. Again, it is a result of the contract negotiations process. When the provider agrees to accept the allowable charge, the difference between the charge and the allowable charge becomes an adjustment in the provider's financial accounting system.

The next data element to discuss is other adjustment. Insurance companies use a variety of labels for this data element. In figure 11.5, the column labeled "Other Adjustment" represents the dollar amount for rejected or denied services. An example would be a noncovered service that is denied. This is how insurance companies identify line items that are not reimbursed.

The next data element is the cost-sharing amount. Payers may use a variety of labels for the cost-sharing data on the EOB. In chapter 2, "Health Insurance," cost sharing was discussed in detail. There are two primary types: coinsurance and copayments. In figure 11.5 the cost-sharing responsibility is represented by the column labeled "Coinsurance."

Figure 11.5.   Explanation of benefits

	Excellent Healthcare Insurance Company				Date: 08/19/202X		
	Patient's Name: Veronica Casto (Member) ID Number 123-45-6789				Date: 07/13/202X		
Line	Service	Charge	Contractual Allowance	Other Adjustment	Allowable Charge	Coinsurance	Benefit Payment
1	Surgery	1,045.00	812.88	0.00	232.12	46.42	185.70
2	Surgery	1,045.00	812.88	0.00	232.12	46.42	185.70
3	Surgery	1,320.00	730.99	0.00	589.01	117.80	471.21
4	Surgery	890.00	693.76	0.00	196.24	39.25	156.99
5	Surgery	765.00	327.84	0.00	437.16	87.43	349.73
Totals		**$5,065.00**	**$3,378.35**	**$0.00**	**$1,686.65**	**$337.32**	**$1,349.33**
$500 of $500 deductible met as of 06/30/202X							

The last data element is the benefit payment. The EOB includes an accounting of the reimbursement made to the provider by line item or service. In figure 11.5 the reimbursement is represented by the label "Benefit Payment." Again, payers will use various terminology for this category. As mentioned earlier, the allowable charge includes the payer portion or benefit payment and the beneficiary cost-sharing portion. This is illustrated in figure 11.5. When the coinsurance amount ($46.42) is added to the benefit payment amount ($185.70) for line 1, the total is $232.12, which is equal to the allowable charge.

Upon receiving the EOB, the guarantor knows how much to pay the provider's billing office. As discussed in chapter 1, "Healthcare Reimbursement and Revenue Cycle Management," guarantors are the people responsible to pay the bill. Guarantors may be the policyholder, the subscriber, or the patient. The example in figure 11.5 shows that the guarantor is responsible for a payment of $337.32 for the services performed.

Claims Reconciliation

After the claim is adjudicated by the insurance company, **remittance advice (RA)** is electronically returned to the provider via the 835A or 835B electronic format. The RA is a report sent to the provider by third-party payers that outlines claim rejections, denials, and payments to the facility (CMS 2021). Payments are typically made in batches, with the RA sent to the facility and payments submitted to the provider through electronic funds transfer. An RA contains the following additional information:

- Names of multiple patients and their account numbers
- Prior approval number (authorization or precertification number)
- Provider or practitioner number (in addition to name and address)
- Tax identification number
- Check number and amount
- Payment date

- *International Classification of Diseases, Tenth Revision, Clinical Modification* (ICD-10-CM) diagnosis code(s)

- *International Classification of Diseases, Tenth Revision, Procedure Coding System* (ICD-10-PCS) procedure code(s) for inpatient claims

- HCPCS code(s) and modifier(s) for provider and outpatient claims

- Units of services

- Claim status (paid, suspended, rejected, denied, or reversed)

- Reason codes for rejections, denials, noncovered charges, reversals, and other allowances

Once the healthcare facility or provider receives the RA, the claims reconciliation process begins. Facilities and providers compare the expected reimbursement for the claim to the reimbursement received by the payer. Claims reconciliation is a crucial component of the revenue cycle. Specialists in this area work to ensure that the provider can recover all warranted reimbursements for services that have been provided to beneficiaries. This is critical for the organization's financial health. By reviewing and monitoring the RAs, providers can determine the efficiency and effectiveness of their claim submission process. Revenue integrity professionals reconcile accounts based on the information provided in the RA with the expected reimbursement calculated by the provider.

Claims that are denied are submitted to the denials management team for evaluation and the appeals process if warranted. Denials management is discussed in detail in chapter 13, "Revenue Compliance." Claims that include rejections are evaluated for correction. Claims are entered into a corrections workflow that typically involves a coding professional who reexamines the medical documentation to ensure that modifications to the claim are in alignment with revenue integrity principles. Claims may then be paid by the payer after the resubmission or may remain as denied, as depicted in figure 11.6. Adjustments are made to the accounts to reflect the outcome of the appeal.

Collections

Healthcare facilities and providers use RA to reconcile accounts. Not only do they ensure that the third-party payer has reimbursed their portion of the allowable charge, they also ensure that the guarantor has paid their cost-sharing amount in full. Providers may have an internal collection unit or may contract with a collection agency to recover cost-sharing amounts. Collections specialists contact the patient to collect outstanding deductibles and cost-sharing amounts.

It is best practice for providers to collect estimated cost-sharing amounts prior to treatment, but often the estimates are not accurate due to assumptions made about the status of the patient's deductible amount or

Figure 11.6.   Denial management process

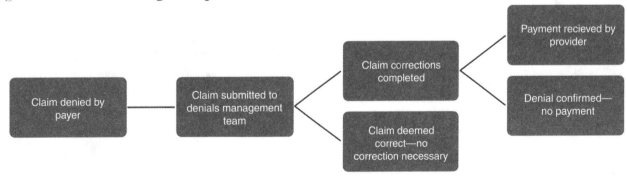

out-of-pocket maximum. If the patient is not able to pay the cost-sharing amount, most providers allow patients to make monthly payments until the amount is settled. Financial counselors, as described in chapter 9, "Revenue Cycle Front-End Processes—Patient Engagement," also assist patients in determining the best strategy to pay the cost-sharing amount if the pretreatment estimate was not accurate.

Revenue Cycle Professions

Part III, "Revenue Cycle Processes," of this text discusses in detail the components of the revenue cycle and their associated tasks. A summary of the revenue cycle and the processes is provided in figure 11.7.

The curriculum of HIM baccalaureate and associate programs provides the necessary educational foundation for graduates to obtain careers in the revenue cycle. In addition to an HIM background, there are several opportunities for HIM professionals to earn credentials specific to the revenue cycle. The American Association of Healthcare Administrative Management (AAHAM) provides the following credentials:

- Certified revenue cycle executive (CRCE)
- Certified revenue cycle professional (CRCP)
- Certified revenue integrity professional (CRIP)
- Certified revenue cycle specialist (CRCS)
- Certified compliance technician (CCT) (AAHAM n.d.)

Figure 11.7.   **Revenue cycle components and tasks**

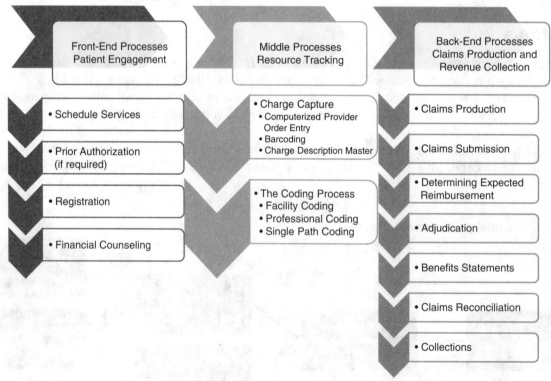

Additionally, the Healthcare Financial Management Association provides the following credentials:

- Certified revenue cycle representative (CRCR)
- Certified specialist payment and reimbursement (CSPR) (HFMA 2023)

These credentials benefit both HIM professionals and their employers. For individuals, an additional credential can help them improve their salary, increase their knowledge base, and navigate their career path (AAHAM n.d.). For employers, credentials increase the competency of staff, increase the productivity and quality of employee performance, and promote an environment of ongoing education and training (AAHAM n.d.).

Patient Connection

Olivia took her new baby boy, Felix, for his two-months visit with Dr. King. Dr. King examined Felix and talked to Olivia about his progress. Dr. King addressed all of Olivia's questions. Dr. King discussed the recommended immunization schedule with Olivia. Before the visit, Olivia reviewed her summary of benefits and coverage (SBC) for coverage for immunizations. The recommended schedule aligned with coverage under Super Payer, so Felix received his shots. Three weeks later, Olivia received an EOB in the mail for the pediatrician visit. Following is the EOB.

The total charges for the well-baby visit were $995. Olivia notices that her coinsurance amount is $0 for the whole visit. She quickly pulls up her Super Payer SBC. (Following is an excerpt from Olivia's SBC.) The SBC indicates that there is no cost sharing for preventive care, screening, or immunization services. Therefore, the coinsurance column on the EOB indicates $0 for all services. Olivia notices how expensive immunizations are, and she is very happy that she chose a health plan from Super Payer that provides excellent coverage for preventive care and immunizations.

Super Payer Insurance Company					Date: 10/02/202X		
Patient's Name: Felix			Member Number: 123-45-8		Service Date: 09/10/202X		
Line	Service	Charge	Contractual Allowance	Other Adjustment	Allowable Charge	Coinsurance	Benefit Payment
1	Immunization adm 1st vaccine	$100.00	$45.00	$0.00	$55.00	$0.00	$55.00
2	Immunization adm each add'l vaccine	$100.00	$45.00	$0.00	$55.00	$0.00	$55.00
3	Immunization adm each add'l vaccine	$100.00	$45.00	$0.00	$55.00	$0.00	$55.00
4	Immunization adm oral	$75.00	$33.75	$0.00	$41.25	$0.00	$41.25
5	Vaccine: Dtap HepB IPV	$105.00	$63.00	$0.00	$42.00	$0.00	$42.00
6	Vaccine: PCV	$170.00	$102.00	$0.00	$68.00	$0.00	$68.00

(continued)

Patient Connection   *(continued)*

7	Vaccine: RV	$65.00	$39.00	$0.00	$26.00	$0.00	$26.00
8	Vaccine: Hib	$30.00	$18.00	$0.00	$12.00	$0.00	$12.00
9	Well-baby visit	$250.00	$112.50	$0.00	$137.50	$0.00	$137.50
Totals		$995.00	$503.25	$0.00	$491.75	$0.00	$491.75
$500 of $500 deductible met as of 03/15/202X							

		What You Will Pay	
Common Medical Event	Services You May Need	Network Provider (You will pay the least)	Out-of-Network Provider (You will pay the most)
If you visit a healthcare provider's office or clinic	Primary care visit to treat an injury or illness	$35 copay/office visit 20% coinsurance for other outpatient services provided during the office visit; deductible does not apply	35% coinsurance
	Specialist visit	$50 copay/visit	50% coinsurance
	Preventive care/ screening/ immunization	No charge	35% coinsurance

Chapter 11 Review Quiz

1. What is a scrubber? When is it used in the revenue cycle process?

2. What electronic format do most facilities use to submit claims to insurance companies?

3. Compare accrual and cash accounting. Why is accrual accounting the better method for healthcare?

4. Which entity performs adjudication—the facility, the provider, or the insurance company?

5. What actions do providers take when a claim or line item is rejected?

6. Provide an example of why a claim would be suspended during the adjudication process.

7. Describe the relationship between the following EOB data elements: charge, allowable charge, and contractual allowance.

8. Fill in the blank. The _____ is the sum of the benefit payment and the cost-sharing amount.

9. The RA indicates line items and claims that are denied. What happens to denied claims?

10. What is the best practice for collection of a patient's cost-sharing amount?

References

AAHAM (American Association of Healthcare Administrative Management). n.d. "Certification." Accessed May 17, 2023. https://aaham.org/page/Certification.

CDC (Centers for Disease Control and Prevention). n.d. "UB-40-P." Accessed February 24, 2023. https://www.cdc.gov/wtc/pdfs/policies/ub-40-P.pdf.

CMS (Centers for Medicare and Medicaid Services). 2023a. "What's a MAC." https://www.cms.gov/Medicare/Medicare-Contracting/Medicare-Administrative-Contractors/What-is-a-MAC.

CMS (Centers for Medicare and Medicaid Services). 2023b. "Who Are the MACs." https://www.cms.gov/Medicare/Medicare-Contracting/Medicare-Administrative-Contractors/Who-are-the-MACs.

CMS (Centers for Medicare and Medicaid Services). 2023c. "Medicare Summary Notice." https://www.cms.gov/Medicare/Medicare-General-Information/MSN.

CMS (Centers for Medicare and Medicaid Services). 2022a. "Transactions Overview." https://www.cms.gov/Regulations-and-Guidance/Administrative-Simplification/Transactions/TransactionsOverview.

CMS (Centers for Medicare and Medicaid Services). 2022b. "Code Sets Overview." https://www.cms.gov/Regulations-and-Guidance/Administrative-Simplification/Code-Sets.

CMS (Centers for Medicare and Medicaid Services). 2021. "Health Care Payment and Remittance Advice." https://www.cms.gov/Medicare/Billing/ElectronicBillingEDITrans/Remittance.

HFMA (Healthcare Financial Management Association). 2023. "Certifications." https://www.hfma.org/education-events/certifications/?gclid=CjwKCAjw9pGjBhB-EiwAa5jl3JZI9sE6oqxjF1_Hi5LedpnNWat07RaouCSfCiUFfCXG0HwrgXMLRhoC7UQQAvD_BwE.

HHS (Department of Health and Human Services). 2003. Health insurance reform: Security standards; Final rule. *Federal Register* 68(34):8333–8399.

White, S. 2018. *Principles of Finance for Health Information and Informatics Professionals*, 2nd ed. Chicago: AHIMA.

Part IV:
Revenue Cycle Management

Chapter 12
Coding and Clinical Documentation Integrity Management

Learning Objectives

❖ Distinguish between different levels of coding professionals' expertise

❖ Describe the process for determining coding productivity standards

❖ Implement coding management responsibilities

❖ Describe tasks included in a clinical documentation integrity program

❖ Execute clinical documentation integrity tasks and functions

Key Terms

Benchmarking
CC/MCC capture rate
Clean claim rate
Clinical documentation integrity (CDI)
Coding compliance plan
Coding management
Computer-assisted coding (CAC)
Denial rate

Discharge status code
Discharged, not final billed (DNFB)
Encoder
Key performance indicator (KPI)
Program for Evaluating Payment Patterns
    Electronic Report (PEPPER)
Query

The coding process is highly regulated and, therefore, sound management practices are mandatory. Although coding is typically a function within the health information management (HIM) department, the support of accurate coding begins with the documentation in the medical record. **Clinical documentation integrity (CDI)** is a program that strives to initiate concurrent and retrospective review of health records to improve the quality of provider documentation. Therefore, both coding management and CDI management are explored in this chapter. Both functions, coding and CDI, require direct and attentive management because they involve diagnosis and procedure codes that directly impact reimbursement amounts for most reimbursement methodologies.

Coding Management

Coding at the highest level of accuracy and efficiency is a key factor in revenue integrity. Therefore, management of the coding function is critical to ensure optimal performance. **Coding management** is the management unit responsible for organizing the coding process so healthcare data can be transformed into the meaningful information required for claims processing (Gentul and Davis 2011, 7). Coding management is carried out by the coding manager. The coding unit is typically comprised of a manager, inpatient and outpatient coding professionals, and data quality analysts. The coding manager is responsible for hiring qualified staff for coding and data quality analyst positions, ensuring proper tools are available, conducting performance assessments, and providing continuing education.

Staffing

The coding manager is responsible for hiring coding professionals. Coding professionals have varying levels of expertise, so it is important for the coding manager to place coding professionals in a position that is compatible with their skill level. Coding professionals can be divided into three levels of expertise: entry-level, experienced, and expert. Figure 12.1 provides characteristics of each level of expertise.

Figure 12.1 indicates that coding credentials express proficiency in coding. However, there are several coding credentials available. It is important for the coding manager to understand the differences among coding credentials so that coding professionals can be placed in the appropriate role. Table 12.1 provides a summary of coding and other applicable HIM credentials.

Determining the appropriate position for a coding professional is a critical function of the coding manager. Placing a coding professional in a role that the individual is not prepared for can lead to frustration, poor performance, and coding turnover. Likewise, placing a coding professional in a role that does not challenge an individual can lead to boredom, lack of interest, and, again, turnover. Throughout the US, coding professionals at all levels of expertise, but especially at the experienced level, are a scarce resource. Therefore, it is essential to keep turnover rates low. With or without a lack of experienced coding professionals, coding managers must invest in entry-level coding professionals to build their team and properly promote them through the progression of coding positions to retain them. Figure 12.2 provides a sample coding position progression. Position responsibilities are provided to give context to the position titles.

It is also important for the coding manager to understand that some coding professionals do not want to have management responsibilities. Good communication with staff members will make clear that their progression may be limited if they do not desire management responsibilities. Regardless of career trajectory, mastery of coding tools is required for all positions within the coding department. The next section will explore common coding tools.

Figure 12.1.   Coding professional characteristics by level of expertise

Entry-Level Coding Professional

- Completed coding coursework in a college or technical program
- Has little experience coding medical records, typically less than 1 year
- Typically uncredentialed
- Requires significant training
- May have slower productivity

Experienced Coding Professional

- Has coded at least 1 year in an area of practice
- Most have a coding credential
- Proficient in same-day surgery/complex ambulatory coding
- Limited exposure to inpatient coding
- Meets productivity and accuracy measures

Expert Coding Professional

- Has mastery skill in multiple code sets
- Numerous years of experience; most likely greater than 5 years
- High level of productivity
- High level of accuracy
- Has one or more coding credentials

Source: Adapted from Gentul and Davis 2011, 5–7.

Table 12.1.   Summary of coding and other applicable HIM credentials

Credential	Title	Granting Organization	Credential Holders Demonstrate
CCA	Certified coding associate	AHIMA	• Coding competency across all settings, including hospitals and physician practices
CCS	Certified coding specialist	AHIMA	• Ability to classify medical data from patient records, often in a hospital setting • Expertise in ICD-10-CM/PCS and CPT coding systems • Knowledge of medical terminology, disease processes, and pharmacology concepts
CCS-P	Certified coding specialist—physician-based	AHIMA	• Specialization in physician-based settings • In-depth knowledge of the CPT coding system and familiarity with the ICD-10-CM and HCPCS Level II coding systems • Expertise in health information documentation, data integrity and quality
CPC	Certified professional coder	AAPC	• Proficiency in the correct application of CPT, HCPCS Level II procedure and supply codes, and ICD-10-CM diagnosis codes • Proficiency across a wide range of services including evaluation and management, anesthesia, surgery, radiology, pathology, and medicine • Knowledge of coding guidelines and regulations to meet compliance requirements
COC	Certified outpatient coder	AAPC	• Proficiency in the correct application of CPT, HCPCS Level II procedure and supply codes, and ICD-10-CM diagnosis codes • Proficiency in assigning accurate medical codes for diagnoses, procedures, and services performed in the outpatient setting and outpatient therapies • Knowledge of coding guidelines and regulations to meet compliance requirements
CIC	Certified inpatient coder	AAPC	• Expertise in assigning accurate ICD-10 medical codes for diagnoses and procedures performed in the inpatient setting • Superior knowledge of current rules, regulations, and issues regarding medical coding, compliance, and reimbursement under MS-DRG system and IPPS • Strong ability to integrate coding and reimbursement rule changes into revenue cycle processes

(continued)

Table 12.1.   *(continued)*

Credential	Title	Granting Organization	Credential Holders Demonstrate
CRC	Certified risk adjustment coder	AAPC	• Proficiency in the correct application of ICD-10-CM diagnosis codes used in risk adjustment payment models • Assign accurate medical codes for diagnosis performed by physicians and other qualified healthcare providers • Understanding of the audit process for risk adjustment models • Ability to identify and communicate documentation deficiencies to providers to improve documentation for accurate risk adjustment coding
RHIA	Registered health information administrator	AHIMA	• Ability to manage people and operational units • Expertise in managing patient health information and medical records, collecting and analyzing patient data • Expertise in using classification systems and medical terminologies • Comprehensive knowledge of medical, administrative, ethical, and legal requirements and standards related to healthcare delivery and privacy of protected patient information
RHIT	Registered health information technician	AHIMA	• Ability to ensure the quality of medical records by verifying their completeness, accuracy, and proper entry into computer systems • Specialization in coding diagnoses and procedures in patient records for reimbursement and research • Compiling and maintaining data on cancer patients as a cancer registrar

Sources: AHIMA n.d.; AAPC n.d.a.

Coding Tools

Coding units rely on coding tools to ensure complete, consistent, and efficient coding. Coding managers may use a variety of, and at times several, coding tools to improve the coding process. As discussed in chapter 10, "Revenue Cycle Middle Processes—Resource Tracking," the code sets designated in the Health Insurance Portability and Accountability Act of 1996 (HIPAA)—*International Classification of Diseases, Tenth Revision, Clinical Modification* (ICD-10-CM), *International Classification of Diseases, Tenth Revision, Procedural Coding System* (ICD-10-PCS), and the Healthcare Common Procedure Coding System (HCPCS)—are a primary tool for coding units. Thus, coding managers should ensure that all coders have access to current code sets through print books or electronic means. Access to the codes sets, however, is not enough. Coding professionals should also have access to the coding guidelines published for each code set, as discussed in chapter 10. In the upcoming sections, three additional key coding tools are discussed: facility-specific coding guidelines, coding and abstraction platforms, and computer-assisted coding (CAC).

Facility-Specific Coding Guidelines

Coding professionals are trained to correctly interpret and apply the ICD-10-CM Official Coding Guidelines for Coding and Reporting and the ICD-10-PCS Official Coding Guidelines for Coding and Reporting. Additionally,

Figure 12.2. Sample coding position progression

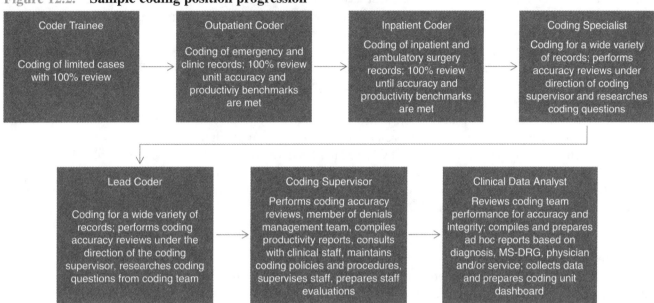

Source: Adapted from Gentul and Davis 2011, 79.

coding professionals follow advice presented in the *AHA Coding Clinic for ICD-10-CM and ICD-10-PCS*, *CPT Assistant*, and *AHA Coding Clinic for HCPCS*. Aside from these national standards, facilities often develop their own internal guidelines. The goals of facility-specific coding guidelines are to (1) encourage complete documentation that supports consistent code assignment and (2) serve as a training tool for newly hired coding professionals. Facility-specific coding guidelines should not duplicate or contradict the official coding guidelines and official coding advice. Rather, the internal guidelines should lead a facility's coding staff to report diagnoses and procedures in a consistent way. Sample facility-specific guideline topics include the following:

- When to query a physician for clarification

- Procedures that are soft coded at the facility

- Procedures that are hard coded at the facility

- Documents that are appropriate to use in the coding process (namely, problem list)

- Appropriate use of unlisted Current Procedural Terminology (CPT) codes

- Appropriate use of ICD-10-CM status codes (namely, amputation status) (Johnson and Rickard 2020)

This topic list illustrates how facility-specific coding guidelines are necessary for training new coding professionals, collecting consistent data, and tracking the changes of data collection from year to year (Johnson and Rickard 2020). Developing facility-specific coding guidelines is a laborious process, and yearly maintenance is required. The American Health Information Management Association (AHIMA) provides a practice brief to assist coding managers with these tasks. Developing Facility-Specific Coding Guidelines was published in 2020 and is available in the AHIMA HIM Body of Knowledge.

Coding and Abstraction Platform

Facilities and physician practices use a variety of coding and abstraction platforms to insert coded data into the electronic health record (EHR). Some platforms may be included in the EHR system used by the facility or practice. Some may be from a different vendor and interface than the EHR system. The sophistication of the platforms varies greatly by vendor and by setting. The most advanced platforms typically include an encoder solution. An **encoder** is a software program used to facilitate the assignment of diagnostic and procedure codes according to the rules of the coding system (Sayles 2020, 87). Using an encoder increases the consistency and efficiency of the coding process. The encoder moves the coding professional through the coding process by prompting them with queries that follow ICD-10-CM and ICD-10-PCS coding conventions and guidelines. Additionally, some encoders allow the user to calculate the reimbursement classification, such as Medicare severity-diagnosis related group (MS-DRG) or ambulatory payment classification (APC), for the encounter.

However, not all coding and abstraction platforms include an encoder, especially those geared toward the physician office setting. Instead, many physician-based EHR systems include search functions that allow the physician or clinician to search for an ICD-10-CM or HCPCS code by clinical terms. For example, the physician can search for diagnosis codes by entering "type 2 diabetes." The system will provide a drop-down list of all type 2 diabetes codes, and the physician can select the correct code. One drawback to this method of coding is that the coding conventions and guidelines for ICD-10-CM are often not utilized, which can lead to incorrect sequencing of codes and poor coding accuracy.

Computer-Assisted Coding

Many facilities use **computer-assisted coding (CAC)** as a tool to improve coding efficiency and support code accuracy. CAC is the process of extracting and translating dictated and then transcribed free-text data (or dictated and then computer-generated discrete data) into diagnostic and procedural codes of varying classifications for billing and coding purposes. The foundation of CAC is natural language processing (NLP). NLP is a technology that converts human language (structured or unstructured) into data that can be translated and then manipulated by computer systems. It is a branch of artificial intelligence. The basic CAC process is displayed in figure 12.3.

As shown in figure 12.3, the CAC process includes the coding professional applying coding principles and then validating CAC-suggested codes. The software "learns" from the coding professional's validation and final code selection and improves on what codes are automatically suggested on future encounters. The more the coding professional works with the CAC system, the more refined the software becomes. It is important to make clear to leadership and staff that CAC is used to *assist* coding professionals, not replace them (Land 2019, 33). If used properly, CAC can improve coding efficiency. A 2013 study showed that coding professionals' use of CAC software resulted in a 22 percent reduction in coding time per record (Dougherty et al. 2013, 54–56). Additionally, the study showed that the use of CAC did not reduce accuracy.

Facilities typically use a staged approach for CAC implementation starting with the outpatient ancillary setting and moving toward the inpatient setting. It is important to closely monitor CAC performance through the implementation phases. The following list of tips can help coding managers ensure optimal use of CAC software:

- Clinicians do not use consistent verbiage. Further, the verbiage doesn't always match CAC's NLP mapping. It is important to incorporate careful validation of auto-suggested codes to prevent incorrect code assignment.

- NLP identifies every instance of a word in the software parameters. Coders must validate the suggested codes and choose the correct code when multiple variations of the same condition are suggested multiple times.

- CAC does not evaluate the quality of documentation and may erroneously auto-suggest codes that require clarification from the physician to support revenue integrity. For example, CAC may suggest a code from the history and physical that has since been resolved.

- CAC may suggest codes from ancillary reports that have not been validated by the clinician. During the validation step, coding professionals must ensure that the documentation is clinically validated. (Land 2019, 32–33)

Figure 12.3. **Basic CAC process**

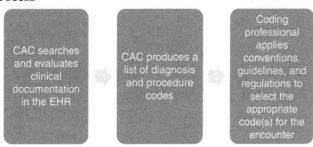

Achieving optimal use of CAC software takes time and patience, but significant payoffs in consistency and efficiency are often worth the effort. In addition to CAC, facility-specific coding guidelines and coding and abstraction platforms enhance coding performance. They allow individual coding professionals and coding units to be more consistent and efficient at coding medical records. Because the diagnosis and procedures often impact reimbursement amounts, optimal performance is desired and closely monitored. In the next section, topics to support performance assessment are discussed.

Performance Assessment

A critical component of coding management is performance assessment. Coding managers must evaluate coding professional performance on an ongoing basis. There are three main performance criteria to consider:

- Productivity: number of medical records coded per hour

- Accuracy: coding is error-free and complete

- Query appropriateness: queries are issued when appropriate, are free of error, and are respectful

Based on the tasks assigned to coding professionals in individual hospitals, more criteria may be warranted. Examples include abstraction accuracy and query production. A **query** is a provider communication tool used concurrently or retrospectively to obtain documentation clarification (AHIMA 2016, 7). In order to assess performance, coding managers need to establish performance measures. Measures can be based on past performance, results of benchmarking, or results of research studies from professional associations such as AHIMA. To determine whether coding professionals' performance meets standards, the coding manager must establish regular monitoring of staff. Monitoring may not need to take place daily, but it must be consistent and in accordance with policies and procedures. In the next sections, the three main performance criteria—productivity, accuracy, and query appropriateness—will be explored.

Productivity

Coding productivity is the expected number of medical records coded per working hour. The coding unit will have multiple productivity measures because a variety of record types are coded. For example, the standard for coding emergency department records will be different than the standard for inpatient records. The coding manager will need to determine how many productivity measures are applicable for the unit. There are several factors to determine when establishing performance standards. The factors can be divided into three categories: facility influencers, coding professional influencers, and medical record influencers. Figure 12.4 provides a summary of the factors by category.

The coding manager must consider which of these influencers are applicable for their facility or practice. For example, if the facility is an 850-bed teaching hospital with a Level I trauma unit, it will probably take longer to code an inpatient record than a 200-bed community hospital. Likewise, if the setting is a cardiology practice that involves

Figure 12.4.   Coding productivity factors by category

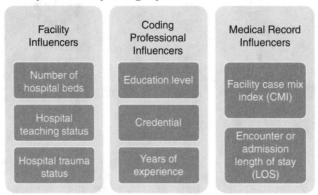

Source: Adapted from Alakrawi et al. 2017, 40–45.

several surgeons, the time it takes to code a record is most likely longer than a record from a family practice that does not include surgeons.

Coding professional influencers are very important. Education, credentials earned, and years of experience can cause productivity rates to significantly vary from coder to coder. Therefore, coding managers may want to include expected productivity levels in the various coding positions included in the unit (see figure 12.2). By doing so, the productivity standard takes into consideration the coding professional influencers. Set productivity standards by coding position also help the coding manager determine when a coding professional is ready to be considered for a promotion. The productivity standard for a coding trainee should differ from an inpatient coder. Not only does the type of medical record vary (outpatient versus inpatient), but the coding professional characteristics vary as well.

Lastly, medical record influencers impact productivity standards at the most granular level, meaning aspects of an individual admission impact the time required to code that record. In a 2017 coding productivity study, researchers found that nearly 13 percent of productivity variability was due to facility case-mix index (CMI) and encounter length of stay (LOS) (Alakrawi et al. 2017, 40–45). CMI is a value that compares the overall complexity of the healthcare organization's mix of patients with the complexity of the average of all hospitals. The more complex the encounter measured by MS-DRG relative weight, the longer it took to code the record. Likewise, the greater the LOS, the longer it took to code the record (Alakrawi et al. 2017, 40–45). Therefore, coding managers may want to consider CMI and LOS when establishing the productivity standard range. Example 12.1 describes the process for the development of a coding productivity standard.

Example 12.1

Kerry is the coding manager at Community Hospital. According to statistics from the coding and abstraction platform, on average it takes 25 minutes to code an inpatient admission. The admission LOS impacts the time. For an admission of one to two days, it takes 14 minutes to code the medical record. For an admission of 9 to 10 days, it takes 41 minutes to code the record. To create a productivity range, Kerry must calculate the number of records that could be coded per day if all records were 9 to 10 LOSs to establish the lower bound. Kerry has determined that her inpatient coder position has 420 minutes per day to code medical records.

420 minutes/41 minutes = 10 records per day

Likewise, Kerry must determine the upper bound by determining how many inpatient records could be coded per day if all of the records had an LOS of one to two days.

420 minutes/14 minutes = 30 records per day

(continued)

Therefore, the acceptable range for an inpatient coder would be 10 to 30 records per day. However, to meet productivity standards, a coding professional that averages 10 per day must have supporting data from the coding and abstraction system that show that the records coded were all 9-to-10-day LOS admissions. If the data do not support this, then the coding professional has not met productivity standards.

The concepts shown in example 12.1 can be applied to CMI as well to further fortify the productivity standard. In today's environment, coding productivity standards cannot be "cookie-cutter" standards. Facility, coding professional, and admission characteristics that influence coding productivity must be taken into consideration to set a standard that is challenging yet applicable to the individual coding unit.

Accuracy

Coding accuracy includes confirmation that the diagnosis and procedure code(s) assigned for an encounter are the correct codes and that all required codes are present. For an inpatient or outpatient encounter reported on a facility claim, this includes the admitting diagnosis, principal diagnosis, secondary diagnoses, principal procedure, and secondary procedure(s). Additionally, for outpatient claims this includes modifiers. For an encounter reported for a provider claim, this includes diagnosis codes with diagnosis pointer, procedure codes, service codes, supply codes, and modifiers. Most coding managers include correct discharge status code in the accuracy measure. **Discharge status code**, also known as discharge disposition, is a code reported on an inpatient claim to identify where the patient is being discharged or transferred to at the end of their stay. Discharge status codes are specific to the UB-04 claim form and only applicable to the inpatient setting. Examples of discharge status codes include the following:

- 01: Discharge to home or self-care (routine discharge)
- 03: Discharged/transferred to a skilled nursing facility (SNF) with Medicare certification in anticipation of skilled care
- 06: Discharged/transferred to home under care of organized home health service organization in anticipation of covered skilled care
- 07: Left against medical advice or discontinued care
- 20: Expired (Noridian 2022)

Most coding managers require an accuracy rate of 95 percent, although this rate can be adjusted for coding trainees or new coding professionals who are working their way to proficiency. It is best practice to have regular, predetermined periods of monitoring to determine accuracy for coding professionals. For example, the coding manager should monitor and determine accuracy for a lead coder at least once per month. During the monitoring period, the coding manager or designated auditor will evaluate coding performance. The auditor would verify the accuracy of codes the coding team member reports. The auditor will keep statistics that, over time, will produce the accuracy rate. At the end of the performance year, the coding manager will combine data from all periods of review to determine the annual accuracy rate.

Some coding staff members may require additional periods of monitoring. For example, a new hire should be monitored more often throughout their probationary period. The coding manager should collect sufficient accuracy data through this 90-day period to determine whether the new coding professional meets the qualification for the position and should continue on after the probation period has ended. Coding team members who have not met accuracy standards during past review periods should be monitored more often.

Periodically, coding managers may have an external auditor conduct a baseline audit to establish coder accuracy. This is typically a retrospective review where the auditor determines if records from the past year or six months were accurately coded. The audit will provide statistics on the accuracy rate, types of errors identified, and suggestions for educational topics needed for the coding team. Coding managers can use this baseline data to establish monitoring periods going forward. Audits are discussed in detail in chapter 13, "Revenue Compliance."

Query Appropriateness

With the proliferation of CDI programs across the US, some of the querying responsibility has been shifted to the CDI staff. CDI staff are a group of professionals who are trained in clinical documentation best practices—most commonly referred to as CDI specialists. Most CDI specialists have a coding background, a nursing background, or both. However, it is important to remember that only a portion of inpatient and outpatient admissions are included in the CDI review process. The admissions not included in the CDI review process may have clinical documentation that requires clarification during the coding process. Further, even admissions that were included in CDI activities may, after discharge, require a query from the coding staff. Therefore, it is important for the coding manager to ensure that queries issued by the coding staff are appropriate. The following criteria can be used to measure if a query is appropriate or compliant:

- It is clear and concise.

- It contains clinical indicators from the medical record.

- It presents only the facts identifying why the clarification is required.

- It does not include impact on reimbursement or quality measures.

- It aligns with facility or practice query policies and procedures that establish who to query, what to query, and how to query. (AHIMA-ACDIS 2019, 3–5)

Writing a compliant query is not an easy task. The coding unit, CDI specialists, and clinicians have a shared goal that everyone who reviews the medical record documentation can understand the clinical and procedural aspects of the admission. Writing queries requires a significant amount of clinical knowledge. In this question, the coding professional should be clear on what information they expect to receive back from the clinician. Some basic tips for writing queries include the following:

- Avoid making the query confusing or convoluted, and be as clear and concise as possible.

- Avoid asking multiple questions in the same query.

- Do not introduce a new diagnosis in the question.

- Do not put response options in the question. Response options, such as a list of potential diagnoses, may be provided in a separate section of the query after the question is introduced. See example 12.3 below.

- Do not lead the physician to an answer.

A good query should contain clinical information from the medical record. Figure 12.5 highlights clinical information, when available, that could be used in the query to assist the clinician in answering the main question. For example, if the coding professional is asking the physician about chronic kidney disease, then the baseline creatinine should be included in the clinical section of the query.

Examples 12.2 and 12.3 provide more insight into creating compliant queries. It is important not to lead the physician or clinician to an answer to the query. The query should be constructed so the physician can review pertinent clinical indicators and provide a more specific diagnosis, if applicable, without influence.

Figure 12.5.   **Clinical information for queries**

Clinical Indicators	Treatment and Monitoring	Related Conditions
• Signs and symptoms suggesting the diagnosis • Vital sign derangements • Abnormalities on physical exam • Abnormal laboratory, imaging, etc.	• Medications, transfusion, therapy, etc. • Planned work-up, procedures • Linkage, cause and effect, etiology	• Risk factors • Comorbidities

Example 12.2 Clinical Scenario

A patient is admitted with pneumonia. The admitting H&P examination reveals a WBC of 14,000; a respiratory rate of 24; a temperature of 102 degrees; a heart rate of 120; hypotension; and altered mental status. The patient is administered an IV antibiotic and IV flue resuscitation.

Leading query: The patient has elevated WBCs, tachycardia, and is given an IV antibiotic for pseudomonas cultured from the blood. Are you treating sepsis?

Nonleading query: Based on your clinical judgement, can you please provide a diagnosis that represents the below-listed indicators?

- Elevated WBCs
- Tachycardia
- IV-antibiotic administration

Please document the condition and causative organism (if known) in the medical record.

Source: AHIMA 2013.

Example 12.3 Clinical Scenario

A patient is admitted for a right hip fracture. The H&P notes that the patient has a history of chronic congestive heart failure. A recent echocardiogram showed left ventricular ejection fraction of 25 percent. The patient's home medications include metoprolol XL, lisinopril, and Lasix.

Leading query: Please document if you agree that the patient has chronic diastolic heart failure.

Nonleading query: It is noted in the impression of the H&P that the patient has chronic congestive heart failure, and a recent echocardiogram noted under the cardiac review of systems reveals an EF of 25 percent. Can you please further specify the type of chronic heart failure?

The following options are available for consideration:

- Chronic systolic heart failure

(continued)

Example 12.3 Clinical Scenario   *(continued)*

- Chronic diastolic heart failure

- Chronic systolic and diastolic heart failure

- Some other type of heart failure

- Undetermined

Please circle an option, if applicable.

Source: AHIMA 2013.

AHIMA and the Association of Clinical Documentation Improvement Specialists (ACDIS) provide several tools, including query templates, free of charge to coding managers to help them develop internal query policies and procedures. The use of queries by the CDI specialists is discussed in detail later in this chapter.

Coding Dashboard

Coding managers assess the performance of individual coding professionals, but they are also responsible for assessing the performance of the coding unit as a whole. The coding manager can develop a coding dashboard to monitor and assess **key performance indicators (KPIs)** for their unit. A KPI is a quantifiable measure of performance over time for a specific objective (Qlik n.d.). Recommended KPIs are included in figure 12.6.

In the inpatient hospital setting, CMI is based on the MS-DRG's relative weight, which is part of the Medicare inpatient prospective payment system. CMI may be used to compare the overall complexity of a healthcare organization's patients with the complexity of the average of all hospitals. It is monitored by the coding manager monthly because coding accuracy has a significant influence on the MS-DRG assignment. If coding accuracy falls below the standard, MS-DRG assignment could be negatively impacted. Therefore, CMI is often used as a measure of how effective coding management is at the facility. Typically, CMI is calculated for a specific period and is derived from the sum of all MS-DRG weights divided by the number of cases for the period under review. See chapter 14, "Healthcare Data in Action: Real-World Analysis," for step-by-step instructions to calculate CMI. CMI reflects the accuracy of coding for diagnoses and procedures that are used to assign the MS-DRG for inpatient encounters. When CMI shifts up or down, the coding manager can perform an analysis to determine the root cause of the variance. The root cause may or may not be related to coding performance. It is important to acknowledge that other factors can impact a facility's CMI, such as shifts in surgery volume, newly purchased equipment such

Figure 12.6.   KPIs recommended for coding dashboard

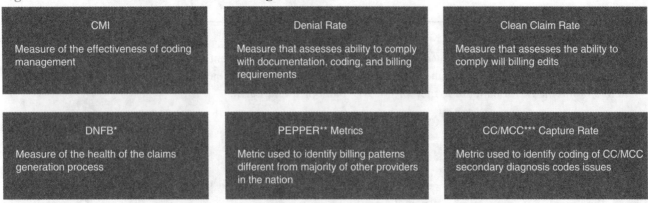

*Discharged, not final billed (DNFB)
**Program for Evaluating Payment Patterns Electronic Report (PEPPER)
***Complication/Comorbidity (CC)/Major Complication/Comorbidity (MCC)

as ventilators, or recently opened or closed service lines. Shifts in volume can have a significant impact on CMI. However, if coding performance is identified as a root cause of the CMI shift, it is important for the coding manager to quickly assess if the shift is following principles of revenue integrity.

Denial rate is a metric used to determine if the coding unit complies with coding requirements. Denial rate is a different measure of coding accuracy. If reimbursement is denied because an admission was incorrectly coded, then the coding error is included in the denial rate. Again, it is important to remember that there are many causes in claims denials, including failure to submit medical documents to the payer, failure to meet medical necessity, performing services in an inappropriate setting, and failure to comply with state or federal regulations. Another aspect of denials to remember is that the appeals process can be quite long. So, the denial rate used in the dashboard should be for encounters where the appeals process has been exhausted or terminated. Denial management is discussed in detail in chapter 13, "Revenue Compliance."

The **clean claim rate** measures the coding unit's ability to comply with billing edits. Clean claim rate is a great metric for outpatient and provider coding where several billing edits have been established by Medicare and other payers. For example, the Medicare National Correct Coding Initiative (NCCI) provides edits for both the outpatient facility and provider settings. The edits are designed to promote correct coding. Other examples include the edits included in the Medicare Code Editor for the inpatient setting and the Medicare Outpatient Code Editor for the outpatient setting. These editing systems are used by the Medicare administrative contractors (MACs) to ensure that claims are accurate and complete prior to reimbursement. These and other coding and billing compliance tools are discussed in detail in chapter 13, "Revenue Compliance."

Discharged, not final billed (DNFB) is a measure of the health of the claims generation process. It can be measured in days or in dollars. This is a different view of coding productivity. If coding productivity is reduced, the DNFB could rise because medical records are not being coded and cannot be released for claim submission to the payer. The opposite is true as well; increases in coding productivity can reduce the DNFB, allowing shorter waiting periods for claims generation after discharge. Coding managers must take DNFB into consideration when granting personal time off for their staff. Likewise, coding managers must take action if illnesses or natural disasters prevent staff from working at full capacity. Like all the other measures, there are other factors that can impact DNFB, such as delays in the pathology department completing pathology reports for specimens removed during surgery, or delays in physician completion of operative reports or other key clinical documentation.

Coding managers can use comparative data sets, such as the **Program for Evaluating Payment Patterns Electronic Report (PEPPER)**, to monitor coding accuracy. This hospital-specific report is produced by the Centers for Medicare and Medicaid Services (CMS) and provides statistics for discharges that are vulnerable to improper payments. Specifically, the reports identify areas that are prone to over- or undercoding based on past improper payment reviews. Typically, these areas of concern arise from complex coding guidelines and ongoing issues with incomplete physician documentation. As part of a dashboard, coding managers can select the PEPPER measure that best applies to their facility at that point in time. PEPPER measures can be rotated based on a schedule or on an as-needed basis. Examples of PEPPER measures include the following:

- Respiratory infections
- Septicemia
- Medical MS-DRGs with CC or MCC
- Ventilator support
- Percutaneous cardiovascular procedures

The PEPPER report is derived from inpatient admissions, and therefore is an indication of inpatient coding accuracy.

Another KPI to include in a coding dashboard is the **CC/MCC capture rate**. CC/MCC capture rate is the percentage of admissions within an MS-DRG family assigned to an MS-DRG with CC, MCC, or both. Figure 12.7 illustrates how to calculate the CC/MCC capture rate for an MS-DRG family.

Figure 12.7.   Calculation for CC/MCC capture rate for an MS-DRG family

MS-DRG Family – Minor Small & Large Bowel Procedures		
MS-DRG 344 – Minor Small & Large Bowel Procedures with MCC Volume = 15	MS-DRG 345 – Minor Small & Large Bowel Procedures with CC Volume = 30	MS-DRG 346 – Minor Small & Large Bowel Procedures without CC/MCC Volume = 18

Calculation		
# cases for MS-DRG 344 divided by the total number of cases in MS-DRGs 344–346 times 100 (15/63)* 100 23.8%	# cases for MS-DRG 345 divided by the total number of cases in MS-DRGs 344–346 times 100 (30/63)* 100 47.6%	# cases for MS-DRG 346 divided by the total number of cases in MS-DRGs 344–346 times 100 (18/63)* 100 28.6%

Add together the percentages for MS-DRGs that include CC and MCC

23.8% + 47.6% = 71.4% CC/MCC Capture Rate

Figure 12.7 illustrates the CC/MCC capture rate for one MS-DRG family. However, this calculation can also be applied by major diagnostic category, surgical or medical status, and overall (for all cases). Once the coding manager has decided which cases they would like to be included in the CC/MCC capture rate, the rate can be trended and monitored over time. CC/MCC capture rate is another metric that can be used to monitor coding accuracy. It specifically examines if the coding unit is correctly coding secondary diagnoses.

Not only does a dashboard allow the coding manager to monitor and assess staff performance, but a dashboard is a good communication tool. Members of the revenue integrity team can view the coding dashboard and understand coding performance at that point in time. Dashboards often include trend lines, which allow leadership to see performance improvement or identify areas of concern that require immediate attention. Figure 12.8 provides a sample dashboard for a coding unit.

Figure 12.8 displays key metrics for a coding unit, including monthly CMI, monthly DNFB, denial rates by month, variance for PEPPER target measures, clean claim rate, and monthly CC/MCC capture rates. The dashboard provides an overview of the coding unit's performance for the coding manager and leadership.

Coding Compliance Plan

The coding manager should develop and maintain a **coding compliance plan**, which focuses on the unique regulations and guidelines to which coding professionals must comply. The coding compliance plan is a component

Figure 12.8. **Sample dashboard for a coding unit**

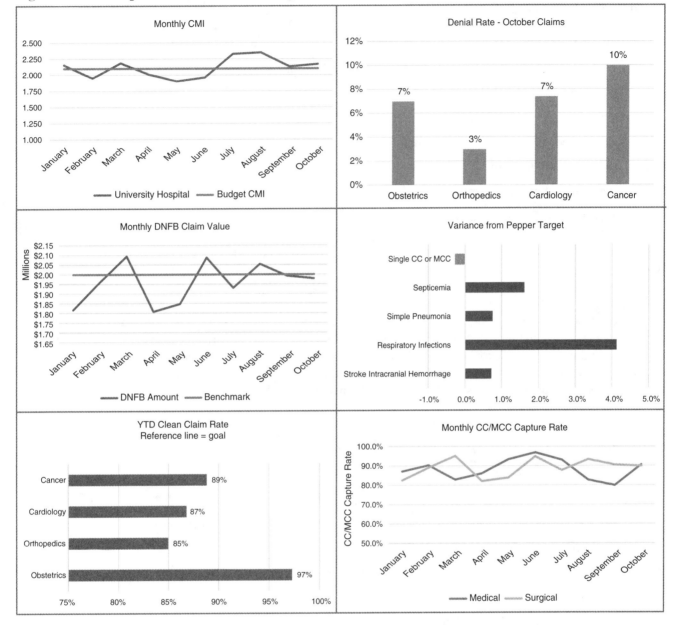

of the HIM department compliance plan and the overall corporate compliance plan at its facility. The AHIMA Standards of Ethical Coding should be a primary component of the coding compliance plan. (The current standards are provided as online resources that accompany this text.) Building a strong compliance plan is essential for establishing a solid coding team. The core areas of the coding compliance plan are policies and procedures, education and training, and auditing and monitoring.

Policies and Procedures

Well-designed and complete policies and procedures provide employees with consistent guidance to perform their assigned tasks. Without such guidance, employees may complete their tasks in different ways, causing confusion, inefficiencies, and possibly noncompliance. Managers should perform a job analysis to ensure every task has an established policy or procedure to govern it. Because coding has so many rules and official guidelines, it is crucial that this section of the coding compliance plan be methodically compiled. Following is a selection of issues that should be included in a coding compliance plan:

- Physician query process
- Coding diagnoses not supported by medical documentation
- Upcoding
- Unbundling
- Coding medical records without complete documentation
- Assignment of discharge status codes
- Correct use of encoding software
- Correct use of CAC software

Although this list is far from exhaustive, it identifies an array of activities the coding compliance plan should cover.

Education and Training

A good education plan is essential to succeeding as a coding team. To be compliant, coding professionals must continually participate in their education. Rules and regulations for public and private payers are released regularly. Billing and coding compliance tools are discussed in more detail in chapter 13, "Revenue Compliance." Recognized means of communication of this vital information must be established in the coding compliance plan. Issues that should be placed on the continuous education schedule include the following:

- Public and private payer guidelines
- *Medicare National Coverage Determinations Manual*
- *Medicare Claims Processing Manual*
- *Medicare Program Integrity Manual*
- Official Coding Guidelines for ICD-10-CM/PCS, CPT, and HCPCS Level II codes
- Quarterly and yearly code changes
- Quarterly and yearly prospective payment system changes
- Office of Inspector General (OIG) work plan issues
- National Correct Coding Initiative (NCCI)

Special attention should be paid to new coding professionals' work. Every coding manager must assess a new employee's compliance level and degree of understanding. Education must be provided to bring deficient coding professionals up to speed with expected guidelines. Completion of required educational sessions should be built into annual evaluations and reviews for all coding, billing, and reimbursement employees. Education can be provided internally and externally. Local, state, and national professional organizations, such as AHIMA, offer a variety of educational sessions throughout the year. Sessions are provided in person and remotely through webinars and online courses.

Auditing and Monitoring

Managers must be diligent at auditing and monitoring compliance in the coding unit. During the auditing phase, the coding manager gathers information about the department's compliance with policies and procedures. Incorporating internal and external auditing into the coding compliance plan has proven to be the best strategy. Internal auditing enables managers to see firsthand where their units' strengths and weaknesses lie. External auditing provides an unbiased view of a department's performance. Together, internal and external audits help coding managers build effective education plans for their units.

The process of comparing performance with preestablished standards or performance of another facility or group is called **benchmarking**. Two forms of benchmarking can help a manager determine the staff's level of compliance: internal and external benchmarking. Internal benchmarking, or trending, allows the manager to examine reporting rates over time. This exercise helps the manager pinpoint the specific period when a compliance issue arose. External benchmarking, or peer comparison, helps managers know how their teams have performed compared with peers. Issues can reveal, for example, whether coding practices put the facility at risk. Benchmarking helps establish reasonable parameters. Target areas for internal and external benchmarking should correlate with those highlighted in the policies and procedures and education and training sections of the coding compliance plan, along with problem areas identified during routine internal and external audits.

Once a compliance program has been established or has been significantly modified, it is important to measure the program's effectiveness. To assist facilities in this task, the OIG has released a resource guide. This document is a result of work completed by the Health Care Compliance Association (HCCA)-OIG Effectiveness Roundtable. *Measuring Compliance Program Effectiveness: A Resource Guide* can be downloaded from the OIG website.

Check Your Understanding 12.1

1. Describe the CCS credential.

2. What is CAC?

3. Which coding KPI measures effectiveness of coding management?

4. What are the basic components of a coding compliance plan?

5. Using the data displayed below, calculate the March 202X CC/MCC capture rate for the chronic obstructive pulmonary disease MS-DRG family.

MS-DRG Family Chronic Obstructive Pulmonary Disease Admission Data for March 202X		
MS-DRG	**MS-DRG Description**	**Admission Volume**
190	Chronic obstructive pulmonary disease with MCC	15
191	Chronic obstructive pulmonary disease with CC	25
192	Chronic obstructive pulmonary disease without CC/MCC	30

Clinical Documentation Integrity

CDI programs are implemented to improve the quality of provider documentation. By improving provider documentation, coding performance and accurate reimbursement for services can be optimized. Therefore, CDI is a valuable component of achieving revenue integrity.

CDI programs have been implemented for inpatient and outpatient care within hospitals for decades. However, they are expanding into healthcare sites outside of the hospital setting, such as home health, inpatient rehabilitation hospitals, and physician offices (Butler 2017, 16). Goals of a CDI program include the following:

- Obtain clinical documentation that captures the patient severity of illness (SOI) and risk of mortality (ROM)

- Identify and clarify missing, conflicting, or nonspecific provider documentation related to diagnoses and procedures
- Support accurate diagnostic and procedural coding, and MS-DRG assignment, leading to appropriate reimbursement
- Promote health record completion during the patient's course of care, which promotes patient safety
- Improve communication between physicians and other members of the healthcare team
- Provide awareness and education
- Improve documentation to reflect quality and outcome scores
- Improve coding professionals' clinical knowledge (AHIMA 2016, 7)

The CDI team's activities are directed to ensure that physician and clinician documentation is timely, complete, and specific so that the coding process can be efficient and accurate. It is important to establish the characteristics of high-quality documentation to really understand the foundation of a CDI program. There are seven universal characteristics of high-quality documentation, as shown in figure 12.9.

Figure 12.9.   Characteristics of high-quality documentation

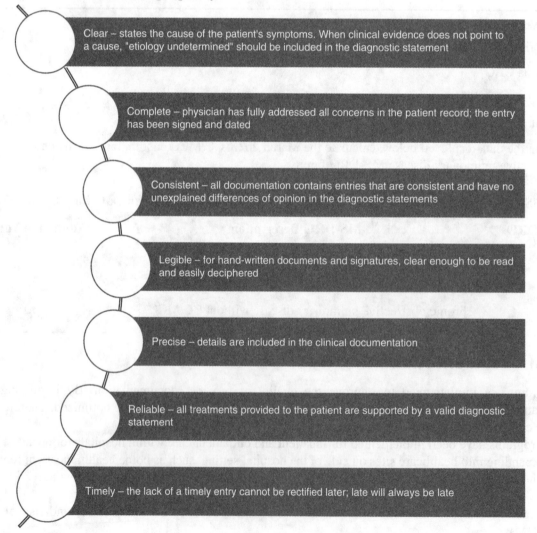

Source: AHIMA-ACDIS 2019.

These characteristics drive the CDI process. In the next section, the CDI process will be discussed in detail.

CDI Process

There is not one standard CDI process that all facilities use. The process must be customized to meet the needs of the facility or practice based on available resources and funding. In this section, a basic process for inpatient CDI will be presented and discussed. The process can be divided into three main functions: record review, query for documentation clarification, and physician education. Figure 12.10 presents these main functions and tasks included for each.

The first medical record review takes place the day after admission. During this first review a working MS-DRG is determined. Additionally, the CDI specialist will set the initial SOI level and the initial ROM level. The working MS-DRG, SOI, and ROM are updated throughout the admission when the CDI specialist reviews the medical record again and more clinical documentation is available.

As part of the initial and subsequent reviews, the CDI specialist determines if there is a need for a query. Queries are crafted and sent electronically or verbally discussed with the physician. CDI specialists use the same query construction guidelines that were discussed earlier in this chapter in the Query Appropriateness section. As queries are answered and physician documentation secured, the CDI specialist updates the working MS-DRG, SOI, and ROM. An unanswered query can be submitted a final time post-discharge. The coding unit can use the query results to finalize the MS-DRG for the admission.

When a physician's documentation needs clarification, it is a good time to educate the physician about documentation. For example, if the physician documents "Infectious disease, will start antibiotics," the CDI specialist can use this opportunity to explain to the physician that to properly code the condition, the coding professionals need to know the specific type of infection and the organism responsible for the infection, if known. Another example is when a physician documents "low sodium." The CDI specialist can educate the physician that the coding professional needs the physician to document hyponatremia instead of low sodium.

It is important to remember that the CDI specialist may review the medical record multiple times throughout the patient admission depending on the admission LOS. When the LOS is long enough for multiple reviews, all three of these functions are repeated multiple times: review, query, educate, repeat.

Figure 12.10. **Main CDI functions**

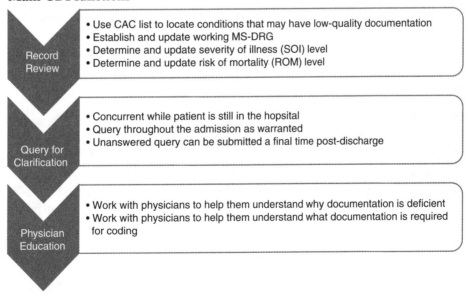

CDI Staffing

A typical CDI position is the clinical documentation improvement specialist. Preferred qualifications for this position include the following:

- Bachelor's degree in healthcare field (such as RN or RHIA)

- Five years' experience in healthcare field such as clinical care, utilization review, or HIM

- Credential such as CDIP or CCDS for inpatient

- Credential such as CDIP, CCDS-O, or CDEO for outpatient

- Critical thinking and problem-solving skills

- Ability to work with little or minimum direct supervision

- Excellent writing skills

- Clear and accurate verbal communication skills

- Experience with medical code sets, Medicare Part A and B programs, and MS-DRG assignment, and knowledge of CC/MCC assignment (AHIMA 2016, 31–32)

Certification is highly preferred if not mandatory. Table 12.2 provides a summary of CDI credentials. Management positions in CDI include CDI quality assurance auditor, CDI manager, and CDI director.

CDI Performance Assessment

Performance assessments must be conducted for CDI professionals as well as for the CDI program. Like coding management, the CDI manager must monitor CDI productivity and accuracy. Remember that not all inpatient records are included in CDI interventions. Certain specialties are chosen for CDI review based on denial rates, past audits, and other metrics. Additionally, each admission has a unique LOS. This can make establishing CDI review standards challenging. For example, the time it takes to review a cardiovascular surgery case with a six-day LOS may be very different from a GI medical case with a six-day LOS. An example of a CDI individual standard would be 10 new reviews and 10 to 15 follow-up reviews per eight-hour shift.

Monitoring accuracy is crucial. Accuracy includes proper review of the medical record, correct assignment of the working MS-DRG, correct establishment of SOI and ROM, appropriate identification of need for and creation of queries, and clear and concise communication with physicians and other clinicians. Writing a compliant query is critical to CDI accuracy and integrity. Recall the criteria used to measure if a query is appropriate or compliant on page 234.

The CDI manager or CDI quality assurance auditor should monitor CDI specialists' performance on a regular schedule throughout the performance year. Annual data should be summarized and used for annual performance reviews and bonuses, if warranted.

CDI Program Metrics

It is important to communicate the health of the CDI program to leadership, physicians, and staff. Several metrics, shown in table 12.3, are available to show performance improvements gained from the CDI program. CDI managers and program directors select metrics to illustrate performance to leadership on a monthly basis through a dashboard and each year through an annual report. An example CDI dashboard is shown in figure 12.11.

AHIMA has published numerous toolkits and practice briefs designed to assist CDI professionals with the development and management of a CDI program. Additionally, AHIMA has compiled Ethical Standards for Clinical Documentation Improvement (CDI) Professionals. This document sets forth professional values and ethical principles that CDI professionals can strive to meet and is provided in the online resources that accompany this text.

Table 12.2. **Summary of CDI credentials**

Credential	Title	Granting Organization	Credential holders demonstrate:
CDIP	Certified documentation improvement practitioner	AHIMA	• Knowledge and competence in high-quality clinical documentation within patient health records • Competence in capturing documentation necessary to fully communicate patients' health status and conditions
CCDS	Certified clinical documentation specialist	ACDIS	• Understanding of a wide range of specialized disciplines, including education in anatomy and physiology, pathophysiology, and pharmacology • Knowledge of official medical coding guidelines, CMS, and private payer regulations related to the inpatient prospective payment system • Ability to analyze and interpret medical record documentation and formulate appropriate physician queries • Ability to benchmark and analyze clinical documentation program performance
CCDS-O	Certified clinical documentation specialist—outpatient	ACDIS	• Competency for CDI in the outpatient setting, which includes physician practices, hospital clinics, emergency department, and others
CDEO	Certified documentation expert outpatient	AAPC	• Expertise in reviewing outpatient documentation for accuracy to support coding, quality measures, and clinical requirements • Ability to identify and communicate documentation deficiencies to providers to improve documentation for accurate risk adjustment coding • Sound knowledge of medical coding guidelines and regulations, including compliance and reimbursement • Thorough understanding of anatomy, pathophysiology, and medical terminology necessary to correctly code using CPT, ICD-10-CM, and HCPCS Level II coding systems

Source: AHIMA n.d.; AAPC n.d.b; ACDIS n.d.

Table 12.3.   CDI performance metrics

Metric	Metric Description
Review rate	Total discharges reviewed divided by number of discharges available to be reviewed by a CDI specialist
Physician clarification impact rate	The number of clarifications placed by a CDI intervention that had an impact on the MS-DRG assignment
Severity clarification rate	The number of clarifications placed by a CDI intervention that resulted in a severity change The number of clarifications placed by a CDI intervention that resulted in a risk of mortality change
Physician response to CDI specialist rate	The number of times a physician responds to a CDI intervention divided by the number of CDI interventions issued
Physician agreement with CDI specialist rate	The number of times a physician agrees with a CDI intervention divided by the number of CDI interventions issued
Working MS-DRG/Final MS-DRG match rate	Number of times the final working MS-DRG is the same as the billed MS-DRG divided by the number of discharges reviewed by a CDI specialist
Physician response to CDI query turnaround time	How long it takes for a physician to respond to a CDI query
CMI trend	Compare baseline CMI to actual CMI and goal CMI. CMI can be broken down by specialty, medical/surgical, etc.
CC/MCC capture rate	Percentage of discharges that include a CC or MCC secondary diagnosis that impact MS-DRG assignment. Can be broken down by specialty, medical/surgical, etc.
Top MS-DRGs reviewed	By discharge volume, a listing of the final MS-DRGs included in CDI reviews
Conditions most often queried	By volume, the conditions that most often lead to a CDI intervention
Clinician/Physician most often queried	By volume, the clinician/physician that has received the most CDI queries

Source: Adapted from AHIMA 2016, 10–12.

Figure 12.11.   Sample CDI dashboard

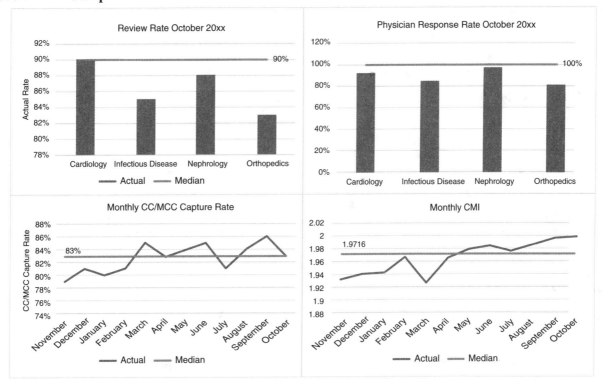

Patient Connection

Sierra is a CDI specialist at Memorial Hospital. She has been assigned to the orthopedics unit, and she reviews medical and surgical visits daily. She reviewed the admission for patient Malakai on day two of his stay. She continues to follow his admission even though an intervention was not warranted during her initial review. On day five she reviews the record and notices that a wound culture was taken because patient Malakai's surgical site is red, sore, and weeping foul-smelling fluid. Dr. Shah orders to start IV antibiotics. Sierra writes a query to the physician asking him to document the reason for the IV antibiotics in the medical record.

Dr. Shah receives the CDI query on day six of patient Malakai's stay. Although the culture results are not ready, Dr. Shah remembers that during CDI training, it was discussed that physicians should always provide clinical validation for treatments. Therefore, Dr. Shah documents "suspected bacterial infection at surgical site on right knee" to provide clinical validation for why the IV antibiotics were ordered. When the laboratory results are released, Dr. Shah will confirm the results in the medical record and list the type of bacteria causing the infection at that time.

Chapter 12 Review Quiz

1. Match each credential on the left with its granting organization on the right.

    CCDS   _____   a.   AAPC

    CCS-P   _____   b.   ACDIS

    CPC   _____   c.   AHIMA

(continued)

Chapter 12 Review Quiz   *(continued)*

2. What are some characteristics of an experienced coding professional?

3. How does the use of an encoder support revenue integrity?

4. What role do coding professionals have in the CAC process?

5. What factors should be considered when determining coding productivity measures?

6. Define DNFB.

7. What are the seven characteristics of high-quality documentation?

8. Describe the three main functions included in CDI.

9. What is the role of queries in the CDI process?

10. Which CDI metric measures the percentage of time a physician responds to a CDI query?

References

AAPC (American Academy of Professional Coders). n.d.a. "Medical Coding Certification Online." Accessed February 26, 2023. https://www.aapc.com/certification/medical-coding-certification.aspx.

AAPC (American Academy of Professional Coders). n.d.b. "Medical Documentation Certification." Accessed February 26, 2023. https://www.aapc.com/certification/cdeo/.

ACDIS (Association of Clinical Documentation Improvement Specialists). n.d. "About ACDIS' Certifications and Certificates." Accessed February 26, 2023. https://acdis.org/certification.

AHIMA (American Health Information Management Association). 2016. *Clinical Documentation Improvement Toolkit.* http://bok.ahima.org/PdfView?oid=301829.http://bok.ahima.org/PdfView?oid=301829.

AHIMA (American Health Information Management Association). 2013. "Physician Query Examples." https://journal.ahima.org/page/physician-query-examples.

AHIMA (American Health Information Management Association). n.d. "Certification." Accessed February 26, 2023. http://www.ahima.org/certification.

AHIMA-ACDIS (American Health Information Management Association and Association of Clinical Documentation Improvement Specialists). 2019. *Guidelines for Achieving a Compliant Query Practice (2019 Update).* https://acdis.org/resources/guidelines-achieving-compliant-query-practice%E2%80%942019-update.

Alakrawi, Z. M., V. J. M. Watzlaf, S. Nemchik, and P. T. Sheridan. 2017. New study illuminates the ongoing road to ICD-10 productivity and optimization. *Journal of AHIMA* 88(3):40–45. http://bok.ahima.org/doc?oid=302058#.XotNYKhKiUk.

Butler, M. 2017. CDI programs expanding outside the hospital. *Journal of AHIMA* 88(7):14–17.

Dougherty, M., S. Seabold, and S. E. White. 2013. Study reveals hard facts on CAC. *Journal of AHIMA* 84(7):54–56. http://library.ahima.org/doc?oid=106668#.Xodx1qhKiUk.

Gentul, M. K. and N. A. Davis. 2011. "Structure and Organization of the Coding Function." Chapter 1 in *Effective Management of Coding Services*, 4th ed., edited by L. A. Schraffenberger and L. Kuehn. Chicago: AHIMA.

Johnson, L. M. and A. Rickard. 2020. Practice Brief: Developing facility-specific coding guidelines. *Journal of AHIMA* 91(1): 44–49.

Land, D. 2019. Tips for getting the most out of computer-assisted coding. *Journal of AHIMA* 90(6):32–33.

Noridian. 2022. "Patient Discharge Status Codes." https://med.noridianmedicare.com/web/jea/topics/claim-submission/patient-discharge-status-codes.

Qlik. n.d. "What Is a KPI?" Accessed February 26, 2023. https://www.qlik.com/us/kpi#:~:text=KPI%20Examples-,What%20is%20a%20KPI%3F,the%20organization%20make%20better%20decisions.

Sayles, N. B. 2020. "Health Information Functions, Purpose, and Users." Chapter 3 in *Health Information Management Technology: An Applied Approach*, 6th ed., edited by N. B. Sayles and L. Gordon. Chicago: AHIMA.

Chapter 13
Revenue Compliance

Learning Objectives

❖ Identify the coding compliance issues that influence reimbursement

❖ Explain the roles of various Medicare improper payment review entities

❖ Structure audits to support revenue integrity

❖ Examine compliance guidance for coding and billing of healthcare services

❖ Organize a denials management program

Key Terms

Abuse
Administrative denial
Audit
Claim denial
Clinical denial
Clinical validation denial
CMS program transmittal
Compliance
Comprehensive Error Rate Testing (CERT) program
Demand letter
False Claims Act
Fraud
Improper payment reviews
Local coverage determination (LCD)

Medically unlikely edit (MUE)
Medicare Code Editor (MCE)
Medicare Integrity Program
Medicare severity diagnosis-related group (MS-DRG) coding denial
National Correct Coding Initiative (NCCI)
National coverage determination (NCD)
Office of Inspector General (OIG)
Procedure-to-procedure (PTP) edit
Recovery audit contractor (RAC)
Recovery Audit Program
Unbundling
Upcoding
Vulnerability

In chapter 1, "Healthcare Reimbursement and Revenue Cycle Management," revenue integrity was introduced. Revenue integrity is performing revenue cycle duties to obtain operational efficiency, compliance adherence, and legitimate reimbursement. In this chapter, compliance adherence is discussed in detail.

For coding, billing, and reimbursement professionals, **compliance** means performing job functions according to the laws, regulations, and guidelines set forth by Medicare and other third-party payers. Today, being compliant with the rules and regulations is just one component of being proficient at a healthcare professional's job. It is an indication that, as a professional, the person will perform at an acceptable skill level and ethical standard. It is the responsibility of coding, billing, and reimbursement professionals to perform their jobs with integrity at all times. The AHIMA Standards of Ethical Coding sets forth guidelines that all coding, billing, and reimbursement professionals should understand and ponder during ethical decision-making. (A copy of the standards is included in the online resources that accompany this text.) In this chapter, we will first explore how Medicare and other payers determine compliance by examining fraud and abuse, oversight of Medicare claims payments, and nongovernment payer reviews. In the second part of the chapter, we explore how facilities and providers can improve compliance with federal and state regulations through audit management, using coding and billing compliance tools and denials management. An **audit** is a systematic and objective review of revenue cycle processes to determine the level of compliance with policies, procedures, and regulations.

Fraud and Abuse

In simple terms, **fraud** in the healthcare arena is a healthcare provider requesting payment or reward when the requester knows it is against healthcare rules and regulations. Medicare includes the following as types of Medicare fraud:

- Knowingly submitting false claims or making misrepresentations of fact to obtain a federal healthcare payment for which no entitlement would otherwise exist

- Knowingly soliciting, receiving, offering, or paying remuneration (for example, kickbacks, bribes, or rebates) to induce or reward referrals for items or services reimbursed by federal healthcare programs

- Making prohibited referrals for certain designated health services (CMS 2021a, 6)

An example of fraud is submitting a claim to Medicare for a service that was not rendered.

Abuse occurs when a healthcare provider unknowingly or unintentionally submits an inaccurate claim for payment. Abuse generally results from unsound medical, business, or fiscal practices that directly or indirectly result in unnecessary costs to the Medicare program. An example of abuse would be inadvertently reporting a procedure code that describes a service that was more extensive than the procedure performed. In Medicare, the most common forms of fraud and abuse include the following:

- Billing unnecessary medical services

- Charging excessively for services or supplies

- Misusing codes on a claim (upcoding or unbundling)

- Knowingly ordering medically unnecessary items or services for patients

- Paying for referrals of federal healthcare program benefits

- Billing Medicare for appointments patients failed to keep (CMS 2021a)

It is important to understand the legislative history of fraud and abuse. The **False Claims Act** was passed during the Civil War to penalize federal contractors of all kinds who knowingly filed a false or fraudulent claim, used a false record or statement, or conspired to defraud the US government (Enriquez 2011, 371). Today, the False Claims Act provides the support for the federal government to rebuke abusers of the Medicare and Medicaid systems. From the mid-1980s through late 1990s, there was a wave of federal legislation that targeted Medicare and Medicaid fraud and abuse. Not only did the revamped and newly created legislation show Congress's commitment to protecting the Medicare Trust Fund, but it gave the Centers for Medicare and Medicaid Services (CMS) the resources and penalties necessary to battle fraud and abuse.

Some acts relevant to Medicare and Medicaid predate these programs, and others were created specifically to support them. The Medicare and Medicaid Patient and Program Protection Act of 1987 supports the use of civil monetary penalties for acts of fraud and abuse against the Medicare and Medicaid programs. This act allows for fines up to $10,000 per violation and exclusions from Medicare participation.

In 1991, the **Office of Inspector General (OIG)** released seven elements that it believed should serve as the foundation of an effective corporate compliance plan (HHS 1998, 8989). The OIG is a division of the Department of Health and Human Services (HHS) that investigates issues of noncompliance in the Medicare and Medicaid programs, such as fraud and abuse. The elements released by the OIG are as follows:

1. Written policies and procedures
2. Designation of a compliance officer
3. Education and training
4. Communication
5. Auditing and monitoring
6. Disciplinary action
7. Corrective action

In response to numerous laboratory investigations for improper coding and billing, Compliance Program Guidance for Clinical Laboratories was released in February 1997 and then revised in August of the following year (1998). The guidance provides principles for compliant documentation and coding practices in laboratories. For example, laboratories were instructed that they must not use diagnostic information from earlier dates of service on current laboratory testing orders. At the time, this was common practice, but it is a compliance risk because whether a patient's condition warrants a procedure may change from visit to visit.

In February 1998, the OIG released Compliance Program Guidance for Hospitals. This document highlighted several coding and billing areas that were at risk for noncompliance. Some examples are reporting services at a higher level than performed, reporting component codes rather than comprehensive codes for services, and reporting an incorrect discharge destination.

Since 1998, numerous other Compliance Program Guidance documents have been released for various healthcare settings, including hospice, home health, physician practices, and skilled nursing facilities. Because hospitals' operations and reimbursement systems have changed since 1998, the OIG decided to revise the Program Guidance. In January 2005, CMS released the Supplemental Compliance Program Guidance for Hospitals in the *Federal Register*. Although expanded, the original seven elements continue to be the basis for an effective hospital compliance plan:

1. Designation of a compliance officer and compliance committee
2. Development of compliance policies and procedures, including standards of conduct
3. Development of open lines of communication
4. Appropriate training and education
5. Internal monitoring and auditing
6. Response to detected deficiencies
7. Enforcement of disciplinary standards (HHS 2005, 4874–4876)

The Supplemental Compliance Program Guidance for Hospitals provides further detail about compliance risk areas for outpatient procedure coding, admissions and discharge criteria, supplemental payment considerations, and use of information technology (HHS 2005, 4860–4862). A copy of the Supplemental Compliance Program Guidance for Hospitals can be found on the OIG website. Even though this program guidance was released several years ago, it continues to be used as the foundation for coding compliance programs.

A joint effort of HHS, OIG, CMS, and the Administration on Aging (AOA), Operation Restore Trust was released in 1995 to target fraud and abuse among healthcare providers. The program originally focused on five states (California, Illinois, Florida, New York, and Texas), where a third of the Medicare and Medicaid population resided. Within the first two years, Operation Restore Trust spent $7.9 million and recovered $188 million—a 24-to-1 return on investment. This major push for accurate coding and billing eventually spread to become a nationwide effort. In addition to fraud and abuse investigations, Operation Restore Trust paved the way for implementation of a national toll-free fraud and abuse hotline, the Voluntary Disclosure Program, and Special Fraud Alert documents.

Although the Health Insurance Portability and Accountability Act of 1996 (HIPAA) is widely known for its security and privacy provisions, a large portion of the act focused on fraud and abuse prevention. HIPAA created the **Medicare Integrity Program**. Not only did Medicare continue to review provider claims for fraud and abuse, but the focus expanded to cost reports, payment determinations, and the need for ongoing compliance education (Enriquez 2011, 372).

One objective of the Balanced Budget Act of 1997 (BBA) was to improve program integrity for Medicare. The provisions within the BBA attempted to educate Medicare beneficiaries about their role in preventing and reporting fraudulent acts. Beneficiaries were advised to review Medicare summary notices (MSNs; formerly explanations of Medicare benefits, or EOMBs) for errors and to report errors to the secretary of HHS. In addition, they were notified of their right to request copies of detailed bills for healthcare services and informed of the implementation of a toll-free fraud and abuse hotline. The BBA also initiated a data collection program to collect fraud and abuse information in the healthcare sector as mandated by HIPAA. As legislation regarding healthcare fraud and abuse became more prevalent, the need for a stronger workforce behind the laws was inevitable. Personnel were added to the Department of Justice (DOJ) and Federal Bureau of Investigation (FBI) to keep up with the warranted reviews.

Since 2002, several laws that focus on improper payment have been enacted. Significant laws include the following:

- The Improper Payments Information Act of 2002 (IPIA; Public Law 107-300)

- The Improper Payments Elimination and Recovery Act of 2010 (IPERA; Public Law 111-204)

- The Improper Payments Elimination and Recovery Improvement Act of 2012 (IPERIA; Public Law 112-248)

- The Fraud Reduction and Data Analytics Act of 2015 (FRDAA; Public Law 114-186)

These laws have been replaced by the most recent improper payment law, the Payment Integrity Information Act of 2019 (PIIA; Public Law 116-117). PIIA charges agencies like CMS with identifying, reporting, and reducing improper payments. The first step is to gather a statistically valid estimate of the annual amount of improper payments. CMS uses the following programs to collect these data:

- **Comprehensive Error Rate Testing (CERT) program** measures improper payments for traditional Medicare

- Medicare Part C Improper Payment Measurement program (Part C IPM) measures improper payments for Medicare Part C, also known as Medicare Advantage

- Medicare Part D Improper Payment Measurement program (Part D IPM) measures improper payments for Medicare Part D, also known as the Medicare prescription drug plan

- Payment Error Rate Measurement Program (PERM) measures improper payments for Medicaid and CHIP

- Exchange Improper Payment Measurement program (EIPM) measures improper payments of the Advance Payment of Premium Tax Credit (APTC) administered by the American Health Benefit Exchanges (CMS 2021b)

CMS must also implement a plan to reduce improper payments and report progress annually in the Agency Financial Report. These acts have greatly affected the Medicare Integrity Program. To learn more about the program, view the *Medicare Program Integrity Manual*, available for download at the CMS website.

Oversight of Medicare Claims Payments

Not only is CMS required to protect the Medicare Trust Fund, but legislative acts such as PIIA also provide specific requirements for reporting and correcting improper payments. To complete the numerous requirements, CMS has established the Medical Review Program. Under this program, CMS uses a variety of Medicare contractors to complete medical reviews, which are also known as **improper payment reviews**. The goal of the program is to reduce payment errors. To reduce payment errors, the contractors identify billing and coverage errors and provide education to providers to prevent future mistakes. Figure 13.1 provides a snapshot of the roles for some of the various entities included in medical reviews or improper payment reviews.

The goal of the program is to reduce Medicare payment errors by identifying and eliminating billing errors made by providers. Medicare contractors focus reviews on preidentified areas that have been determined by contractor data analysis. Contractors use a variety of edits to identify claims for prepayment and post-payment reviews. Medical reviews consist of the Medicare contractors collecting information and performing a clinical review to determine whether Medicare's coverage, coding, and medical necessity requirements are met.

The major causes of improper payments include physician orders missing, signatures being illegible or missing, and medical records documentation not supporting medical necessity. Additionally, review entities look for unbundling and upcoding of services. **Unbundling** is the process in which individual component codes are submitted for reimbursement rather than a single comprehensive code. **Upcoding** is the fraudulent process of submitting codes for reimbursement that indicate more complex or higher-paying services than the patient actually received.

Provider education is a key component of this program. After areas of concern or vulnerabilities are identified, Medicare contractors are expected to publish guidance to the medical community regarding coverage, coding, and medical necessity requirements. In addition, Medicare Learning Network (MLN) articles should be created on behalf of CMS to improve transparency of the medical review process. Several programs provide guidance and education for facilities and providers to improve compliance. Four key programs—CERT, the Medical Review Program, OIG General Reports, and the National Recovery Audit Program—are explored in the text that follows.

Figure 13.1.   Examples of Medicare and Medicaid medical review entities

Medical Review Entity	Types of Claims	Purpose of Review
A/B MAC	Parts A & B claims	Identify and prevent improper payments
Recovery Audit Contractor (RAC)	Parts A, B, C and D claims Medicaid claims	Identify and correct improper payments
Supplemental Medical Review Contractor (SMRC)	Medicaid claims Medicare Part A & B claims Durable medical equipment, prosthetics, orthotics, and supplies (DMEPOS) claims	Lower improper payment rates

Source: CMS 2023a.

Comprehensive Error Rate Testing Program

As mentioned earlier, the CERT program measures improper payments in various healthcare settings for Medicare. It was first a responsibility of the OIG, and national error rates were calculated by the OIG from 1996 to 2002. The program was transitioned to Medicare beginning in 2001. The IPIA of 2002 solidified the program, and Medicare released its first report in 2003. The purpose of CERT is to measure improper payments, not to measure fraud. During each reporting period, claims are randomly selected for review from each of the types of Medicare contractors, as illustrated in figure 13.2.

CERT identifies improper payments as follows:

- Payment that should not have been made

- Payment made in an incorrect amount

- Payment to an ineligible recipient

- Payment for an ineligible service

- Duplicate payment

- Payment for service that was not received

- Payment for an incorrect amount

National error rates are calculated each year and are published with the associated financial effect of improper payments. The error rate has varied from year to year, and the error rate for fiscal year (FY) 2022 was 7.46 percent ($31.46 billion). The primary error identified by CERT was insufficient documentation to support reported services. The second largest error category was failure to meet medical necessity (CMS 2022a, 2). The 2022 error rate is considerably lower than the error rate for FY 2016, which was 11 percent ($41.08 billion). However, with improper payment figures remaining in the billions, there continues to be a need for this program as well as for continued Medicare claims reviews.

Figure 13.2.   The CERT process

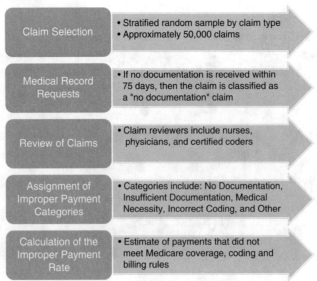

Source: Adapted from CMS 2016a.

Office of Inspector General Reports

Although the OIG no longer executes CERT, the agency provides relevant reports to the Medicare Review Program for continued use in improper payment reviews. Significant OIG reports are communicated via Medicare transmittals to Medicare contractors for use in their medical review activities. Each year, the OIG provides its Work Plan, which outlines the areas of focus for the upcoming year. Providers and facilities can use the Work Plan to construct their own compliance reviews on these topics of interest. In addition to the annual Work Plan, the OIG provides a listing of all active Work Plan items on the website. It can be found on the OIG website under the "Reports and Publications" tab. For example, a 2022 issue is Medicare Payments for Trauma Claims (OIG n.d.). Specifically, this issue targets facilities that improperly billed for trauma team activation that is not medically necessary. Additionally, the OIG will ensure that providers that have received trauma team activation payments are designated or verified as trauma centers. The OIG review will examine if payments to facilities were properly made. Healthcare facilities can be proactive by performing reviews based on Work Plan issues on their own. If documentation, coding, or billing issues are identified, facilities can rectify them immediately.

Recovery Audit Program

What began as a demonstration project is now a fully implemented CMS program that encompasses all areas of Medicare and Medicaid. The **Recovery Audit Program** is executed under the Medicare Integrity Program and is designed as another CMS avenue to prevent improper payments and ultimately to protect the Medicare Trust Fund. A main component of the Recovery Audit Program is to prevent future improper payments.

A **recovery audit contractor (RAC)** is a federal contractor that carries out the provisions of the National Recovery Audit Program. Because of the direct interaction between RACs and providers, most refer to the entire program as RACs instead of by the program name. Unlike other improper payment review entities, RACs are reimbursed via a contingency fee based on the amount of improper payments identified and successfully collected. Contingency fees range from 9 percent to 12.5 percent for most claim types. Durable medical equipment (DME) contingency fees have a higher range at 14 to 17.5 percent. RACs must successfully collect improper payments to retain the contingency fees. RACs must return contingency fees if improper payment determinations are overturned at any level of the appeals process (CMS 2016b, 4). Figure 13.3 shows the RACs and their assigned jurisdictions.

The RAC program has five key program components that are used to measure its success:

1. Ensure accuracy

2. Implement effective and efficient program operations

3. Maximize transparency

4. Minimize provider burden

5. Develop robust provider education (CMS 2016b, 9–13)

The first component is to ensure accuracy. It is imperative that the RACs accurately identify improper payments. RACs must have a physician medical director as well as certified coding professionals on staff. For medical necessity reviews, many RACs use registered nurses or other clinical staff. Additionally, a RAC must have review issues, also known as vulnerabilities, approved by the recovery audit validation contractor before performing audits. A **vulnerability** is a claim type that poses a financial risk to the Medicare program because the claim type is susceptible to improper payments (CMS 2016b, 22). The RACs must publish all vulnerabilities on their websites before the vulnerabilities can be used in audits. Table 13.1 provides sample RAC vulnerabilities.

To ensure the accuracy of the RACs, CMS uses an independent contractor to review and validate a monthly random sample of claims where an improper payment has been identified. In FY 2019, each RAC achieved an overall accuracy score of 94 percent or higher (CMS 2019, 17).

Figure 13.3.   RAC jurisdictions

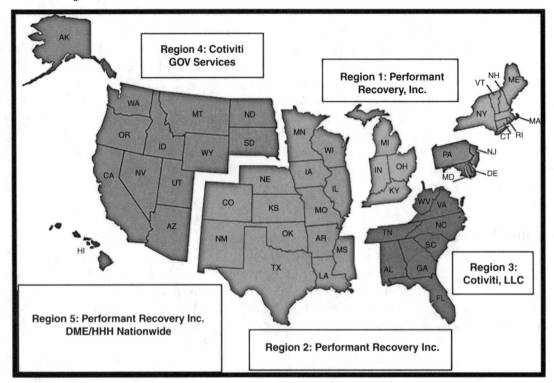

Source: CMS 2023b.

Table 13.1.   Sample RAC vulnerabilities

Issue Number and Name	Review Type	Provider Type
0001 – Inpatient Hospital MS-DRG Coding Validation	Complex	Inpatient Hospital
0003 – Sacral Neurostimulation: Medical Necessity and Documentation Requirements	Complex	Ambulatory Surgical Center, Inpatient Hospital, Outpatient Hospital, Professional Services (Physicians)
0019 – Durable Medical Equipment Billed While Inpatient	Automated	DME Physician/DME Supplier
0147 – Magnetic Resonance Imaging Procedures: Excessive Units	Automated	Professional Services (Physician), Outpatient Hospital

Source: CMS 2022b.

The second component of the program is that the RAC must ensure the program operates efficiently and effectively. This key component is in place to ensure consistent and high-quality communication among all stakeholders. During communication, stakeholders share information about identified program vulnerabilities, coding and billing guidelines, and Medicare and Medicaid regulations. Additionally, the program works to improve the RAC Data Warehouse and the use of Electronic Submission of Medical Documents (esMD) for medical records requests.

The third key component is to maximize transparency. The RACs prepare and post online quarterly newsletters that provide the fiscal impact of overpayments and underpayments for each RAC by quarter. Each RAC's top issue is also provided. RACs also use web portals so providers can review the status of claims and track the progress of the auditing process. Some RACs use the portals to send messages to providers about audits and to request additional information.

The fourth key component is to minimize provider burden. Any given medical record or encounter may be reviewed by only one improper payment review entity for a given issue. Therefore, if a Medicare administrative contractor (MAC) has reviewed an encounter for medical necessity, the encounter cannot be reviewed by the RAC. However, the encounter may be reviewed by the RAC for another issue, such as improper coding. CMS has imposed request limits of 45 days on RACs to lessen provider burden. The limits are provider-specific and are based on the provider's total number of paid Medicare claims from the previous 12-month period. Adjustments are made to the limit based on the provider's denial rate. Therefore, if the provider has a high denial rate, then the RAC can request a greater number of records. Additionally, if a provider operates multiple types of facilities (inpatient, outpatient, rehabilitation), then there is a maximum percentage limit per type of claim that can be targeted for review. This ensures only the most at-risk vulnerabilities are reviewed and that providers can adequately prepare for the process. Lastly, RACs must establish a customer service center to answer queries from facilities and practices.

The final key component is to develop robust provider education. The RACs and MACs collaborate to ensure policies are correctly interpreted. There are scheduled conference calls between RACs, MACs, CMS policy staff, and CMS clinical staff to ensure uniformity in policy application across improper payment review entities. CMS regularly partners with state and national hospital associations to provide RAC updates. These interactions are designed for two-way communication. CMS gains knowledge from the provider community, and the providers receive updates and feedback from CMS.

The RAC process begins with the RACs determining a set of vulnerabilities to review for the period. Once the vulnerabilities are set, the RACs begin to review claims to identify potential improper payments. There are three types of reviews:

1. *Automated*: RACs use claims data analysis to identify improper payments.

2. *Semiautomated*: RACs initiate the review through claims data analysis but then require the submission of the medical record documents to substantiate the improper payment.

3. *Complex*: RACs require the review of clinical medical record documents to confirm the improper payment.

For a semiautomated review or complex review, the RAC will request medical records from the facility or provider. The provider must follow a strict timetable when submitting records to the RAC. Documents can be submitted through esMD, or hard copies can be mailed to the RAC. After the RAC review is completed and an improper payment has been identified, the RAC passes the information to the provider via a notification. After notification, the provider has 30 days to request a discussion with the RAC regarding the claim determination. This discussion period allows the provider to submit additional documentation to support their case for the claim in question. However, if an appeal is made on the notification, then the discussion period is terminated, and the appeal process begins. RACs pass the overpayment and underpayment information to the MAC, and the MAC issues a **demand letter** to the facility or provider. The demand letter requests a specific amount to be repaid, provides a detailed rationale for the improper payment, and includes instructions for adjudication or appeal. Facilities or providers that disagree with the improper payment can appeal the RAC decision. The appeal process can be a five-level process for Medicare Part A and B claims as displayed in table 13.2.

Dollar thresholds are enforced for the administrative law judge (ALJ) ($160 for calendar year) and judicial review ($1,600) appeals levels. Appeals can be time consuming and costly to the facility or provider. However, successful appeals provide valuable information that can be used to improve medical record documentation and to support future appeals.

Table 13.2.   RAC appeal process for Medicare Parts A and B

Appeal Type	Appeal Presiding Party	Time Frame
Redetermination	MACs	Appeal received by the MAC within 120 calendar days of initial determination; the MAC transmits written notice of redetermination within 60 calendar days of receipt of the request for redetermination.
Reconsideration	Qualified independent contractors (QICs)	Appeal must be filed within 180 calendar days of receipt of the redetermination. QICs must transmit notice of reconsideration within 60 calendar days of receipt of the request for reconsideration.
Hearing or Review by Office of Medicare Hearings and Appeals (OMHA)	Administrative law judge (ALJ) or attorney adjudicator	Appeal must be filed within 60 calendar days of receipt of the reconsideration notice. ALJs must issue a decision, dismissal order, or remand to QIC within 90 days. Failure to do so results in the provider escalating to the next level of the appeal process.
Medicare Appeals Council	Appeals council	Appeal must be filed within 60 calendar days of the ALJ decision or dismissal. The appeals council generally issues a decision, dismissal order, or remand to ALJ within 90 days. Failure to do so results in the provider escalating to the next level of the appeal process. Due to volume of appeals pursued by providers, the 90-day time frame has historically been exceeded because the appeals court cannot meet the demand.
Judicial Review	Federal district court	Appeal must be filed within 60 days of notice of the appeals council's decision. The federal court does not have a deadline to issue its decisions.

Source: CMS 2016b.

For FY 2019, the RACs collected $162.03 million in improper payments (CMS 2019, 5). CMS paid the recovery auditors $25.58 million, and there was $34.64 million in CMS administrative costs. This resulted in $34.64 million returned to the Medicare Trust Funds for FY 2019 (CMS 2019, 5). The RACs completed a complex review for 42,274 claims, which resulted in over $124 million in corrections (both underpayments and overpayments). Additionally, RACs completed an automated review for 140,944 claims, resulting in over $42 million in corrections. There were significantly fewer semiautomated reviews in 2019, with only 1,254 claims reviewed and just over $324,000 in corrections (CMS 2019). As shown in figure 13.4 most of the corrected payments were from the inpatient facility setting (28.70 percent), closely followed by the outpatient facility setting (28.65 percent).

In FY 2019, over 17,468 appeals were overturned or partially overturned in the provider's favor (CMS 2019, 17–20). With this level of appeal success, facilities must continue to closely monitor their RAC determinations and take action if medical record documentation, coding guidelines, or Medicare regulations support the initial coding of the claim. Facilities must incorporate vulnerabilities and issues identified by RACs and other Medicare contractors into their coding compliance plans to prevent future improper payments.

Figure 13.4.   RAC corrections by provider type

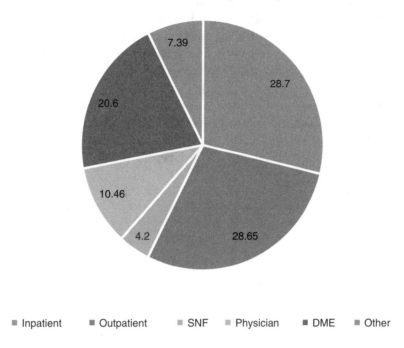

RAC Corrections by Setting

■ Inpatient   ■ Outpatient   ■ SNF   ■ Physician   ■ DME   ■ Other

Source: CMS 2019, 11.

Nongovernment Payer Reviews

As with CMS, other payers have developed medical review programs to ensure payments are warranted and accurate. However, unlike with Medicare—for which the review programs, issues under review, and review results for the regions and nation are available for the healthcare community to review online—commercial payers typically do not publish such information for all to see. Individual payers develop review criteria based on their historical data and prior reviews. Commercial payers may incorporate issues that have previously been identified by Medicare but that are applicable to their beneficiary profile into their own review portfolio. For example, commercial payers may use excisional debridement vulnerabilities identified by RACs. However, commercial payers would need to develop criteria for newborn or pregnancy reviews because the volume for these cases is low for the Medicare population. When commercial payer reviews are executed at a healthcare facility, the review topics, as well as the findings, should be incorporated into the coding compliance plans.

Check Your Understanding 13.1

1. The new coding assistant at the Good Physicians Group office coded and submitted a claim to Blue Cross for an initial evaluation and management office visit when, in fact, the patient was established with the practice and was seen strictly for a follow-up medical check. The resulting error was an example of

   _____.

2. List three ways Medicare contractors strive to meet their goal of reducing improper payments.

3. List three improper payment review entities and the purpose of their reviews.

4. What differentiates recovery auditors from other entities performing improper payment reviews?

5. How can healthcare facilities use the OIG Work Plan to enhance their compliance efforts?

Audit Management

Audits are functions that allow retrospective reconstruction of events, including who executed the events in question, why, and what changes were made as a result (Foltz and Lankisch 2020, 513). When audits are inserted into the revenue cycle arena, they are utilized to provide a systematic and objective review of revenue cycle processes to determine the level of compliance with policies, procedures, and regulations. Audits can be internal or external. An internal audit is initiated by the healthcare facility or provider practice. An internal audit can be conducted by a staff member or contracted out to a consulting firm. Internal audits are valuable quality assurance tools that support revenue integrity. An example of an internal audit would be a coding audit to establish a baseline compliance rate for the coding unit. An external audit is initiated by a third-party payer and performed by employees of that insurance company. An example of an external audit is a MAC conducting an audit on behalf of Medicare. Internal audits, also referred to as self-audits, are valuable tools to reduce a facility's level of noncompliance. Internal audits can help in the following ways:

- Reduce coding and billing fraud and improper payments
- Improve patient care
- Lower the chances of an external audit by third-party payers
- Create a robust culture of compliance (CMS 2016c)

It is important to have good audit management to get the most out of an audit. Audit management includes creating and executing an internal audit program, as well as managing external audit requests.

Internal audit programs provide a framework for how to achieve revenue integrity or a high level of revenue cycle compliance. A key standard is to develop a program that will review 3.5 to 5 percent of total medical record volume per month (Humbert 2018, 18). For audits to meet this standard, they should be planned so they are ongoing and consistent throughout the various revenue cycle processes. The internal audit plan will determine the annual focus areas. The compliance department works with the coding manager, clinical documentation integrity (CDI) manager, and ancillary department managers to determine compliance issues. Additionally, the compliance department, along with the previously mentioned managers, will review recent compliance topics identified through the internal coding analytics dashboard, OIG Work Plan, RAC vulnerabilities lists, high-volume or high-dollar denials, and past audits. Figure 13.5 provides sample focus areas for revenue cycle internal audit plans. Once the revenue cycle team establishes the focus areas for the year, an audit plan can be developed for each audit and an audit schedule set.

Figure 13.5.   Sample focus areas for revenue cycle internal audit plans

Reimbursement	Coding	CDI
Top MS-DRGs	Low/high CC/MCC capture rates	Medical necessity denials
Late charges	Principle diagnosis assignment	Decreased query rate
Charge description master (CDM) errors	ICD-10-PCS coding	Decreased physician agreement rate
Charge capture	POA assignment	Working MS-DRG–Final MS-DRG agreement rate
One-day stays	Discharge disposition (status) assignment	Query compliance

An audit plan predetermines the who, what, where, when, why, and how for the audit. It is a critical communication tool that ensures that all stakeholders agree to and understand the goals and scope for the audit. Figure 13.6 outlines the components of an audit plan.

As outlined in figure 13.6, there are numerous components to ensuring an audit is fully vetted and ready for execution. As mentioned in the How section of figure 13.6, it is important to select the best sampling technique for the audit. Because it is not feasible to review all medical records or encounters, sampling is used to provide a representation of the population in the audit time frame. There are generally two types of sampling techniques: probability sampling and nonprobability sampling. Probability sampling techniques include the following:

- Simple random sampling (SRS): In this sampling technique, each admission in the population has an equal chance of being selected. An example is numbering every admission in the time frame and using a random number generator to select the audit sample.

- Systematic random sampling: In this sampling technique, the medical records for the audit are identified by selecting every nth unit on the list. An example is taking a list of medical records for the month of May and selecting the first record and then every fourth record thereafter.

- Stratified random sampling: In this sampling technique, the medical records are divided into similar groups or strata based on a criterion. Each medical record is assigned to only one stratum. Once the strata are established, the medical records are randomly selected from each stratum. An example of this concept is basing strata by Medicare severity diagnosis-related group (MS-DRG). Then a set number of medical records is randomly selected from each MS-DRG stratum.

- Cluster sampling: In this sampling technique, the medical record population is divided into groups before the sample is selected. Each medical record is assigned to only one cluster. An example of this technique is to assign clusters by discharge date for the month of August. Then the discharge dates are randomly selected. All medical records for the discharge dates randomly selected are included in the audit.

Nonprobability sampling does not involve a random sampling of the population. Nonprobability sampling includes the following:

- Judgment sampling: In this technique, the subject matter expert relies on their own judgment to select the sample for the audit. An example of when judgment sampling would be used is when the healthcare facility is aware of an issue based on previous studies and uses that as a guide to sample cases.

- Quota sampling: In this sampling technique, the medical records are stratified, and then the subject matter expert selects the number of medical records based on a specified proportion. An example of this technique is to divide medical records by surgeon. Then the sample is selected based on the percentage of total surgeries performed during the study period for each surgeon.

- Convenience sampling: In this sampling technique, selection for the audit is based on the availability of the medical record that is "conveniently" available to be included in the audit. An example would be when the data quality auditor present in the coding unit that day specializes in neoplasm coding, so the coding manager identifies only neoplasm cases to be audited that day. The convenience of the type of auditor present drives the content of the audit. (White 2020, 238–239)

It is very important to select the correct sampling technique to meet the goals of the audit. For example, if the goal of the audit is to establish a coding quality performance baseline and be sure that each coder is represented proportionately in the sample, then the best sampling technique is stratified random sampling. Another example would be, if the goal of the audit is to assess the quality of medical record documentation for cardiac surgery admissions, then the best sampling technique is SRS of the population of cardiac surgery admissions only.

Figure 13.6   Components of an audit plan

Who

- Who is the client or audience for the audit? This is the area or group that will receive the audit results.
- Who will conduct the audit? This may be an individual or a team. The audit plan will establish the expertise required for the audit.

What

- What is the focus of the audit? This section outlines the criteria that will be evaluated for compliance with rules, policies and procedures, and regulations.
- What documents and data points will be audited? This section specifies which documents within the medical record will be reviewed. It also includes documents or data outside of the medical record such as CDI queries and UB-04 billing forms.

Where

- Where will the audit be performed? This component discusses if the audit will take place at the medical facility or if it will be performed offsite. The electronic health record allows for audits to be performed offsite by remote coders or external consulting firms.

When

- What is the time frame for the medical records or data elements included in the audit? This section specifies the time frame for the sample selection. For example, medical records with a discharge date of 1/1/20XX-6/30/20XX.
- When will the audit take place? This is a critical piece of information. Management will plan to provide training and education and set monitoring protocol to take place after the audit. It is important to know when the audit will be performed and when the final report will be provided to the client.

Why

- Why is the audit being conducted? In addition to the focus of the audit, it is important to understand the goals of the audit. Audits can be performed to establish a baseline metric, to assess compliance, or to ensure that risk areas previously audited have been corrected. Establishing goals for the audit is a critical component of the audit plan.

How

- How will the audit sample be selected? There are multiple types of samples to be considered for an audit. The audit plan should identify which technique is best for the audit.
- How will the audit be conducted? Each audit should have a data collection tool so consistent data points are captured for each encounter. Data collection tools can be in paper forms or can be in electronic format.
- How will the compliance/error rate be calculated? For medical recording coding audits the plan should establish if code over code or record over record methodology should be used.
- How will the results be communicated? It is important to specify the final deliverable for the audit. For example, the final deliverable may consist of a formal presentation to stakeholders followed by a written report and when the final report will be provided to the client.

At the completion of the audit, all parties involved will want to know how well the facility performed. Therefore, it is important to establish how the compliance rate will be calculated. There are four basic methodologies for compliance rate calculation:

1. Code over code: In this methodology, all codes are assigned a weight of 1. Emphasis is placed on the correct assignment of each code.

2. Weighted code over code: In this methodology, select categories of codes, such as principal diagnosis and complication or comorbidity (CC)/major complication or comorbidity (MCC) codes, are given a greater weight than other codes. The greater the assigned weight, the greater emphasis the facility places on the correct assignment of the code.

3. Record over record: In this methodology, each record is assigned a weight of 1. Emphasis is placed on the correct assignment for all codes for the entire record.

4. Weighted record over record: In this methodology, various coding criteria are assigned a weight for each code. For example, correct assignment of principal diagnosis, CC/MCC secondary diagnosis codes, POA indicator, and principal procedure and discharge disposition codes that impact patient classification assignment are given the highest weights. Secondary diagnoses that change severity of illness (SOI) or risk of mortality (ROM), or are CMS hierarchical condition categories (HCCs), are assigned a modest weight. Non-CC/MCC secondary diagnosis codes, secondary procedure codes, and discharge disposition codes that do not impact patient classification assignment are given the lowest weight. In this methodology, varying degrees of emphasis are placed on types of coded data. (Stanfill 2019, 31)

Code over code and record over record are the simplest and most used compliance rate methodologies. Weighted code over code and weighted record over record are becoming more popular as coding managers strive to ensure revenue integrity around reimbursement methodologies (Stanfill 2019, 30). For example, great emphasis is placed on assigning the correct MS-DRG, as discussed chapter 5, "Medicare Hospital Acute Inpatient Payment System." Using either of the weighted compliance rate methodologies emphasizes the coded data elements that contribute to the MS-DRG assignment. The weighted compliance rate methodologies can also be used to define a more detailed performance review for coding professionals. Figure 13.7 provides the compliance rate formulas for each type of methodology.

Compliance rates for coding audits can be complex. However, in general terms the compliance rate is how many times something happened divided by how many times something could have happened. Example 13.1 provides sample audit results with the compliance rates calculated for each type of methodology.

Figure 13.7.   Compliance rate formulas

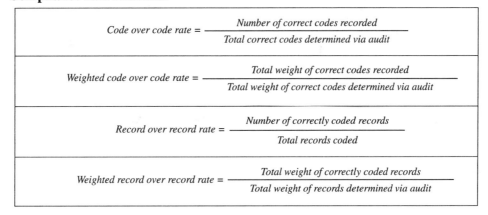

$$\text{Code over code rate} = \frac{\textit{Number of correct codes recorded}}{\textit{Total correct codes determined via audit}}$$

$$\text{Weighted code over code rate} = \frac{\textit{Total weight of correct codes recorded}}{\textit{Total weight of correct codes determined via audit}}$$

$$\text{Record over record rate} = \frac{\textit{Number of correctly coded records}}{\textit{Total records coded}}$$

$$\text{Weighted record over record rate} = \frac{\textit{Total weight of correctly coded records}}{\textit{Total weight of records determined via audit}}$$

Example 13.1

Record		A	B	C	D	Totals
Total Codes		5	8	7	3	23.0
Principal Dx	Coded	1	1	1	1	4.0
	Error	0	0	1	0	1.0
Coded MCCs	Coded	0	2	2	1	5.0
	Error	1	0	0	0	1.0
Total MCCs—via audit		1	2	2	1	6.0
Other Codes	Coded	2	3	4	1	10.0
	Error	1	0	0	0	1.0
Total Other Codes—via audit		1	3	4	1	9.0
PDX Weight		2	2	2	2	8.0
MCC Weight		1.5	1.5	1.5	1.5	6.0
Other Code Weight		1	1	1	1	4.0
Total Weight		4.5	8	9	4.5	26.0
Correct Number of Codes		3	6	7	3	19.0
Correct Code Count		1	6	6	3	16.0
Correct Code Weight		3	8	6	4.5	21.5

In this scenario, the principal diagnosis is weighted as 2, MCCs are weighted as 1.5, and all other codes are weighted as 1. Using this scenario, one may calculate the following rates:

$$\text{Code over code rate} = \frac{\text{Number of correct codes recorded}}{\text{Total correct codes determined via audit}}$$

$$= \frac{1+6+6+3}{3+6+7+3} = \frac{16}{19} = 84.2\%$$

$$\text{Weighted code over code rate} = \frac{\text{Total weight of correct codes recorded}}{\text{Total weight of correct codes determined via audit}}$$

$$= \frac{3+8+6+4.5}{4.5+8+9+4.5} = \frac{21.5}{26.0} = 82.7\%$$

$$\text{Record over recod rate} = \frac{\text{Number of correctly coded records}}{\text{Total records coded}}$$

$$= \frac{2}{4} = 50\%$$

(continued)

$$\textit{Weighted record over record rate} = \cfrac{\textit{Total weight of correctly coded records}}{\textit{Total weight of records determined via audit}}$$

$$= \frac{8 + 4.5}{26} = \frac{12.5}{26} = 48\%$$

It is important to note that correct codes are codes that are not revised (replaced, adjusted, or re-sequenced), added, or deleted. Since nonweighted approaches are still the most prevalent methodologies, these compliance rate methodologies are better for internal and external benchmarking. For a weighted approach to be relevant, all parties need to use the same weighting scheme to make the data comparable. Regardless of the methodology chosen, it is imperative to take this into consideration when developing the audit data collection tool. If a weighted methodology is chosen, the ability to assign codes to a weighted category should be present on the data collection tool. Data collection tools are discussed in more detail in the next section.

Another key component of the audit plan is the data collection tool. Considerable thought must go into developing an audit tool that provides data to support the goals of the audit. For example, if the goal is to audit the charge capture of services provided during an intensity-modulated radiation therapy (IMRT) protocol used for patients undergoing radiation therapy treatment for cancer, then the data collection tool should include all services that could be provided during the course of treatment. An example of a data collection tool for IMRT protocol is provided in figure 13.8.

As illustrated in figure 13.8, the data collection tool is very detailed. It goes beyond ensuring that what was captured on the claim is correct and also allows the auditor to identify if charges were missed during the charge capture process. The tool also incorporates key compliance guidance prompting the auditor to see if the facility followed these rules. This data collection tool allows the auditor to report at the completion of the audit (1) if the charges that were captured are correct and (2) if the facility failed to capture charges for the course of treatment.

Audit deliverables convey the results of the audit to the revenue cycle team. It is best practice to request a presentation of the results as well as a written report with supporting data files. The presentation should include a review of the audit scope and highlight the main areas of concern. This provides the revenue cycle team with an overview of the audit results. It is best practice to design a value-added audit where insights and next steps are provided by the auditor. The final report should provide more details about the audit including an account of all inaccuracies identified during the audit. A manager or subject matter expert should review the audit report details and confirm agreement with the issues the auditor identified. The revenue cycle team should request references for coding and billing advice. External auditors are not held accountable by third-party payers about advice provided in auditing reports. Rather, the hospital or physicians are held accountable for compliance. Therefore, the hospital or physician must research advice provided by external consultants to ensure it is accurate and complies with state and federal regulations.

Audits are only beneficial if one acts on the information included in the final report. Based on the audit findings, the revenue cycle team will develop education and training to target risk areas. For example, if the coding audit identifies that the coding professionals are incorrectly coding coronary artery bypass procedure *International Classification of Diseases, Tenth Revision, Procedure Coding System* (ICD-10-PCS) codes, then education and training should be provided for the inpatient coding staff. Another example would be if the audit identified that 8 percent of the CDI queries for the month of July were leading the physician to document a CC or MCC secondary diagnosis code, then the education and training would target CDI professionals. Along with education and training, the staff manager may need to initiate performance improvement plans for staff members that fall below quality or performance standards or key performance indicators. For example, if the key performance indicator for coding accuracy is 95 percent, and coder A has a performance rate of 80 percent in the audit, then the coding manager should develop and initiate a performance improvement plan for this coding professional.

After education and training are provided, the appropriate manager should incorporate monitoring to review staff performance for compliance with the training. Managers can review the professionals' work, such as a review of coding or CDI query writing. The manager may also use metrics such as dashboards to review number of records coded per day, number of denials by coding professional, or number of queries written by CDI professional (see chapter 10, "Revenue Cycle Middle Processes—Resource Tracking," for an example of a coding management dashboard). Based on the monitoring results, an additional audit may be considered to ensure compliance.

Figure 13.8.   Sample data collection tool for IMRT audit

IMRT - Instensity Modulated Radiation Therapy

Patient
MRN

Check box when billed	Section One - Services Typically Performed Once per Course of Treatment	
	Images	
	77014	Report for images obtained prior to planning
	Simulation	
	77290	Confirm that physician order is present
	77332-77334	Confirm that devices are documented in the simulation note/report
# units		Use modifier -59 if provided on the same date of service as 77301
	77338	77338 new code 2010 for MLC devices for IMRT
# units		
	C1716	Use code C1716 when gold seeds are utilized
	77280	Confirm that verification simulation was ordered and performed
	Treatment Planning	
	77301	Report once per course of treatment
		NCCI Edits:
		Do not report 3D simulation separately
		Do not report isodose separately
		Do not report dosimetry or physics verification separately
		Do not report special treatment plan separately
	Basic Radiation Dosimetry	
	77300 # units	Report one unit for each IMRT beam
	Special Physics Consultation	
	77370	Confirm that the consultation is requested by radiation oncologist
		Confirm that a patient specific issue is addressed and documented
		Confirm that the results are documented in a report
	Boost Plan	
	77307	Bill each service performed
	77300	Verify that there is a new plan code
	77332-77334	Confirm that devices are documented in the simulation note/report
	Treatment Delivery	
See table	77385-77386	Report once per treatment session
		If provided BID, use modifier 76/77 for second session
		If conventional radiation is provided in addition to IMRT, it is bundled and is not separately reported.
See table	77417	Port films - report once per 5 treatment sessions
See table	77336	Weekly physics check - report once per 5 treatment sessions
		If initial chart check is performed prior to treatment delivery, **do not bill**

(continued)

Figure 13.8.   *(continued)*

IMRT - Instensity Modulated Radiation Therapy

Treatment Date	Port Films (77417)		Weekly Physics Check (77336)	
	Performed (Y for Yes; N for No)	Billed (Y for Yes; N for No)	Performed (Y for Yes; N for No)	Billed (Y for Yes; N for No)

Section Two - Reoccurring Services within a Course of Treatment

Coding and Billing Compliance Tools

In today's healthcare environment, every facility has a compliance plan. It is important for clinical, ancillary, and business operations departments to have policies and procedures that align with the facility's compliance plan. Because coding and billing affect reimbursement, this is a highly regulated area (Bowman 2008, 115). Leadership teams for coding and billing functions must develop protocols to ensure compliance with the laws, regulations, and requirements for all payers, both government and private. It is a challenge to stay up to date with all compliance guidance. Making compliance guidance a part of regular activities will help ensure that the coding and billing teams stay focused on compliance. Likewise, a good working relationship with the facility's compliance department will help the teams address and resolve difficult compliance issues.

Numerous publications and policy documents must be reviewed and assessed throughout the year to keep the revenue cycle operations compliant with coding and billing regulations. This section provides an overview of many publications that affect revenue compliance. Though many of these documents pertain to Medicare, private payer regulations should not be forgotten. Many private payers have adopted compliance guidelines similar to Medicare, but the specifics for each payer should be closely examined and incorporated into the facility's compliance plan. Several types of compliance guidance are explored in the following sections, including *Medicare Claims Processing Manual*, CMS transmittals, national and local coverage determinations, National Correct Coding Initiative (NCCI), Outpatient Code Editor (OCE), and payer-specific edits.

Medicare Claims Processing Manual

The *Medicare Claims Processing Manual* (Publication 100-04) is one of the many manuals included in the CMS Internet-Only Manuals System. The Internet-Only Manuals System is used by CMS program components, partners, contracts, and other agencies to administer CMS programs. Day-to-day operating instructions, policies, and procedures based on statutes, regulations, guidelines, models, and directives are included in the manuals (CMS n.d.).

The *Medicare Claims Processing Manual* has 39 chapters and provides guidance for producing claims for all healthcare settings (inpatient, outpatient rehabilitation, and the like). General billing regulations, as well as service area–specific requirements are provided. Revenue cycle coordinators should be familiar with many of the chapters and may study more closely the requirements outlined for the service areas included in the hospital's own book of business. For example, the revenue cycle coordinator may have a cursory understanding of ambulatory surgical center regulations but may have a detailed understanding of hospital inpatient requirements.

The *Medicare Claims Processing Manual* is updated throughout the year based on changes made to the various prospective payment systems. For example, changes brought about by the final inpatient prospective payment system (IPPS) rule in August would be incorporated in the *Medicare Claims Processing Manual* by October 1. Likewise, the modifications from the final outpatient prospective payment system (OPPS) rule in November would be incorporated by January 1. One excellent feature is that CMS displays changes to the *Medicare Claims Processing Manual* in red, allowing users to browse the individual chapters and easily locate recent changes.

CMS Transmittals

CMS program transmittals are used by CMS to communicate policies and procedures for the various payment systems' program manuals to the MACs. Current and historic transmittals dating back to 2000 can be found under the "Regulations and Guidance" tab at the CMS website (CMS 2021c).

Revenue cycle professionals should stay up to date with transmittals released for Part A and Part B Medicare payment systems. They should read transmittals carefully and communicate the information effectively to the compliance department and applicable department representatives on the revenue cycle team. Any issues related to the charge description master (CDM) should be incorporated into the facility's active CDM as warranted. The CDM coordinator should keep an audit trail of changes made to the CDM based on transmittal guidance.

National and Local Coverage Determinations

National coverage determinations (NCDs) are rules that are released by CMS that describe the circumstances under which medical supplies, services, or procedures are covered nationwide by Medicare under Title XVIII of the Social Security Act of 1935 and other medical regulations and rulings. After the NCD has been published, it is binding for all Medicare contractors (MACs, durable medical equipment regional contractors [DMERCS], quality improvement organizations [QIOs], and so on). Contractors are responsible for notifying the provider community of an NCD release. Contractors do not have the authority to deviate from an NCD when absolute words such as "never" or "only if" are used in the policy. When reviewing coverage issues, the contractors may cover services at their own discretion based on a **local coverage determination (LCD)** if an NCD has not been established.

LCDs provide facilities and physicians with the circumstances under which a service, procedure, or supply is considered medically necessary (CMS 2023c). An LCD is used to determine coverage within the jurisdiction of the MAC, rather than nationwide, as with an NCD. There are regional differences in medical necessity, and, thus, differences in coverage for Medicare supplies, services, and procedures. LCDs are educational materials intended to assist facilities and providers with correct billing and claim processing. Within the LCD is a listing of *International Classification of Diseases, Tenth Revision, Clinical Modification* (ICD-10-CM) codes that indicate which conditions are covered and which conditions are not covered. Additionally, there may be a list of the Healthcare Common Procedure Coding System (HCPCS) codes for which the LCD applies.

It is important to understand the difference between coverage and medical necessity. For example, chest x-rays are covered by Medicare. However, the service is only reimbursed by Medicare when it is deemed medically necessary. This means that the physician must provide sufficient medical documentation to support ICD-10-CM diagnosis coding of the condition, to substantiate that the service is warranted for diagnostic or therapeutic treatment of the patient. Medicare does not pay for services that are not medically necessary.

The *Medicare National Coverage Determinations Manual* (NCD Manual) is an Internet-Only Manual (also called IOM) published by CMS. This manual lists all topics included in the numerous active NCDs. The publication number for the NCD manual is 100-03.

To gain a clear understanding of coverage issues, examine NCD 140.2, shown in figure 13.9. From the information provided in this NCD, the Medicare program will not reimburse breast reconstruction procedures for cosmetic reasons. Cosmetic surgery is excluded from coverage under Section 1862(a)(10) of the act. However, breast reconstruction following the removal of a breast for any medical reason is a covered procedure. This coverage determination applies to both the affected and the contralateral unaffected breast (CMS 2023d, section 140.2).

Additional information regarding LCDs is located in the *Medicare Program Integrity Manual* (Publication 100-08), chapter 13, "Local Coverage Determinations." Chapter 13 outlines Medicare policy regarding NCDs and LCDs and then provides the regulations for LCD creation, modification, distribution, execution, and appeals.

Figure 13.9.   NCD 140.2—Breast reconstruction following mastectomy

---

140.2 Breast reconstruction following mastectomy

(Rev. 1, 10-03-03)

CIM 35-47

During recent years, there has been a considerable change in the treatment of diseases of the breasts such as fibrocystic disease and cancer. While extirpation of the disease remains of primary importance, the quality of life following initial treatment is increasingly recognized as of great concern. The increased use of breast reconstruction procedures is due to several factors:

- A change in epidemiology of breast cancer, including an apparent increase in incidence;
- Improved surgical skills and techniques;
- The continuing development of better prostheses; and
- Increasing awareness by physicians of the importance of postsurgical psychological adjustment.

Reconstruction of the affected and the contralateral unaffected breast following a medically necessary mastectomy is considered a relatively safe and effective noncosmetic procedure. Accordingly, program payment may be made for breast reconstruction surgery following removal of a breast for any medical reason.

Program payment may not be made for breast reconstruction for cosmetic reasons. (Cosmetic surgery is excluded from coverage under §1862(a)(10) of the Act.)

Source: CMS 2023d, 41–42.

When examining LCDs, it is important to understand the difference between policies and articles. An LCD policy contains only the reasonable and necessary provisions regarding a supply, procedure, or service. For example, an LCD policy may provide a list of codes describing which conditions warrant medical necessity and which conditions do not.

MACs use an article to provide guidelines about the benefit category, statutory exclusions, and coding provisions. For example, coding guidelines relating to diagnosis codes in the medical necessity code list would be provided in an article, not in the LCD policy itself. Thus, to fully understand an LCD and effectively implement it, a revenue cycle professional must read the policy as well as any associated articles.

To find NCDs and LCDs for a specific geographic area, revenue cycle professionals can access the Medicare Coverage Database at the CMS website. This search engine allows the user to search documents of national coverage or local coverage. Additionally, the user can search articles and policies by geographic area or MAC. It also allows the user to enter search criteria, such as Current Procedural Terminology (CPT) or HCPCS code, keywords, ICD-10-CM codes, coverage topics, and date criteria.

National Correct Coding Initiative

The **National Correct Coding Initiative (NCCI)** is a set of edits that was designed to promote national correct coding practices and to control improper coding that results in inappropriate payment for Part B claims. NCCI edits have been in place for outpatient claim editing since January 1, 1996. There are two sets of NCCI edits, one for the physician setting and one for the hospital outpatient setting. The hospital outpatient setting edits are embedded in the editing system used by MACs to process claims under OPPS.

The purpose of the NCCI edits is to ensure proper CPT and HCPCS coding for Medicare Part B services. These edits are not medical necessity denial edits, but rather they are in place to ensure correct coding and payment. The edits are designed to audit CPT codes based on the CPT coding conventions, national and local policies and edits, coding guidelines developed by national societies, analysis of standard medical and surgical practices, and a review of current coding practices (CMS 2023e).

Within the set of edits, there are two types: **procedure-to-procedure (PTP) edits** and **medically unlikely edits (MUEs)**. The PTP edits identify instances in which two procedure codes should not be reported together on the same date of service for a single beneficiary unless it is appropriate to append a modifier. Typically, PTP edits are for errors in comprehensive coding. Some edits represent the failure to report a comprehensive code. Instead, the facility has inappropriately reported components of the service. Some PTP edits represent unbundling. In these cases, a comprehensive code and a component code are reported together. PTP edits also contain mutually exclusive edits. These code combinations consist of codes that would not reasonably be reported together or that should not be reported together. There are two versions of PTP edits, one for practitioners (physicians, clinicians, and ambulatory surgical centers) and one for hospital-based facilities (hospital outpatient, home health, physical therapy, occupational therapy, speech-language pathology, comprehensive rehabilitation facilities, and skilled nursing facilities).

MUEs identify the maximum number of units of service that are allowable for a HCPCS code for a single beneficiary on a single date of service. When the unit of service is higher than the allowable amount, then the line item is flagged for rejection, or denial. There are three versions of MUE: practitioner (physician and clinicians), DME supplier, and facility outpatient (hospital outpatient and critical access hospitals).

All PTP edits and MUEs are released quarterly on the CMS website. Figure 13.10 provides an example of a PTP NCCI edit for a laboratory panel.

CMS publishes the *National Correct Coding Initiative Policy Manual for Medicare Services*, available on the CMS website. Additionally, the *Medicare Claims Processing Manual* contains information regarding NCCI edits in chapter 23, section 20.9. Chapter 23, section 20.9.1, "Correct Coding Modifier Indicators and HCPCS Codes Modifiers," discusses the NCCI edits that allow providers to use modifiers to indicate special circumstances when the code edit should be bypassed based on the patient's specific course of treatment (CMS n.d.). Several modifiers have specific usage guidelines to prevent fraud and abuse situations.

Figure 13.10.   NCCI edit

CPT code 80061 (lipid panel) includes the following tests:

CPT code 82465—Cholesterol, serum or whole blood, total

CPT code 83718—Lipoprotein, direct; HDL cholesterol

CPT code 84478—Triglycerides

When all tests are performed, the panel test, CPT code 80061, should be reported in place of the individual tests.

Source: CMS 2023e.

Medicare Code Editor and Medicare Outpatient Code Editor

The **Medicare Code Editor (MCE)** is software that detects and reports errors identified on Medicare inpatient claims. The edits use coded data, mainly ICD-10-CM and ICD-10-PCS codes, to identify errors. The MCE definitions are published annually in conjunction with the IPPS final rule. MCE v40.1, applicable for FY 2023, included 15 active edits. Examples of MCE edits include the following:

- Invalid diagnosis or procedure code
- Age conflict
- Unacceptable principal diagnosis
- Noncovered procedure
- Manifestation code as principal diagnosis (CMS 2023f)

Revenue cycle professionals identify which codes or data elements are applicable for each edit in the "Definitions of Medicare Code Edits" document released by CMS.

The Medicare Outpatient Code Editor (OCE) is a software program designed to process data for the Medicare hospital outpatient payment system pricing and to audit facility claims data. The processing function prepares submitted claims data for the Medicare Pricer software by doing the following:

- Editing the claims for accuracy
- Assigning appropriate ambulatory payment classifications (APCs)
- Assigning CMS-designated status indicators
- Assigning payment indicators
- Computing applicable discounts
- Determining a claim disposition based on generated edits
- Determining whether packaging is applicable
- Determining applicable payment adjustments (CMS 2022c)

The editing function audits claims for coding and data entry errors. The extensive edits in the OCE are applied to claims, individual diagnoses and procedures, and code sets. Table 13.3 provides a sample of edits included in the

Table 13.3.   **Sample of the edits included in the OCE**

Edit	Generated When....
1. Invalid diagnosis code	The principal diagnosis field is blank, there are no diagnoses entered on the claim, or the entered diagnosis code is not valid.
2. Diagnosis and age conflict	The diagnosis code includes an age range, and the age is outside that range.
8. Procedure and sex conflict	The sex of the patient does not match the sex designated for the procedure code reported. This edit is bypassed if condition code 45 is present on the claim.
28. Code not recognized by Medicare; alternate code for same service may be available	The procedure code has "Not recognized by Medicare" indicator.
41. Invalid revenue code	The revenue code is not in the list of valid revenue code entries.

Source: CMS 2023g, 54–68.

OCE. When activated, OCE edits have an associated line or claim disposition attached to them. Table 13.4 provides a listing of the edit dispositions and their definitions.

Depending on the claim disposition, providers or facilities may correct the claim or process adjustments based on facility policy. It is crucial that facilities monitor and analyze claim disposition. Possible reasons for claim errors should be investigated, with corrective action taken when applicable. Most revenue cycle teams have an ongoing quality monitoring process in place so resolutions to claim errors can be incorporated into the process. Example 13.2 walks through a simple analysis for OCE edit number 48.

Example 13.2

In January, the reconciliation unit at Hospital A begins to see Medicare bills with rejections for OCE edit number 48, revenue center requires HCPCS. Upon investigation, it is found that a line item for a newly added charge code is missing the CPT code in the CDM. When the claim is generated, the line-item data for this service are included on the claim. However, for this service the revenue code is present, but the CPT code is not. Perhaps during the annual update, the line item was created, but the CPT code was not added to the line item. Though this is a somewhat simple fix to the CDM—the CPT code is added to the line item—it is a wake-up call to the CDM unit that quality review of the CDM annual update may need to be revisited and the process improved.

The edits are updated quarterly and posted under the "Medicare" tab on the CMS website. Revenue cycle professionals should review the edits annually to ensure all requirements of claims processing are applied in the middle processes, resource tracking component of the revenue cycle.

Payer Policy Manuals

Most commercial payers release payer policy manuals. Typically, the manuals are released or updated annually in coordination with the payer's FY. The payer policy manuals outline billing rules and regulations like the CMS online manuals. In addition to policy manuals, commercial payers will issue policy alerts that highlight a new or highly monitored coding and billing topic. The policy manuals also include payer-specific edits. These edits should

Table 13.4.   Listing of the edit dispositions and their definitions

Disposition	Definition
Claim rejection	There are one or more edits present that cause the whole claim to be rejected. A claim rejection means that the provider can correct and resubmit the claim but cannot appeal the claim rejection.
Claim denial	There are one or more edits present that cause the whole claim to be denied. A claim denial means that the provider cannot resubmit the claim but can appeal the claim denial.
Claim return to provider (RTP)	There are one or more edits present that cause the whole claim to be returned to the provider. A claim returned to the provider means that the provider can resubmit the claim once the problems are corrected.
Claim suspension	There are one or more edits present that cause the whole claim to be suspended. A claim suspension means that the claim is not returned to the provider; the claim is not processed for payment until the MAC decides or obtains more information.
Line item rejection	There are one or more edits present that cause one or more individual line items to be rejected. A line item rejection means that the claim can be processed for payment with some line items rejected for payment. The line item can be corrected and resubmitted but cannot be appealed.
Line item denial	There are one or more edits present that cause one or more individual line items to be denied. A line item denial means that the claim can be processed for payment with some line items denied for payment. The line item cannot be resubmitted but can be appealed.

Source: CMS 2023g, 43–44.

be analyzed by the compliance department and adhered to by coding and billing teams. For example, state workers' compensation (WC) provisions may not cover preventive immunizations. However, they may cover tetanus shots postinjury and have advised facilities to report these charges in revenue code 0450 via a policy alert. The claims processing system used by WC contains an edit to deny claim line items reported with revenue codes 0770 to 0779, preventive care services. Thus, when a tetanus administration is provided to a WC patient in the emergency department, the code should be reported with revenue code 0450, rather than 0771, for patients with a WC financial class.

Check Your Understanding 13.2

1. Define internal audit and external audit.

2. Maria is the coding manager at Community Hospital. She is preparing an inpatient medical record audit plan. She has a list of the inpatient discharges from January to March 202X. She has elected to include the fourth record and then every eighth medical record thereafter for inclusion in her review. Which type of probability sampling did Maria use to choose records for the audit?

3. Provide three examples of the types of information that are included in the *Medicare Claims Processing Manual*.

4. Medicare issues national coverage determinations (NCDs) and MACs release local coverage determinations (LCDs). Compare and contrast these two types of documents.

5. Discuss the two types of edits included in the National Correct Coding Initiative (NCCI).

Denials Management

Claims that healthcare providers and facilities submit to health insurance companies are not always approved and paid. A **claim denial** is "the refusal of an insurance company or carrier to honor a request by an individual (or his or her provider) to pay for health care services obtained from a health care professional" (Healthinsurance. org n.d.). Even though a considerable amount of reimbursement is at risk for denial, there are estimates that 90 percent of claim denials are preventable (Humbert 2019). Therefore, to mitigate the financial risk associated with claims denials, healthcare facilities support denials management. The goals of a denials management program are to decrease the volume of denials and associated lost reimbursement for the denials, to convert initial denials into payable claims, and to improve processes to prevent future denials.

There are two types of denials, administrative and clinical. An **administrative denial** occurs when the insurance provider finds fault with the claim. This includes incorrect coding, failure to obtain preauthorization, registration issues, failure to submit medical record documentation or an itemized claim when requested by the insurance provider, and duplicate charge or claim. These types of denials could also be called *technical denials*. A **clinical denial** is issued when the insurance provider questions a clinical aspect of the admission, such as the length of stay (LOS) of the admission, the level of service, if the encounter meets medical necessity parameters, the site of the service, or if clinical validation is not passed. A **clinical validation denial** indicates that there are insufficient clinical indicators or discussion points within the health record documentation to support the diagnosis assigned to the patient (Powers 2019, 18). External auditors examine medical record documentation for a combination of the following to assess if a patient's disease or condition is appropriately supported:

- Clinical evaluation
- Therapeutic treatment
- Diagnostic procedure
- Increased nursing care
- Extended LOS (Combs 2018, 38)

If evidence of more than one of these criteria is not located in the documentation, then the encounter is at risk for a clinical validation denial. When clinical validation denials are issued, a facility should bring together case management, CDI, and coding representatives to review the case and determine the next steps. Another type of clinical denial that involves CDI and coding is the **MS-DRG coding denial**. An MS-DRG coding denial is one where the payer believes there is a coding error that impacts the MS-DRG assignment based on the *Official Guidelines for Coding and Reporting* or *Coding Clinic* guidance (Parker 2022). For MS-DRG coding denials, the coding manager, data quality analyst manager, and CDI manager can work together with the clinical denial specialist to determine if the denial is valid and if not, which party will complete the appeal. A clinical denial specialist is a health information professional who has a background in coding and has become proficient with addressing and correcting coding and billing edits (Humbert 2019, 48).

Within the facility setting the clinical denial specialist and the coding and CDI departments focus on clinical denials. But it is important to consider that medical coding denials only account for 5 percent of denials (Change Healthcare 2022). Front-end revenue cycle issues represent most denials at 41 percent. The types of front-end denials are registration and eligibility, authorization and precertification, and medical necessity (Change Healthcare 2022). Back-end revenue cycle issues account for 34 percent of denials and include missing or invalid claim data, medical record documentation requested but not provided, and untimely filing. Middle revenue cycle issues represent only 17 percent of denials. These include medical coding, noncovered services, and avoidable care denials (Change Healthcare 2022).

Many facilities create a denials management team, which consists of representatives from the following work areas:

- Health information management department
- Physicians, including a physician advisor
- Coding unit
- CDI team
- Case management
- Managed care contracts unit
- Revenue cycle team
- Legal department
- Finance department
- Compliance office (Powers 2019, 19)

A popular alternative name is the edit and denials team. Team members work together to assess and monitor denials. The team establishes goals and sets metrics and key performance indicators to support them. Three key goals of a denials management team are as follows:

- Reduce the number of denials (lower denial rate)
- Identify the source of denials
- Develop physician and staff knowledge of documentation, coding, and billing regulations

The team also works to promote communication and collaboration among its members. For example, as mentioned earlier, collaboration between case management, coding, and CDI is required to address clinical validation denials. A transparent metrics approach, which is discussed in an upcoming section, helps to foster communication and collaboration as well.

A key member of the denials management team is the clinical denial specialist. A clinical denial specialist actively works to resolve denials by performing the required claim research, collaborating with subject matter experts, determining if an appeal is warranted, writing the denial appeal when applicable, and resubmitting the claim when appropriate. For example, the denial specialist may research clinical indicators for common denials. Organizations such as Kidney Disease: Improving Global Outcomes (KDIGO) and the Surviving Sepsis Campaign provide guidelines, reference keys, and common abbreviations and acronyms used by clinicians and providers to treat patients and document care. The clinical denial specialist can use these guidelines to help them assess the pathway for clinical denials (to appeal or not appeal). The clinical denial specialist will follow the denial to completion. Similar to the RAC denial process discussed earlier in this chapter, each payer will have a denials process. Denials processes are similar among payers, but the clinical denial specialist will need to pay close attention to payer-specific appeal time frames to ensure responses and other key documents are filed in a timely manner.

In addition to actively resolving denials, the denial management team works to understand the reasons for denials so that they can prevent future denials. A three-step approach is used to meet this goal:

1. Track denials
2. Perform root cause analysis
3. Provide ongoing training and education

A best practice for a denials management team is to track denials. Teams may purchase a tracking system or develop one in-house. Key data elements to track include the following:

- Payer
- Denial type
- Date of denial
- Billing amount
- Amount denied
- If appeal was submitted
- Amount recovered

With the data collected in the denial tracking system, the team can create a dashboard to monitor metrics or key performance indicators such as denial rate. Denial rate is a measure of how well a facility or practice complies with billing rules and regulations for all payers (HFMA n.d.). It is calculated by dividing the total number of claims denied by the total number of claims remitted (HFMA n.d.). Additional metrics include top reasons for denial by payer, appeal success rate, top targeted MS-DRGs, and Medicare return to provider (RTP) rate. Figure 13.11 is a sample dashboard of denials management metrics.

Once denials are tracked and assessed, teams should initiate a root cause analysis. An alternative term used is *variance analysis*. Root cause analysis is a technique used to discover the underlying causes of a problem (Carter and Palmer 2020, 565). The basis of root cause analysis is to use problem-solving methods to improve performance. Examples of analysis tools include Pareto charts, five whys, fishbone diagrams, scatter diagrams, and failure mode and effects analysis (FMEA). Each of these tools helps the team identify portions of the billing and coding process that may be revised to reduce the denial rate.

Figure 13.11.   Sample dashboard of denial management metrics

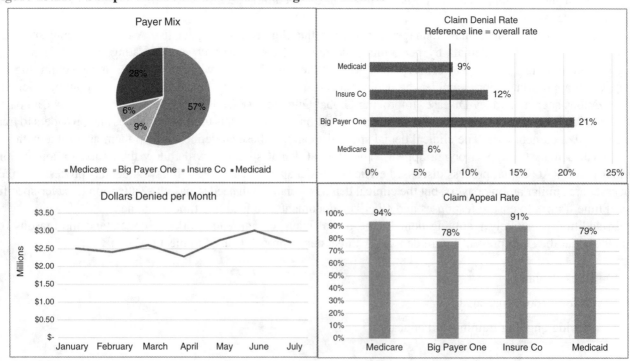

After the reasons for the denials have been identified, the denials management team should develop training and education programs. Training and education should be tailored and targeted toward the appropriate audience based on the root cause analysis findings. For example, if the analysis identifies that the coders are inappropriately coding CC and MCC diagnosis codes for cardiovascular surgery cases, then the education should be directed to the coding professionals and include specific examples of inaccurate and accurate coding for cardiac encounters. After training and education is provided, it is best practice for the denials management team to monitor performance. This can be accomplished through second-level reviews prior to claim submission. The additional review by denial specialists will ensure that claims are properly assembled prior to a request for payment. Any issues with the claim identified during the review, such as incomplete documentation, can be addressed prior to submission, saving the facility the cost of processing claim denials. Lastly, the denials management team can utilize the results of the root cause analysis to modify their claim editing system, which is also known as a scrubber. By altering the editing system, the denials management team can flag claims for review based on specific payer rules. Again, the focus is to prevent an errored claim from being submitted to the payer.

Patient Connection

Kris is the coding manager at Memorial Hospital. She is designing an audit to be performed in January 202X. She begins preparing her plan by addressing who, what, where, when, why, and how.

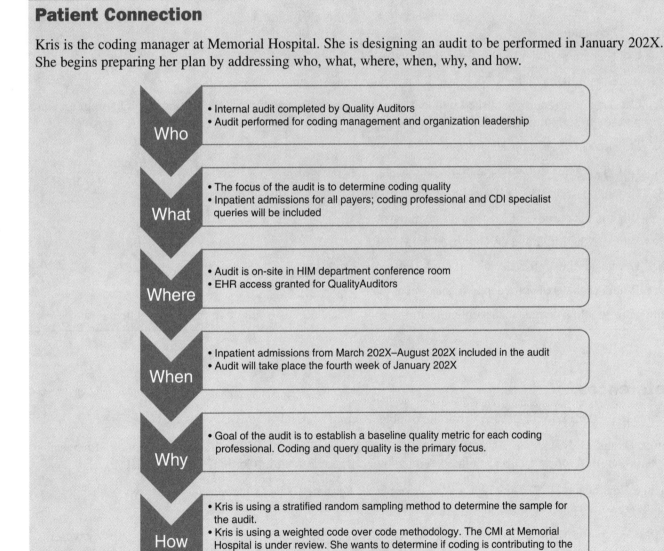

Who
- Internal audit completed by Quality Auditors
- Audit performed for coding management and organization leadership

What
- The focus of the audit is to determine coding quality
- Inpatient admissions for all payers; coding professional and CDI specialist queries will be included

Where
- Audit is on-site in HIM department conference room
- EHR access granted for QualityAuditors

When
- Inpatient admissions from March 202X–August 202X included in the audit
- Audit will take place the fourth week of January 202X

Why
- Goal of the audit is to establish a baseline quality metric for each coding professional. Coding and query quality is the primary focus.

How
- Kris is using a stratified random sampling method to determine the sample for the audit.
- Kris is using a weighted code over code methodology. The CMI at Memorial Hospital is under review. She wants to determine if coding is contributing to the downward trend.

(continued)

Patient Connection   *(continued)*

Although patient Malakai and patient Olivia will never know, both their records were chosen for the internal coding audit through the stratified random sampling method. Take a moment to think about internal hospital processes. Do you think patients are aware of internal compliance processes that may involve their medical records? Facilities and providers perform numerous tasks to ensure that revenue integrity is met. Some of those tasks involve auditing patients' medical records for accuracy. It is one way to ensure efficient and quality healthcare is provided to patients.

Chapter 13 Review Quiz

1. Which of the following is not a common form of fraud and abuse?

    a. Upcoding

    b. Unbundling

    c. Using a modifier to circumnavigate an NCCI edit

    d. Submitting a claim to Medicare for a service that was not rendered

2. Describe how reports published by the Medicare Comprehensive Error Rate Testing (CERT) program can be used to support improper payment reviews.

3. Describe the RAC appeals process.

4. List three goals of internal audits.

5. List and describe the components of an audit plan.

6. What is the purpose of Medicare transmittals?

7. Why are the MCE and OCE utilized by MACs?

8. Define administrative denial and clinical denial.

9. What are the goals of a denial management team?

10. How would a denials management team use root cause analysis to improve the facility's denial rate?

References

Bowman, S. 2008. Why ICD-10 is worth the trouble. *Journal of AHIMA* 79(3): 24–29.

Carter, D. and M. N. Palmer. 2020. "Performance Improvement." Chapter 18 in *Health Information Management Technology: An Applied Approach*, 6th ed., edited by N. B. Sayles and L. Gordon. Chicago: AHIMA.

Change Healthcare. 2022. *The Change Healthcare 2022 Revenue Cycle Denials Index*. https://www.change healthcare.com/insights/denials-index.

CMS (Centers for Medicare and Medicaid Services). 2023a. "Medical Review and Education." https://www.cms .gov/research-statistics-data-and-systems/monitoring-programs/medicare-ffs-compliance-programs/medical -review.

CMS (Centers for Medicare and Medicaid Services). 2023b. "Medicare Fee for Service Recovery Audit Program." https://www.cms.gov/research-statistics-data-and-systems/monitoring-programs/medicare-ffs -compliance-programs/recovery-audit-program.

CMS (Centers for Medicare and Medicaid Services). 2023c "Local Coverage Determinations." https://www.cms .gov/medicare/coverage/determinationprocess/lcds.

CMS (Centers for Medicare and Medicaid Services). 2023d. "Medicare National Coverage Determinations Manual CMS 100-03." https://www.cms.gov/regulations-and-guidance/guidance/manuals/downloads/ncd103c1 _part2.pdf.

CMS (Centers for Medicare and Medicaid Services). 2023e. "National Correct Coding Initiative Edits." https://www.cms.gov/medicare-medicaid-coordination/national-correct-coding-initiative-ncci/ncci-medicare.

CMS (Centers for Medicare and Medicaid Services). 2023f. "Definitions of Medicare Code Edits (v40.1)." https://www.cms.gov/medicare/medicare-fee-for-service-payment/acuteinpatientpps/ms-drg-classifications -and-software.

CMS (Centers for Medicare and Medicaid Services). 2023g. "OCE Quarterly Release Files: IOCE Quarterly Data Files V240.R1." https://www.cms.gov/medicare/coding/outpatientcodeedit/oceqtrreleasespecs.

CMS (Centers for Medicare and Medicaid Services). 2022a. 2022 Medicare Fee-for-Service Supplemental Improper Payment Data. https://www.cms.gov/files/document/2022-medicare-fee-service-supplemental-improper -payment-data.pdf.

CMS (Centers for Medicare and Medicaid Services). 2022b. "Approved RAC Topics." https://www.cms.gov /research-statistics-data-and-systems/monitoring-programs/medicare-ffs-compliance-programs/recovery-audit -program/approved-rac-topics?combine=&items_per_page=10&page=0.

CMS (Centers for Medicare and Medicaid Services). 2022c. "I/OCE Purpose & Background." https://www.cms .gov/medicare/coding/outpatientcodeedit.

CMS (Centers for Medicare and Medicaid Services). 2021a. Medicare Fraud & Abuse: Prevent, Detect, Report. Medicare Learning Network ICN MLN4649244. https://www.cms.gov/Outreach-and-Education/Medicare -Learning-Network-MLN/MLNProducts/Downloads/Fraud-Abuse-MLN4649244.pdf.

CMS (Centers for Medicare and Medicaid Services). 2021b. "Improper Payments Measurement Programs." https://www.cms.gov/Research-Statistics-Data-and-Systems/Monitoring-Programs/Improper-Payment -Measurement-Programs.

CMS (Centers for Medicare and Medicaid Services). 2021c. "Transmittals." https://www.cms.gov/es/node /172701.

CMS (Centers for Medicare and Medicaid Services). 2019. FY 2019 Medicare FFS RAC Report to Congress. https://www.cms.gov/files/document/fy-2019-medicare-ffs-rac-report-congress-appendices.pdf.

CMS (Centers for Medicare and Medicaid Services). 2016a. "Introduction to CERT." https://www.cms.gov/ Research-Statistics-Data-and-Systems/Monitoring-Programs/Medicare-FFS-Compliance-Programs/CERT /Downloads/IntroductiontoCERT_January2016.pdf.

CMS (Centers for Medicare and Medicaid Services). 2016b. Recovery Auditing in Medicare Fee-For-Service for Fiscal Year 2015. https://www.cms.gov/Research-Statistics-Data-and-Systems/Monitoring-Programs/Medicare -FFS-Compliance-Programs/Recovery-Audit-Program/Downloads/FY2015-Medicare-FFS-RAC-Report-to -Congress.pdf.

CMS (Centers for Medicare and Medicaid Services). 2016c. Self-Audit Snapshot. https://www.cms.gov /Medicare-Medicaid-Coordination/Fraud-Prevention/Medicaid-Integrity-Education/Downloads/ebulletins-self -audit.pdf.

CMS (Centers for Medicare and Medicaid Services). n.d. Medicare Claims Processing Manual Publication 100-04. Accessed March 9, 2023. https://www.cms.gov/Regulations-and-Guidance/Guidance/Manuals/Internet -Only-Manuals-IOMs-Items/CMS018912.

Combs, T. 2018. "A Summary of the AHIMA CDI and Coding Collaboration in Denials Management Toolkit, 36–38." https://library.ahima.org/doc?oid=302440#.X3CwyWhKiUk.

Enriquez, K. D. 2011. "Compliance." Chapter 11 in *Effective Management of Coding Services*, edited by L. A. Schraffenberger and L. Kuehn. Chicago: AHIMA.

Foltz, D. A. and K. M. Lankisch. 2020. "Fraud and Abuse Compliance." Chapter 16 in *Health Information Management Technology: An Applied Approach*, 6th ed., edited by N. B. Sayles and L. L. Gordon. Chicago: AHIMA.

Healthinsurance.org. n.d. "Denial of claim." Glossary. Accessed March 9, 2023. https://www.healthinsurance.org /glossary/denial-of-claim/.

HFMA (Healthcare Financial Management Association). n.d. "Map Keys." Accessed March 9, 2023. https://www.hfma.org/data-and-insights/map-initiative/map-keys/.

HHS (Department of Health and Human Services). 2005. OIG supplemental compliance program guidance for hospitals. *Federal Register* 70(19):4858–4876.

HHS (Department of Health and Human Services). 1998. Publication of the OIG Compliance Program Guidance for Hospitals. *Federal Register* 63(35):8987–8998.

Humbert, S. 2019. Denial prevention: Understanding common culprits and how to avoid them. *Journal of AHIMA* 90(5):48–49.

Humbert, S. 2018. How to choose the right coding audit method. *Journal of AHIMA* 89(3):18–19.

OIG (Office of Inspector General). n.d. "Review of Medicare Payments for Trauma Claims." Accessed March 8, 2023. https://oig.hhs.gov/reports-and-publications/workplan/summary/wp-summary-0000742.asp.

Parker, S. 2022. How CDI professionals can lead the clinical validation denials process. *Journal of AHIMA*. https://journal.ahima.org/AMP_EDN/383/How-CDI-Professionals-Can-Lead-the-Clinical-Validation-Denials -Process-1638.amp.html.

Powers, M. 2019. How to battle coding denial trends: Creating a proactive appeal strategy. *Journal of AHIMA* 90(3):16–19.

Stanfill, M. 2019. In pursuit of comparable coding audit benchmarks. *Journal of AHIMA* 90(1):30–31, 47.

White, S. 2020. *Calculating and Reporting Healthcare Statistics*, 6th ed. Chicago: AHIMA.

Part V:
Revenue Cycle
Analysis

Chapter 14
Healthcare Data in Action: Real-World Analysis

Revenue cycle analysis is the examination of health data with the intent to improve the administrative and clinical functions that contribute to the capture, management, and collection of patient service reimbursement. As discussed in chapter 1, revenue integrity principles include operational efficiency, compliance adherence, and legitimate reimbursement. Revenue cycle analysis supports these principles and promotes health data and information transparency. Establishing good focus areas for revenue cycle analysis takes a considerable amount of research by the analytics team. Team members must stay up to date on compliance issues published and discussed in various government and other third-party payer documents. As discussed in chapter 13, "Revenue Compliance," compliance guidance such as the Office of Inspector General (OIG) Work Plan, Comprehensive Error Rate Testing (CERT) report, and National Recovery Audit Program annual report should be reviewed each year. These documents provide insight into the directions the Medicare improper payment review entities, such as Medicare administrative contractors (MACs) and recovery audit contractors (RACs), are taking and highlight potential vulnerabilities and risk areas. This chapter is designed to provide the student with a variety of examples of revenue cycle analysis. This chapter examines eleven case studies:

1. Case-mix index (CMI) analysis

2. Outpatient service-mix index (SMI) calculation

3. Medicare severity diagnosis-related group (MS-DRG) relationship analysis

4. Medicare reimbursement variation analysis

5. Site of service analysis: Inpatient versus outpatient

6. Evaluation and management (E/M) facility coding in the emergency department (ED)

7. Physician coding analysis

8. Outpatient Code Editor (OCE) review for hospital outpatient services

9. Physician productivity analysis

10. Clinical documentation integrity (CDI) program analysis

11. MS-DRG denials

These case studies highlight the most common revenue cycle areas that data analysts examine in order to support revenue integrity.

The eleven case studies presented in this chapter show the wide variety of analyses that are needed to support revenue integrity in healthcare organizations. Both facilities and physician practices can use analysis to improve their operational efficiency. Likewise, analysis is extremely helpful in identifying risk areas. Investigating and engaging in performance improvement processes will help hospitals and physician practices ensure they are adhering to compliance guidelines, rules, and regulations and only receiving reimbursement that is legitimate for the services and supplies provided to patients.

Case-Mix Index Calculation

Case-mix index (CMI) is one of the most common focus areas for healthcare analysis. CMI is a value that compares the overall complexity of the healthcare organization's patients with the average complexity of patients for all hospitals. Before analysis begins, it is important to understand how CMI is calculated. CMI includes all MS-DRG admissions for a specified period of time. But only three MS-DRGs will be used to illustrate CMI calculation in this chapter. The calculation begins with basic admission data elements as shown in table 14.1.

The CMI calculation uses the following formula:

$$CMI = \frac{sum\,of\,MS - DRG\,relative\,weights}{number\,of\,discharges}$$

This is typically computed as a weighted average using the following steps. The first step in CMI calculation is to calculate the weighted volume for each MS-DRG. The weighted volume is calculated by multiplying the MS-DRG relative weight (RW) by the MS-DRG volume. This calculation is performed for each row as shown in table 14.2. For example, the weighted volume for MS-DRG 405 is 15 times 5.5419, or 83.1285. The next step is to sum the weighted volumes. The result for this example is 417.8666 as shown in table 14.2. The calculated values appear in italics in the tables.

The last step is to divide the total weighted volume (417.8666) by the total volume of admissions (148) as shown in table 14.3. The result is a CMI of 2.8234.

The full calculation is as follows:

$$CMI = \frac{15 \times 5.5419 + 55 \times 2.9297 + 78 \times 2.2257}{15 + 55 + 78}$$

$$CMI = \frac{83.1285 + 161.1335 + 173.6046}{148} = \frac{417.866}{148} = 2.8234$$

The MS-DRG RW and volume play a significant role in CMI analysis. Therefore, it is important to understand how they interact with each other. Table 14.4 shows the CMI calculation for three cardiac surgery MS-DRGs.

The CMI for this set of MS-DRGs is 2.4334. In table 14.5, the volume for the highest-weighted MS-DRG, 034, has increased from 20 to 35 cases. Cases from MS-DRG 035 were moved to MS-DRG 034.

Table 14.1.   **MS-DRG data elements for CMI calculation**

MS-DRG	MDC	TYPE	MS-DRG Title	2023 RW	Vol	Weighted Volume
405	07	SURG	PANCREAS, LIVER & SHUNT PROCEDURES W MCC	5.5419	15	
406	07	SURG	PANCREAS, LIVER & SHUNT PROCEDURES W CC	2.9297	55	
407	07	SURG	PANCREAS, LIVER & SHUNT PROCEDURES W/O CC/MCC	2.2257	78	
				Total Volumes	148	
						CMI

Source: CMS 2022, table 5.

Table 14.2.   **First two steps of CMI calculation**

MS-DRG	MDC	TYPE	MS-DRG Title	2023 RW	Vol	Weighted Volume (Calculated)
405	07	SURG	PANCREAS, LIVER & SHUNT PROCEDURES W MCC	5.5419	15	83.1285
406	07	SURG	PANCREAS, LIVER & SHUNT PROCEDURES W CC	2.9297	55	161.1335
407	07	SURG	PANCREAS, LIVER & SHUNT PROCEDURES W/O CC/MCC	2.2257	78	173.6046
Total Volumes					148	417.8666
					CMI	

Source: CMS 2022, table 5.

Table 14.3.   **Last step of CMI calculation**

MS-DRG	MDC	TYPE	MS-DRG Title	2023 RW	Vol	Weighted Volume
405	07	SURG	PANCREAS, LIVER & SHUNT PROCEDURES W MCC	5.5419	15	83.1285
406	07	SURG	PANCREAS, LIVER & SHUNT PROCEDURES W CC	2.9297	55	161.1335
407	07	SURG	PANCREAS, LIVER & SHUNT PROCEDURES W/O CC/MCC	2.2257	78	173.6046
Total Volumes					148	417.8666
					CMI	2.8234

Source: CMS 2022, table 5.

Table 14.4.   **CMI calculation for MS-DRGs 034–036**

MS-DRG	MDC	TYPE	MS-DRG Title	2023 RW	Vol	Weighted Volume
034	01	SURG	CAROTID ARTERY STENT PROCEDURE WITH MCC	3.9994	20	79.9880
035	01	SURG	CAROTID ARTERY STENT PROCEDURES W CC	2.2838	80	182.7040
036	01	SURG	CAROTID ARTERY STENT PROCEDURES W/O CC/MCC	1.8807	35	65.8245
				Total Volumes	135	328.5165
				CMI		2.4334

Source: CMS 2022, table 5.

Table 14.5. **CMI calculation for MS-DRGs with volume increase for the highest-weighted MS-DRG**

MS-DRG	MDC	TYPE	MS-DRG Title	2023 RW	Vol	Weighted Volume
034	01	SURG	CAROTID ARTERY STENT PROCEDURE WITH MCC	3.9994	35	139.9790
035	01	SURG	CAROTID ARTERY STENT PROCEDURES W CC	2.2838	65	148.4470
036	01	SURG	CAROTID ARTERY STENT PROCEDURES W/O CC/MCC	1.8807	35	65.8245
				Total Volumes	135	354.2505
					CMI	2.6240

Source: CMS 2022, table 5.

Table 14.6. **CMI calculation for MS-DRGs with volume increase for the lowest-weighted MS-DRG**

MS-DRG	MDC	TYPE	MS-DRG Title	2023 RW	Vol	Weighted Volume
034	01	SURG	CAROTID ARTERY STENT PROCEDURE WITH MCC	3.9994	20	79.9880
035	01	SURG	CAROTID ARTERY STENT PROCEDURES W CC	2.2838	65	148.4470
036	01	SURG	CAROTID ARTERY STENT PROCEDURES W/O CC/MCC	1.8807	50	94.0350
				Total Volumes	135	322.5000
					CMI	2.3888

Source: CMS 2022, table 5.

The CMI increased from 2.4334 to 2.6240 when the volume increased for MS-DRG 034, which has the highest RW, and decreased for the MS-DRG 035, which has the middle RW. When volume for this MS-DRG with the highest RW increases, the CMI increases. Next, as shown in table 14.6, the volume for MS-DRG 034 returns to 20. The shift in volume is instead moved from MS-DRG 035 to MS-DRG 036, which has the lowest RW.

Table 14.6 illustrates how moving the volume increase to the MS-DRG with the lowest RW (MS-DRG 036) decreased the CMI from 2.4334 to 2.3888. When volume increases for an MS-DRG with an RW greater than the CMI, the CMI will increase. When volume increases for an MS-DRG with an RW less than the CMI, the CMI will decrease. Therefore, increasing volume is not always the solution to a CMI issue. Increased volume in a lower-weighted MS-DRG can significantly contribute to a downward CMI trend.

Case-Mix Index Analysis

Analyzing the growth or decline of a facility's CMI is the beginning phase for assessing the quality of coding and billing practices for hospital acute inpatient encounters. Healthcare analysts begin by comparing the CMI of the facility to that of its peers and the state or nation. Questions the analysts pose for analysis include the following:

- Is the CMI steady?

- Does it increase steadily or drastically?

- Is there a sharp or sudden decline?

To analyze CMI, analysts begin at the CMI level and then drill down to the major diagnostic category (MDC) level. Next, they drill down even further to the MS-DRG level. The following case study describes the analysis process for a CMI trend.

Case study 1: CMI trend analysis process

University Hospital is an 800-bed academic medical center. Financial leadership noticed that the inpatient revenue was below budget and trending lower. The revenue cycle analysis team was tasked with investigating and determining what types of cases were driving the decrease in revenue.

The team started by analyzing the CMI trend over the last four years versus benchmarks from other academic medical centers and community hospitals to see if the same trend could be observed in those providers. The results of the analysis are displayed in the figure that follows.

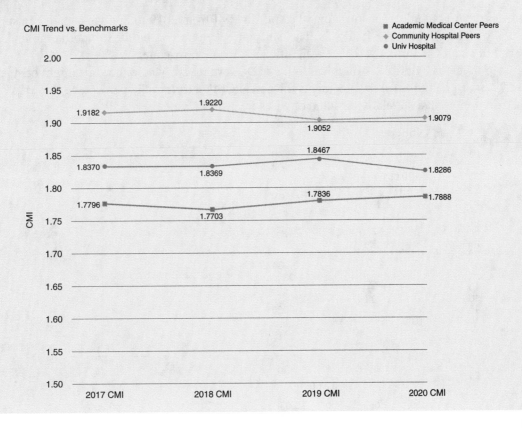

(continued)

Case study 1   *(continued)*

This figure demonstrates that the CMI trend experienced by University Hospital is different than the two peer groups. Only University Hospital experienced a drop in 2020. The next step in this analysis is to divide the admissions for University Hospital into medical and surgical MS-DRGs to determine if one of those subsets of cases is causing the movement in CMI. The statistic used is the percent change in CMI by case type as shown below.

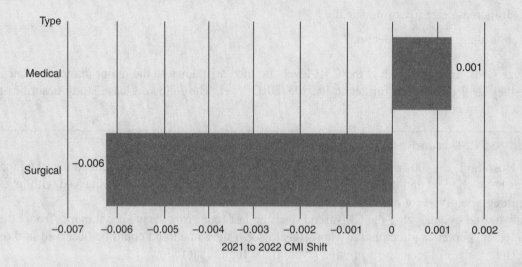

This figure is a bar graph that illustrates that the shift in CMI from 2019 to 2020 is negative in surgical MS-DRGs and positive in medical MS-DRGs. This shift may seem minor, but it is important to understand that the impact of small CMI shifts can have a significant impact on revenue.

The next step in the analysis is to drill down to the MDC level to see where the shift might be most pronounced. The bar graph that follows segments the actual CMI shift (not the percentage) by MDC. The width of the bars represents the relative volume of cases in each MDC.

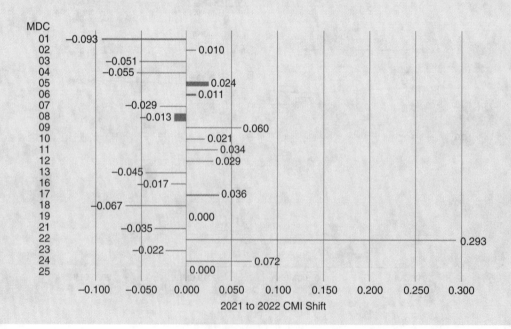

(continued)

MDC 8, Diseases and Disorders of the Musculoskeletal System and Connective Tissue, is the most significant category when both shift and volume are combined. One cannot tell from the data alone what has caused this increase. However, by performing a thorough investigation, the issue(s) can be identified. Several areas to consider in the investigation include the following:

- Coding and billing errors
- Changes in MS-DRG assignment methodology
- Equipment purchases
- New or expanded service areas
- Acquisition of new facilities
- Changes in physician personnel

Regardless of the root cause of the trend, compliance with established rules and regulations must be verified. If coding practices are questionable, then a medical record review should be performed to identify whether a compliance infraction has occurred. Managers should follow established procedures for correcting and reporting a compliance lapse.

Outpatient Service-Mix Index Analysis

CMI is used for acute-care inpatient hospital admissions. But facilities also want to monitor their outpatient encounter population. Therefore, a facility can calculate its outpatient service-mix index (SMI). SMI is the sum of the weights of ambulatory payment classification (APC) groups for patients treated during a given period divided by the total volume of patients treated. The steps in calculating the SMI are as follows:

1. Determine the volume and RW for each APC.
2. Multiply the RW and volume for each APC to calculate the total weight for that APC.
3. Add up the total volume, add up the total weight.
4. Divide the total weight by the total volume.

As illustrated, this is the same calculation that was used earlier to calculate CMI. Facilities can calculate an overall SMI, and they can divide APCs by service areas and calculate SMI at that level. An example of SMI calculation is demonstrated in the following case study.

Case study 2: SMI calculation

Community Hospital would like to calculate its SMI for the ED. The table below shows the volumes for the emergency visit APCs for Community Hospital. Each APC has an RW that determines the payment for the service. Analyzing the SMI for a hospital helps to determine the root cause for increases or decreases in outpatient revenue.

(continued)

Case study 2   *(continued)*

APC	APC short descriptor	Relative weight	Volume	Total Weight
5021	Level 1 emergency visits	0.8617	540	*465.318*
5022	Level 2 emergency visits	1.5838	2,698	*4,273.092*
5023	Level 3 emergency visits	2.7643	4,857	*13,426.210*
5024	Level 4 emergency visits	4.3542	3,068	*13,358.690*
5025	Level 5 emergency visits	6.2445	2,428	*15,162.650*
		Total Volumes	*13,591*	*46,684.947*
		APC Service-Mix Index (SMI)		*3.435*

Source: CMS 2023b.

Once the steps for SMI calculation are completed, the APC SMI equals 3.435.

MS-DRG Relationships Analysis

Within the MS-DRG system, there are MS-DRG families. An MS-DRG family is a group of MS-DRGs that have the same base set of principal diagnoses with or without operating room procedures, which are divided into levels to represent severity of illness. Within MS-DRG families, the presence or absence of a complication or comorbidity (CC) diagnosis or major complication or comorbidity (MCC) diagnosis assigns the case to a higher- or lower-severity MS-DRG. MS-DRG families may contain two or three MS-DRGs.

These MS-DRG relationships pose a revenue integrity concern because the medical record documentation used to support coding the principal diagnosis, complications, and comorbidities may not always be clear or used appropriately by the coding professional. Facilities want the MS-DRG to be correct, not overreported or underreported because of documentation or coding quality.

Included in many Medicare and third-party payer audits is the comparison of the reporting rates for MS-DRG families. For example, the simple pneumonia MS-DRG family is often audited. MS-DRG 193, Simple Pneumonia and Pleurisy with MCC, has a higher RW than the other MS-DRGs in this relationship and should be closely monitored (table 14.7). Hospital reporting of MCCs is closely monitored to ensure all coding rules and regulations have been followed. Furthermore, the medical record documentation is scrutinized to ensure its adequacy for coding purposes. Reporting MS-DRG 193 at a higher rate than warranted will cause the facility to receive reimbursement to which it is not entitled, creating noncompliance.

Table 14.7.   **Simple pneumonia MS-DRG family**

MS-DRG Number	DRG Title	FY 2020 Relative Weight
193	Simple Pneumonia and Pleurisy with MCC	1.3335
194	Simple Pneumonia and Pleurisy with CC	0.8886
195	Simple Pneumonia and Pleurisy without MCC/CC	0.6821

Source: CMS 2022, table 5.

MS-DRG relationship analysis is a drill-down analysis of the CC/MCC capture rate, which was discussed in chapter 12. This analysis is more granular because the analyst is examining the severity of illness (SOI)–level assignment within a single MS-DRG family. The following case study illustrates MS-DRG family analysis.

Case study 3: MS-DRG family analysis

University Hospital is investigating the relative frequency within the simple pneumonia MS-DRG family. The data analyst uses a stacked bar chart to compare University Hospital's reporting percentage for each MS-DRG in the simple pneumonia family to both academic medical center and community hospital peers during the study period. University Hospital's percentage for MS-DRG 193, 48.92 percent, is much higher than either peer group. Since this is the highest weighted member of the MS-DRG family, a medical record review is warranted to determine whether inaccurate coding practices, also referred to as upcoding, are the root cause of the reporting differences. Medical records assigned to MS-DRG 193 should be reviewed to determine whether the assignment of this MS-DRG is supported through documentation in the medical records. Again, established procedures for compliance issues should be followed.

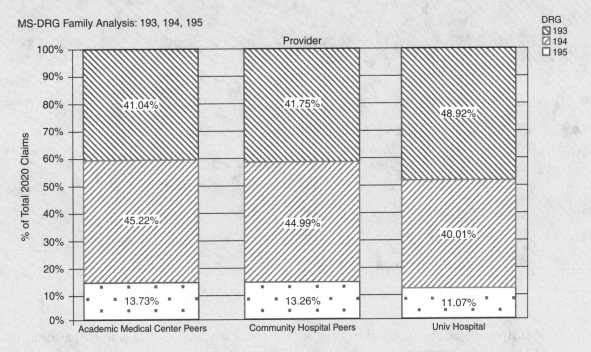

Poor documentation identified during intensive medical record reviews should be addressed with CDI management and medical staff, and incorrect code assignments should be immediately discussed with the coding manager.

Medicare Reimbursement Variation Analysis

Medicare inpatient reimbursement rates are set at the beginning of the fiscal year and remain the same through the rate period. However, there are provisions of the Medicare hospital acute inpatient payment system that, when activated, will result in a reimbursement amount that is different than the expected (typical) amount. Healthcare and financial analysts have in-depth analytic skill and knowledge; however, they might not be well-versed in Medicare reimbursement policies and adjustments. Therefore, collaboration between analysts and coding or reimbursement specialists is often required to answer leadership's question. An example of collaboration between a financial analyst and coding professional is provided in case study 4.

Case study 4: Medicare reimbursement analysis

A financial analyst is charged with the examining the Medicare payment variations for MS-DRG 474, Amputation for Musculoskeletal System and Connective Tissue Disorders with MCC. Last year, City Hospital performed 14 cases. Of the 14, 6 had a reimbursement amount different from the expected payment rate. The expected payment rate for MS-DRG 474 is $30,426.75. The financial analyst reviewed the cases and collaborated with the coding manager to determine the cause of the reimbursement variation for the six cases.

Account Number	Date of Service	MS-DRG	Medicare Reimbursement	Variation Cause
164875	January 1, 202X	474	$30,426.75	
596784	February 3, 202X	474	$23,150.82	PACT Transfer
257469	February 4, 202X	474	$30,426.75	
364821	March 8, 202X	474	$33,972.90	Outlier
674219	April 10, 202X	474	$30,426.75	
682493	May 13, 202X	474	$30,426.75	
249855	June 15, 202X	474	$19,843.56	PACT Transfer
497865	July 16, 202X	474	$30,426.75	
574198	August 23, 202X	474	$31,641.75	New Technology
197865	August 24, 202X	474	$31,641.75	New Technology
794861	September 25, 202X	474	$30,426.75	
893249	October 27, 202X	474	$30,426.75	
912765	October 29, 202X	474	$30,426.75	
976463	December 30, 202X	474	$35,078.47	Outlier

The financial analyst and the coding manager identified that the policy that resulted in lower payments than expected is the post-acute-care transfer (PACT) transfer policy (which was discussed in chapter 5, "Medicare Hospital Acute Inpatient Payment System"). When the PACT transfer policy is activated, the facility receives a per diem payment instead of the full MS-DRG payment, which results in a lower payment than is typical for the admission. Next, the financial analyst and coding manager investigated the four cases where the Medicare reimbursement amount was higher than expected. They identified that for two of the admissions, City Hospital received an outlier add-on amount due to the extremely high costs of treating patients with account numbers 364821 and 976436. The last two cases were linked to one physician, Dr. Patel. After review of supplies data, the financial analyst discovered that a new type of joint implant was used for accounts 574198 and 197865. With that information, the coding manager confirmed that a new technology add-on payment was received for each of the admissions. Further confirmation was received from Dr. Patel. She was trying out a new device for amputations. Collaboration between financial analysts and coding and reimbursement professionals can help resolve queries about Medicare reimbursement variations.

Site of Service Analysis: Inpatient versus Outpatient

A major focus of improper payment reviews is the site of service. In chapter 2, "Health Insurance," utilization reviews were discussed. **Utilization review** is the process of determining whether a patient's medical care is necessary according to established guidelines and regulations. It is also a managed care cost containment measure that assesses the appropriateness of the setting for the healthcare service in the continuum of care and the level of service. Therefore, most utilization reviews include two pathways. First is ensuring that the service is medically necessary, and second is ensuring that the appropriate setting is used to deliver treatment to the patient. Site of service reviews are another name for the second pathway of utilization review and include examining the clinical documentation for the encounter to determine if admission criteria were met to warrant an inpatient admission. If established criteria were not met, then the insurance company deems that the site of service should have been the outpatient setting. This results in a reimbursement adjustment for the encounter.

Several MS-DRGs are under a site of service review by improper payment review entities, such as the MACs and RACs. Documentation and admission criteria are reviewed to determine whether the inpatient setting is the most efficient and effective treatment area for patients. One focus area is diabetes: MS-DRGs 637, Diabetes with MCC; 638, Diabetes with CC; and 639, Diabetes without MCC or CC. The following case study illustrates the concept of a site of service review focused on MS-DRGs prone to utilization review problems.

Case study 5: Site of service analysis

Compliance investigators examine the reporting rates for MS-DRG 637 at University Hospital. The table that follows shows the reporting rate for MS-DRG 637 or the percentage of MS-DRG 637 cases to total discharges for the facility in the study period. University Hospital reported MS-DRG 637 at a similar rate to both peer groups used in the analysis.

MS-DRG 637 reporting rates

Provider/Peer Group	MS-DRG 637 Percentage
University Hospital	0.30%
Academic Medical Center Peers	0.29%
Community Hospital Peers	0.30%

Although the percentage of cases in MS-DRG 637 look similar to peers, examiners look more deeply and examine the frequency of length of stay (LOS) values for MS-DRG 637. The following bar graph displays the average length of stay (ALOS) distribution for MS-DRG 637 within the study period time frame. Again, the data show that the LOS reporting for this MS-DRG is consistent with the national expected ALOS of 5.0. Investigators review encounters in the one-day stay category to verify that admission criteria and medical necessity were met. After drill-down analysis, it appears that this MS-DRG is being appropriately reported at this facility.

(continued)

Case study 5 *(continued)*

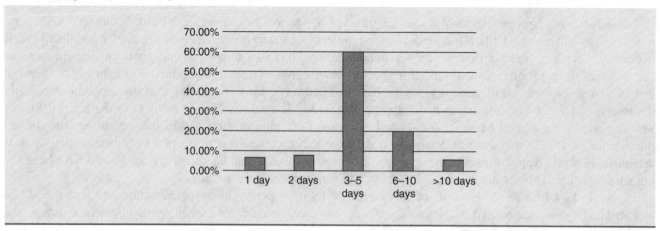

In this case study, no issues were identified with site of service for MS-DRG 637. However, if other MS-DRGs show deviation, they should be investigated by the utilization review committee consisting of representatives from health information management (HIM), quality, utilization, and medical staff. Together, this interdisciplinary team can determine whether the site of service was appropriate for the encounters under review.

Evaluation and Management Facility Coding in the Emergency Department

The implementation of prospective reimbursement methodologies in the Medicare hospital outpatient payment system has brought about new compliance challenges for hospitals. One area under review is evaluation and management (E/M) coding. E/M codes are used to report levels of service for various settings. Facilities typically use the E/M codes for the following facility-based settings:

- Office or other outpatient services, new patient

- Office or other outpatient services, established patient

- ED services

- Critical care services provided in the ED

Because the Healthcare Common Procedure Coding System (HCPCS) code reported on a Medicare outpatient claim drives the APC assignment and hence the level of reimbursement, the code assignment should be closely monitored. Currently, each facility determines hospital-specific criteria to be applied for E/M level of service determination for ED visits. Thus, auditing is necessary to validate that the levels are correctly assigned based on the established criteria. Additionally, auditing will confirm that the criteria reflect the resource consumption experienced at that facility for the services rendered. Table 14.8 provides the E/M HCPCS codes, APCs, RWs, and unadjusted payment amounts for ED encounters. Remember the HCPCS includes CPT codes and HCPCS Level II. The following case study discusses E/M-level analysis.

Table 14.8.   E/M ED HCPCS codes and APC groupings 2023

	99281	99282	99283	99284	99285
APC Group	5021—Level 1 Emergency Visit	5022—Level 2 Emergency Visit	5023—Level 3 Emergency Visit	5024—Level 4 Emergency Visit	5025—Level 5 Emergency Visit
APC Relative Weight	0.8774	1.6322	2.863	4.4589	6.4043
APC Payment (unadjusted)	$75.09	$139.69	$245.03	$381.61	$548.11

Source: CMS 2021.

Case study 6: E/M-level analysis

E/M code distribution is compared across a medium-sized not-for-profit hospital, two peer facilities, and the nation. The data analyst uses a stacked bar chart to show the E/M code distribution during the study period. The data show that hospitals A and B reported codes 99284 and 99285 (high-level ED visits) at a much higher percentage than hospital C and the nation. The Centers for Medicare and Medicaid Services (CMS) has suggested that ED APC distribution should follow somewhat of a bell-shaped curve. Clearly, hospital A deviates far from this configuration even though hospital A has a similar reporting pattern to hospital B.

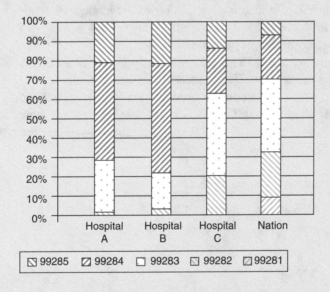

The data analyst must further examine the trend for hospital A. Again, she uses a stacked bar graph to display trending data for the past four years. The data show that hospital A's reporting of higher-level E/M codes has increased from 25 percent of the total cases in year one to 80 percent of the total cases in year four. This drastic increase in the reporting of levels 4 and 5 E/M codes should be addressed by this facility. A medical record audit should be performed to verify that hospital-specific E/M criteria and medical record documentation support the assignment of these higher-level HCPCS codes.

(continued)

Case study 6 *(continued)*

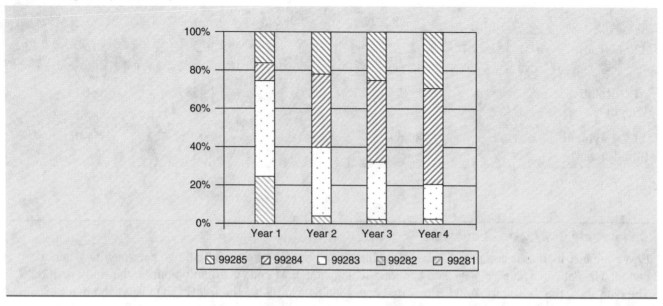

Physician Coding Analysis

Like facilities, physician practices use data analysis to ensure revenue integrity principles are being met. A big difference between facility E/M coding and physician practice E/M coding is that physicians are not able to use "practice-specific" criteria to assign E/M codes like facilities. Instead, they must follow strict E/M coding guidelines that are nationally recognized. Therefore, third-party payers often compare providers or group practices to each other to identify areas of variation. These areas of variation could be risk areas for the third-party payer. Payers perform audits to ensure that E/M coding is compliant with established coding guidelines.

The concept of a bell-shaped curve for HCPCS codes that are natural levels may also be used when comparing the coding practices of physicians. There are several E/M categories available for physician use. Some examples include the following:

- Office or other outpatient services, new patient

- Office or other outpatient services, established patient

- Initial observation care

- Subsequent observation care

- Inpatient consultations

- Initial hospital care

- Subsequent hospital care

The following case study uses E/M codes for clinic visits for new patients and demonstrates distribution and analysis of E/M levels.

Case study 7: Distribution and analysis of E/M levels for physician practice

Super Payer insurance company monitors the E/M coding for all of the primary care physicians that treat their beneficiaries. The Super Payer analysis team creates bell-shaped curves as displayed in the figures that follow. Dr. Rapido's bar graph exhibits the type of bell-shaped curve that Super Payer expects to see in their patient population. Unfortunately, Dr. Queue's bar graph shows a skew toward the higher level of visit.

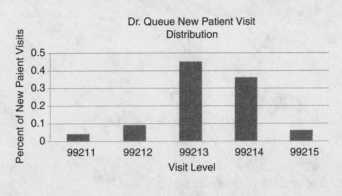

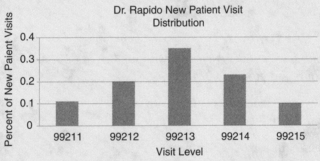

Based on the E/M-level distribution for Dr. Queue, Super Payer may request medical records for an audit. As discussed in chapter 13, "Revenue Compliance," third-party payers perform audits to ensure that data reported on claims are in alignment with coding rules and regulations. During the audit, Super Payer reviewers will examine medical record documentation to assess if Dr. Queue is correctly assigning E/M-level HCPCS codes.

Outpatient Code Editor Review for Hospital Outpatient Services

In chapter 13, "Revenue Compliance," the functionality of the Medicare **Outpatient Code Editor (OCE)** was discussed. The OCE is a software program designed to process data for outpatient prospective payment system (OPPS) pricing and edit claims data based on coding and billing requirements. Ongoing analysis of OCE results can improve a facility's revenue cycle performance. Resolving OCE edit issues increases the efficiency and accuracy of the revenue cycle because more clean claims are produced and sent to third-party payers for adjudication. In the following case study, Community Hospital engages in root cause analysis to identify potential causes of OCE edit activation.

Case study 8: OCE edit analysis for hospital outpatient services

Community Hospital submitted one month of Medicare outpatient claims for auditing by the Medicare OCE. The data set contained 2,530 claims, 17,710 line items, and $5,457,513 in charges. The results of an OCE audit are displayed in the table that follows.

OCE Edit	Edit Description	Violations	Claims Processing Area
01	Invalid diagnosis code	23	Coding
06	Invalid procedure code	21	Coding/CDM
27	Only incidental services reported	16	CPOE/coding/CDM
28	Code not recognized by Medicare; alternate code for same service may be available	14	Coding/CDM
38	Inconsistency between implanted device or administered substance and implantation or associated procedure	17	CPOE/CDM
41	Invalid revenue code	65	CDM
43	Transfusion or blood product exchange without specification of blood product	15	CPOE/CDM
44	Observation revenue code on line item with nonobservation HCPCS code	49	CPOE/CDM
48	Revenue center requires HCPCS code	29	CDM
61	Service can only be billed to the DMERC	14	CPOE/CDM
68	Service provided before date of national coverage determination (NCD) approval	12	Coding/CDM
71	Claim lacks required device code	18	CPOE/CDM

Several edits were evoked during the audit. To improve the revenue cycle process, the RCM team investigated each edit to uncover its root problems. Michael, a revenue cycle analyst, was charged with investigating OCE edits 41 and 48.

OCE edit 41, invalid revenue code, was evoked 65 times during the month. This edit is activated when the revenue code reported on the claim is not in the list of valid revenue codes for OPPS. When this edit is activated, the claim is returned to the provider for correction. Therefore, this error is delaying payment of several claims and is also costing the facility staff time in rework. Each claim must be corrected and resubmitted to the MAC for payment. Clearly, this situation raises revenue code issues. Revenue codes are stored in the charge description master (CDM). Thus, a CDM review is warranted because several line items are stored with incorrect revenue codes. Perhaps a program transmittal was incorrectly interpreted, or a typing mistake was made during data entry in the CDM.

Michael spearheaded a review of the 65 error claims, which showed that two line items in the ancillary section of physical therapy have incorrect information. These two line items represent physical therapy evaluation services, which should be reported using revenue code 0424. However, these line items were assigned revenue code 042, which is not a valid revenue code. This was a simple data entry mistake, but it

(continued)

resulted in delayed payment for several claims. This error is easy to correct, but it reveals the need for the CDM update process to be reviewed to identify risk areas for typing errors. Community Hospital subsequently implemented an additional review component as part of its CDM update process.

OCE edit 48 (revenue center requires HCPCS code) is triggered when an HCPCS code is not reported with a revenue code on the claim, and the revenue center status indicator is not bundled. This edit is not applicable for revenue codes 010X, 021X, 0310X, 0099X, 0905 to 0907, 0500, 0509, 0583, 0660 to 0663, 0669, 0931 to 0932, 0521 to 0522, 0524 to 0525, 0527 to 0528, 0637, or 0948. Note that the X in the revenue code listing means that the revenue code with any last digit is included. Because this edit is activated, claims are being returned to the facility for correction. Like OCE edit 41, this error is also delaying the payment of several claims and is costing Community Hospital staff time for rework. This edit was activated 29 times during the month under review.

Michael conducted a review of these 29 claims, which revealed that they all included the line item number 3268916, used to report lithotripsy. Community Hospital had recently hard coded the lithotripsy services in the CDM, so Michael and the RCM team could not understand why the HCPCS code was not appearing on the claim. Furthermore, the lithotripsy unit was contacted, and its staff confirmed that they performed 35 procedures last month, so why did only 29 claims evoke this edit? What happened to the other six claims? Then, Michael worked with the CDM coordinator to review all line items for lithotripsy services.

The CDM review revealed that there were duplicate line items for this service. Apparently, the previous line item for this service was not marked as inactive when the hard-coding update for lithotripsy services occurred; thus, the CDM contained two active line items for the same service. However, Michael was still puzzled, thinking the RCM team had thoroughly educated the charge entry staff about the line item changes. After further investigation, the RCM team discovered that one charge entry staff member had been on vacation during the training, and, upon returning to work, she was not informed about the line item changes. Thus, she had continued to use the previous line item number.

Two fixes were implemented. First, line item number 3268916 was marked inactive. Second, the charge entry staff member was scheduled for training immediately. Additionally, the RCM team and coding manager learned two lessons. An additional component was needed in the hard-coding conversion plan to review all previous line items for inactive status, and a sign-in sheet was needed for use during training sessions and following up on missing attendees to ensure the education of all staff members in the future.

Physician Productivity Analysis

The concept of relative value units (RVUs) and their role in the Medicare physician fee schedule was introduced in chapter 8, "Medicare Physician and Other Health Professional Payment System." The WORK element of the resource-based relative value scale (RBRVS) system may be used to determine physician productivity. As a refresher, the WORK element is based on the time the physician spends providing a service and the intensity with which that time is spent. The four aspects of intensity are mental effort and judgment, technical skill, physical effort, and psychological stress. The following case study illustrates how the WORK element RVUs (wRVUs) may be used for physician productivity analysis.

Case study 9: Measuring physician productivity

Healthy Physician Clinic is a practice that includes four physicians. Dr. Anderson works full-time. Dr. Burns and Dr. Cruz both work 30 hours per week. Finally, Dr. Dudley works only 20 hours per week. The practice manager set up a wRVU goal of 2,000 per month for each physician full-time equivalent (FTE). She created a physician scorecard to measure the productivity of each of the physicians against the benchmark for this month. The scorecard is shown in the table below.

(continued)

Case study 9 *(continued)*

Healthy Physician Clinic Productivity Scorecard				
	Dr. Anderson	**Dr. Burns**	**Dr. Cruz**	**Dr. Dudley**
Goal RVUs	2,000.00	2,000.00	2,000.00	2,000.00
FTE Status	1.00	0.80	0.80	0.50
Physician Goal	2,000.00	1,600.00	1,600.00	1000.00
Encounters	1,139.00	608.00	1,245.00	342.00
wRVUs Billed	2,173.39	1,759.00	1,201.23	732.41
wRVU Delta	173.39	159.00	(398.77)	(267.59)
wRVU per Encounter	1.91	2.89	0.96	2.14

The practice manager adjusted each physician's goal to reflect the hours worked per week at the clinic in the "Physician Goal" row. For example, Dr. Anderson is expected to achieve the full 2,000 wRVUs because she works full-time at the clinic, but Dr. Dudley's goal is 1,000 wRVUs because he only works half-time, or 20 hours per week, at the clinic. The practice manager notes that only Dr. Anderson and Dr. Burns are achieving their wRVU goal as shown in row "wRVU Delta." This row represents the difference between the physician goal and the actual wRVU billed.

The practice manager was surprised that Dr. Cruz did not meet her wRVU goal. She has a full schedule, as demonstrated by the fact that she has more encounters than any other physician at the clinic. The average wRVU for Dr. Cruz (see row "wRVU per Encounter") is significantly lower than any of the other clinicians. If she is going to continue to perform lower-weighted encounters, then her volume must increase to meet the clinic benchmark. An alternative pathway would be for Dr. Cruz to work with leadership to have a lower physician goal assigned for her.

Clinical Documentation Integrity Program Analysis

A successful clinical documentation integrity (CDI) program includes engagement from both CDI professionals and clinicians. As a refresher, CDI programs strive to initiate concurrent and retrospective reviews of medical records to improve the quality of procedure documentation. In chapter 12, "Coding and Clinical Documentation Integrity Management," metrics used to manage a CDI program were introduced. The following case study examines the relationship between CDI query response rate and physician specialty at Community Hospital.

Case study 10: CDI program analysis

Letha, the CDI director at Community Hospital, was concerned that the rate that physicians responded to queries from the CDI team varied widely by specialty. Letha created a bar graph that depicts the response rates by specialty at Community Hospital.

(continued)

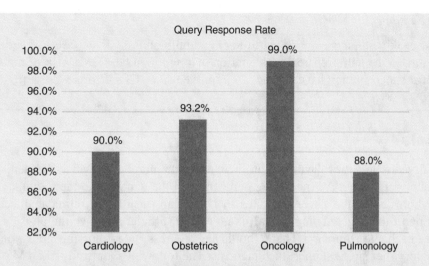

As part of her investigation, Letha interviewed physicians from the four specialties shown in the previous figure. After interviewing the physicians in the pulmonology and cardiology departments, she found that the physicians felt as though the number of queries and the type of questions asked were not perceived to be valuable. The clinicians in those departments were very busy and considered the CDI queries to be a nuisance. Letha thought it was interesting that this type of feedback was primarily provided by those two departments. Physicians in the oncology department provided feedback that they appreciated CDI queries and were conscientious about responding because Dr. Shapiro, the head of the cancer department, is the physician champion of the CDI program. Physicians in the obstetrics department indicated that they are very busy but try to always respond to CDI queries. Letha decided to do an analysis to look at the relationship between the query rate in each of the departments and the corresponding response rate. Letha created a scatterplot to show the results of her analysis.

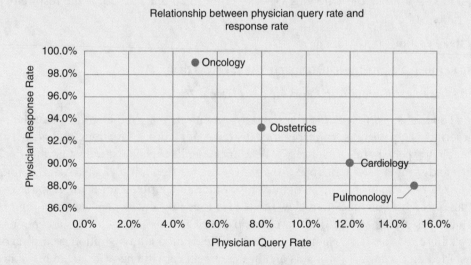

The scatterplot depicted in the above figure compares the physician query rate and response rate for four specialties. Cardiology and pulmonology both have a lower query rate and higher response rate compared to the other specialties. The obstetrics query rate is in the middle and so is the response rate. Cancer has the best response rate, and this is not a surprise considering the feedback received during physician interviews. However, the analysis shows a significant negative relationship between the query rate and the response rate for cardiology and pulmonology. Letha decides to discuss the results of the analysis with Dr. Shapiro. She

(continued)

Case study 10   *(continued)*

plans to ask him to speak with physicians in cardiology and pulmonology in an effort to get them on board with the CDI program. Letha will prepare a presentation that highlights the CMI, risk of mortality, and severity of illness statistics for cancer, which have drastically improved since CDI efforts were introduced in this specialty.

MS-DRG Denials

Over the past several years, facilities have seen an increase in the number of MS-DRG denials. A portion of the denials are due to incorrect coding. An increasing percentage of the denials are due to clinical validation denials. For a clinical validation denial, the payer indicates that there are insufficient clinical indicators present in the medical record to support the targeted diagnosis. It is no longer sufficient to have the physician simply document the condition in the discharge summary. There should be progress notes, nursing notes, and ancillary therapy notes, such as respiratory therapy, to support the diagnosis. The following case study of an MS-DRG denial will be showcased. This case study is a fictional denial and is intended to demonstrate how to identify supporting clinical indicators in the medical record documentation.

Case study 11: MS-DRG denial

A patient is admitted to City Hospital with acute systolic congestive heart failure (CHF) exacerbation. The patient has chronic systolic CHF, a history of breast cancer, and is status post two coronary artery stent placements. On day two of the admission, the patient experiences acute respiratory failure. The MS-DRG reported by City Hospital is 291, Heart Failure and Shock with MCC. The payer has downgraded the MS-DRG to 293, Heart Failure and Shock without CC/MCC by changing the coding for the respiratory failure to hypoxemia. The clinical denials specialist is charged with reviewing the admission to determine whether the patient has acute respiratory failure or hypoxemia.

City Hospital has established the following criteria for a formal diagnosis of acute respiratory failure. Two of the three criteria must be met:

- pO2 less than 60 mmHg (hypoxemia)
- PCO2 greater than 50 mmHg (hypercapnia) with pH less than 7.35
- Signs and symptoms of acute respiratory distress (Decaro 2019)

The clinical denial specialist starts with the signs and symptoms criteria. She identifies that the progress note from day two describes the patient as "in respiratory distress with labored breathing and nostrils flaring. The patient is unable to speak in full sentences." The clinical denials specialist feels that this documentation supports the signs and symptoms criteria. Next, she moves to the arterial blood gas (ABG) laboratory results. The patient has a pO2 of 51 mmHg. This laboratory result meets the criteria for acute respiratory failure. But the clinical denials specialist continues to review the medical record. She locates another progress note that indicates the patient was placed on BiPAP (bilevel positive airway pressure), which is a common treatment for acute respiratory failure. Further, she examines the MAR (Medication administration record) and notes that the patient was started on prednisone, which is another treatment for patients with acute respiratory failure. A progress note on day three states that "the patient is breathing easier, but will continue on BiPAP for the remainder of the day and will complete the course of steroids."

The clinical denials specialist decides to appeal the denial. She believes that the documentation in the medical record is sufficient to support the diagnosis of acute respiratory failure as recorded by the attending physician in the discharge summary. She prepares her denial letter and includes copies of the documentation from the medical record that supports the criteria for acute respiratory failure.

Patient Connection

In chapter 1's Patient Connection, we learned that Dr. King is Olivia's daughter's pediatrician. Dr. King works at City Pediatrician Group. She is one of four pediatricians. Yvonne, the practice manager, tracks physician productivity monthly, similar to the physician productivity analysis included earlier in this chapter. Let's examine the physician productivity for the month of May for City Pediatrician Group. The majority of encounters in the pediatricians' office are for clinic visits. There are very few procedures, other than vaccinations, that are provided in the office. Therefore, Yvonne examined the wRVU levels for HCPCS codes 99202 to 99205 and 99211 to 99215 on the Medicare physician fee schedule search located on the CMS website (CMS 2023a) to develop the monthly goal RVUs.

HCPCS Code	Internal Code Description	wRVU
99202	Level 2 new	0.93
99203	Level 3 new	1.60
99204	Level 4 new	2.60
99205	Level 5 new	3.50
99211	Level 1 est	0.18
99212	Level 2 est	0.70
99213	Level 3 est	1.30
99214	Level 4 est	1.92
99215	Level 5 est	2.80

The majority of the visits at City Pediatrician Group are for established patients at levels 2 and 3. Based on last year's volume, she set the monthly goal RVU for a 1.0 FTE to be 210.

City Pediatrician Group Productivity Scorecard				
	Dr. King	Dr. Aguta	Dr. Torres	Dr. Perez
Goal RVUs	210.00	210.00	210.00	210.00
FTE Status	1.00	1.00	1.00	0.50
Physician Goal	210.00	210.00	210.00	105.00
Encounters	240	250	238	115
wRVUs Billed	264.39	198.00	215.23	108.41
wRVU Delta	54.39	(12.00)	5.25	3.41
wRVU per Encounter	1.10	0.792	0.904	0.942

(continued)

Patient Connection   *(continued)*

The only pediatrician that didn't meet the productivity goal was Dr. Aguta. Dr. Torres and Dr. Perez just met the standard. Only Dr. King has a wRVU per encounter over 1.0. Yvonne wants to encourage the physicians to increase productivity, but she does not want to sacrifice quality or compromise revenue integrity. City Pediatrician Group has a community rating of five stars primarily because patients appreciate the time the physicians spend with patients. Additionally, their last internal audit showed a coding compliance rating of 97 percent. What would you do if you were in Yvonne's position?

References

CMS (Centers for Medicare and Medicaid Services). 2023a. "Physician Fee Schedule." https://www.cms.gov /medicare/physician-fee-schedule/search/overview.

CMS (Centers for Medicare and Medicaid Services). 2023b "Addendum A." https://www.cms.gov/medicare /medicare-fee-service-payment/hospitaloutpatientpps/addendum-and-addendum-b-updates/april-2023-1.

CMS (Centers for Medicare and Medicaid Services). 2022. "FY 2023 Final Rule and Correction Notice Tables: Table 5." https://www.cms.gov/medicare/acute-inpatient-pps/fy-2023-ipps-final-rule-home-page#Tables.

Decaro, S. O. 2019. Documentation tips: Acute respiratory failure. *The Hospitalist*. https://www.the-hospitalist .org/hospitalist/article/212735/pulmonology/documentation-tips-acute-respiratory-failure.

Appendix A
Abbreviation List

AAAHC	Accreditation Association for Ambulatory Health Care	BNI	beneficiary notices initiative
AAHAM	American Association of Healthcare Administrative Management	CAA	Care Area Assessment
		CAC	computer-assisted coding
ABN	advance beneficiary notification of noncoverage	CAH	critical access hospital
		CAHPS	Consumer Assessment of Healthcare Providers and Systems
ACA	Affordable Care Act		
ACDIS	Association of Clinical Documentation Improvement Specialists	C-APC	comprehensive ambulatory payment classification
		CBSA	core-based statistical area
ACO	accountable care organization	CC	complication and comorbidity
ADA	American Dental Association	CCR	cost-to-charge ratio
ADFM	active-duty family member	CCT	certified compliance technician
ADL	activities of daily living	CDC	Centers for Disease Control and Prevention
ADSM	active-duty service member		
AHA	American Hospital Association	CDI	clinical documentation integrity
AHIMA	American Health Information Management Association	CDM	charge description master
		CDT	Code on Dental Procedures and Nomenclature
AHRQ	Agency for Healthcare Research and Quality		
		CEHRT	certified electronic health record technology
ALJ	administrative law judge		
ALOS	average length of stay	CERT	Comprehensive Error Rate Testing
AMA	American Medical Association	CF	conversion factor
AMLOS	arithmetic mean length of stay	CHAMPUS	Civilian Health and Medical Program of the Uniformed Services
AOA	Administration on Aging		
APC	ambulatory payment classification	CHAMPVA	Civilian Health and Medical Program of the Department of Veterans Affairs
APM	advanced payment model		
APM	alternative payment model		
APTC	Advance Payment of Premium Tax Credit	CHIP	Children's Health Insurance Program
		CJR	Comprehensive Care for Joint Replacement
AR	accounts recievable		
ASCQR	Ambulatory Surgical Center Quality Reporting	CLFS	Medicare Clinical Lab Fee Schedule
		CMG	case-mix group
		CMHC	community mental health center
ASP	average sales price	CMI	case-mix index
BBA	Balanced Budget Act of 1997	CMS	Centers for Medicare and Medicaid Services
BBRA	Balanced Budget Refinement Act		

CMS PSI	Centers for Medicare and Medicaid Services Recalibrated Patient Safety Indicator	FDA	US Food and Drug Administration
CMS-HCC	Centers for Medicare and Medicaid Services hierarchical condition categories	FECA	Federal Employees' Compensation Act of 1916
COB	coordination of benefits	FMEA	failure mode and effects analysis
COBRA	Consolidated Omnibus Budget Reconciliation Act	FPL	federal poverty level
		FRDAA	Fraud Reduction and Data Analytics Act of 2015
COLA	cost-of-living adjustment	FTE	full-time equivalent
CoP	Conditions of Participation	FY	fiscal year
CPI	consumer price index	GDP	gross domestic product
CPOE	computerized provider order entry	GMLOS	geometric mean length of stay
CPT	Current Procedural Terminology	GPCI	geographic practice cost index
CRCE	certified revenue cycle executive	HAC	hospital-acquired condition
CRCP	certified revenue cycle professional	HAC POA	hospital-acquired conditions present on admission
CRCR	certified revenue cycle representative	HACRP	Hospital-Acquired Condition Reduction Program
CRCS	certified revenue cycle specialist	HAI	healthcare-associated infection
CRIP	certified revenue integrity professional	HCAHPS	Hospital Consumer Assessment of Healthcare Providers and Systems
CRNA	certified registered nurse anesthetist	HCC	hierarchical condition category
C-SNP	chronic condition special needs plan	HCCA	Health Care Compliance Association
CSPR	certified specialist payment and reimbursement	HCPCS	Healthcare Common Procedure Coding System
DEERS	Defense Enrollment Eligibility Reporting System	HCRIS	Health Provider Cost Reporting Information System
DME	durable medical equipment	HEALTHY KIDS	Helping Ensure Access for Little Ones, Toddlers, and Hopeful Youth by Keeping Insurance Delivery Stable Act
DMERC	durable medical equipment regional contractor		
DNFB	discharged, not final billed		
DOJ	Department of Justice		
DRA	Deficit Reduction Act of 2005	HEDIS	Healthcare Effectiveness Data and Information Set
DSH	disproportionate share hospital		
D-SNP	dual-eligible special needs plan	HFMA	Healthcare Financial Management Association
DTC	discharge to community		
E/M	evaluation and management	HHA	home health agency
EACH	essential access community hospital	HHCAHPS	Home Health Care Consumer Assessment of Healthcare Providers and Systems Survey
ECT	electroconvulsive therapy		
ED	emergency department		
EHR	electronic health record	HH PPS	home health prospective payment system
EIPM	Exchange Improper Payment Measurement		
		HHRGs	home health resource groups
EOB	explanation of benefits	HHS	Department of Health and Human Services
EOMB	explanation of Medicare benefits		
EPSDT	Early and Periodic Screening, Diagnostic and Treatment	HIM	health information management
		HINN	hospital-issued notice of noncoverage
esMD	Electronic Submission of Medical Documents		
		HIPAA	Health Insurance Portability and Accountability Act of 1996
FBI	Federal Bureau of Investigation		

HIPPS	health insurance prospective payment system	LTC-MS-DRG	long-term care Medicare severity diagnosis-related group
HMO	health maintenance organization	LUPA	low-utilization payment adjustment
HPSA	health professional shortage area	MA	Medicare Advantage
HRRP	Hospital Readmissions Reduction Program	MAC	Medicare administrative contractor
HRSA	US Health Resources and Services Administration	MACRA	Medicare Access and CHIP Reauthorization Act
ICD	International Classification of Diseases	MAR	medication administration record
		MCC	major complication and comorbidity
ICD-10-CM	*International Classification of Diseases, Tenth Revision, Clinical Modification*	MCE	Medicare Code Editor
		MCO	managed care organization
		MDC	major diagnostic category
ICD-10-PCS	*International Classification of Diseases, Tenth Revision, Procedure Coding System*	MDS	Minimum Data Set
		MedPAC	Medicare Payment Advisory Commission
IHS	Indian Health Service	MIPS	Merit-Based Incentive Payment System
IMD	institution for mental disease	MLN	Medicare Learning Network
IME	indirect medical education	MMA	Medicare Prescription Drug, Improvement, and Modernization Act of 2003
IPERA	Improper Payments Elimination and Recovery Act of 2010		
IPERIA	Improper Payments Elimination and Recovery Improvement Act of 2012	MMTA	medication management, teaching, and assessment
IPF	inpatient psychiatric facility	MOH	medal of honor
IPF PPS	inpatient psychiatric facility prospective payment system	MP	malpractice
		MPFS	Medicare physician fee schedule
IPFQR	Inpatient Psychiatric Facility Quality Reporting	MS-DRG	Medicare severity diagnosis-related group
IPIA	Improper Payments Information Act of 2002	MSN	Medicare summary notice
		MSSP	Medicare Shared Savings Program
IPM	Improper Payment Measurement	MUE	medically unlikely edit
IPO	inpatient only	NCCI	National Correct Coding Initiative
IPPS	inpatient prospective payment system	NCD	national coverage determination
		NCHS	National Center for Health Statistics
IQR	Hospital Inpatient Quality Reporting	NCQA	National Committee for Quality Assurance
IRC	integrated revenue cycle		
IRF	inpatient rehabilitation facility	NDC	National Drug Code
IRF PAI	inpatient rehabilitation facility patient assessment instrument	NHSN	National Healthcare Safety Network
		NLP	natural language processing
IRF PPS	inpatient rehabilitation facility prospective payment system	nonPAR	nonparticipating physician
		NPI	national patient identifier
IRVEN	Inpatient Rehabilitation Validation and Entry	NPP	nonphysician provider
		NTA	nontherapy ancillary
I-SNP	institutional special needs plan	OASIS	Outcome Assessment Information Set
KPI	key performance indicator		
LCD	local coverage determination	OCE	Outpatient Code Editor
LIP	low-income patient	OCESAA	Omnibus Consolidated and Emergency Supplemental Appropriations Act of 1999
LOS	length of stay		
LTCH	long-term care hospital		

OIG	Office of the Inspector General	RC	Reserve Component
OPL	other party liability	RCM	revenue cycle management
OPPS	outpatient prospective payment system	ResDAC	Research Data Assistance Center
OR	operating room	RIC	rehabilitation impairment category
OT	occupational therapy	ROM	risk of mortality
OWCP	Office of Workers' Compensation Programs	RTP	return to provider
		RUC	Relative Value Scale Update Committee
PA	prior authorization		
PACE	Programs of All-Inclusive Care for the Elderly	RUG	resource utilization group
		RVU	relative value unit
PACT	Post-acute-care transfer	RW	relative weight
PAMA	Protecting Access to Medicare Act of 2014	RxHCC	Medicare Prescription Drug Hierarchical Condition Categories
PAR	participating physician	SBC	summary of benefits and coverage
PBM	pharmacy benefit manager	SCH	sole-community hospital
PCM	primary care manager	SI	status indicator
PCP	primary care physician	SLP	speech-language pathology
PCP	primary care provider	SMI	service-mix index
PCR	payment-to-cost ratio	SMRC	Supplemental Medical Review Contractor
PDPM	patient-driven payment model		
PE	practice expense	SMS	Socioeconomic Monitoring System
PEPPER	Program for Evaluating Payment Patterns Electronic Report	SNF	skilled nursing facility
		SNF HAI	Skilled Nursing Facility Healthcare-Associated Infections
PERM	Payment Error Rate Measurement		
PGDM	patient-driven groupings model	SNF VBP	skilled nursing facility value-based purchasing program
PHP	partial hospitalization program		
PIIA	Payment Integrity Information Act of 2019	SNFRM	skilled nursing facility 30-day all-cause readmission after hospital measures
PMPM	per member per month		
POA	present on admission	SNP	special needs plan
POS	point-of-service	SOI	severity of illness
POW	prisoner of war	SRS	simple random sampling
PPO	prefered provider organization	TFL	TRICARE for Life
PPS	prospective payment system	TIN	taxpayer identification number
PT	physical therapy	TPS	total performance score
PTP	procedure-to-procedure	URAC	Utilization Review Accreditation Commission
QIC	qualified independent contractor		
QLE	qualifying life event	USPSTF	US Preventive Services Task Force
QPP	Quality Payment Program	VA	Veterans Health Administration
RA	remittance advice	VBP	value-based purchasing
RAC	recovery audit contractor	WC	workers' compensation
RAI	resident assessment instrument	WHO	World Health Organization
RBRVS	resource-based relative value scale	WORK	physician work element

Appendix B
Glossary

Abuse Unknowing or unintentional submission of an inaccurate claim for payment.

Accountable care organization (ACO) Population-based model for healthcare delivery and payment.

Accounts receivable (AR) The amounts owed to a facility by patients or insurance companies who receive services but whose payments will be made at a later date.

Accrual accounting Method of accounting where an accounts receivable amount is recorded when services are provided to a patient.

Adjudication The determination of the reimbursement amount based on the beneficiary's insurance plan benefits.

Administrative denial Type of denial issued when the insurance provider finds fault with the claim. Errors include incorrect coding, failure to obtain preauthorization, registration issues, failure to submit medical record documentation or an itemized claim when requested by the insurance provider, and duplicate charge or claim.

Advance beneficiary notification of noncoverage (ABN) Patient financial responsibility form specific to the Medicare outpatient setting that must be provided to Medicare beneficiaries prior to healthcare service delivery.

Adverse selection Enrollment of an excessive proportion of persons with poor health status in a healthcare plan or healthcare organization.

AHA Coding Clinic for HCPCS Newsletter that provides official coding guidance for users of Healthcare Common Procedure Coding System (HCPCS) Level II procedure, service, and supply codes.

AHA Coding Clinic for ICD-10-CM and ICD-10-PCS A publication issued quarterly by the American Hospital Association and approved by the Centers for Medicare and Medicaid Services (CMS) to give coding advice and direction for *International Classification of Diseases, Tenth Revision, Clinical Modification* (ICD-10-CM) and *International Classification of Diseases, Tenth Revision, Procedure Coding System* (ICD-10-PCS).

Allowable charge Amount the third-party payer or insurance company will pay for a service.

Alternative payment model (APM) Payment approach that provides added incentives to deliver high-quality and cost-efficient care.

Ambulatory payment classification (APC) Resource-based system used in the Medicare Hospital Outpatient Prospective Payment System (OPPS). The APC system combines procedures and services that are clinically comparable, with respect to resource use, into groups which are used to determine reimbursement levels.

Appeal Request for reconsideration of denial of coverage or rejection of claim.

Arithmetic mean length of stay (AMLOS) Sum of all lengths of stay in a set of cases divided by the number of cases.

Assignment of benefits A contract between a physician and Medicare in which the physician agrees to bill Medicare directly for covered services, to bill the beneficiary only for any coinsurance or deductible that may be applicable, and to accept the Medicare payment as payment in full. Medicare usually pays 80 percent of the approved amount directly to the provider of services after the beneficiary meets the annual Part B deductible. The beneficiary pays the other 20 percent (coinsurance).

Attribution Assignment of a beneficiary to a particular organization. The organization may be an accountable care organization (ACO).

Audit A systematic and objective review of revenue cycle processes to determine the level of compliance with policies, procedures, and regulations.

Base payment rate (1) Rate per discharge for operating and capital-related components for an acute-care hospital. (2) Prospectively set payment rate made for services that Medicare beneficiaries receive in healthcare settings. The base rate is adjusted for geographic location, inflation, case mix, and other factors.

Benchmarking The process of comparing performance with a preestablished standard or performance of another facility or group.

Beneficiary An individual who is eligible for benefits from a health plan.

Benefit Healthcare service for which the healthcare insurance company will pay. *See* Covered service.

Benefit period Length of time that a health insurance policy will pay benefits for the member, family, and dependents (if applicable).

Bundled payment Reimbursement methodology in which different healthcare providers who are treating the patient for the same or related conditions are paid an overall sum for taking care of the patient's condition rather than being paid for each individual treatment, test, or procedure. Providers are rewarded for coordinating care, preventing complications and errors, and reducing unnecessary or duplicative tests and treatments.

Bundling Occurs when payment for multiple significant procedures or multiple units of the same type of procedure related to an outpatient encounter or to an episode-of-care is combined into a single unit of payment.

Capitation Method of payment for health services in which an individual or institutional provider is paid a fixed, per capita amount for a period.

Case mix Set of categories of patients (type and volume) treated by a healthcare organization and representing the complexity of the organization's caseload.

Case-mix group (CMG) Classification system used in the Medicare Skilled Nursing Facility Services Payment System's patient-driven payment model to group residents into groups based on clinical reason for stay and function level.

Case-mix index (CMI) Single number that compares the overall complexity of the healthcare organization's mix of patients with the complexity of the average of all hospitals. Typically, the CMI is for a specific period and is derived from the sum of all diagnosis-related group (DRG) weights divided by the number of cases.

Case-rate methodology Type of prospective payment method in which the third-party payer reimburses the provider a fixed, preestablished payment for each case.

Cash accounting Method of accounting where all amounts are recorded when the cash or funds are exchanged.

Category I CPT code A Current Procedural Terminology CPT code that represents a procedure or service that is consistent with contemporary medical practice and that is performed by many physicians in clinical practice in multiple locations.

Category II CPT code A Current Procedural Terminology (CPT) code that represents services or test results contributing to positive health outcomes and high-quality patient care.

Category III CPT code A Current Procedural Terminology (CPT) code that represents emerging technologies for which a Category I code has yet to be established.

CC/MCC capture rate Using the MS-DRG system, it is the percent of admissions within an MS-DRG family assigned to an MS-DRG with CC, MCC, or both.

CC/MCC exclusion list Set of principal diagnosis codes that is closely related to a CC or MCC code that takes away the refinement power of the CC or MCC code for an encounter.

Certificate of insurance Formal contract between a healthcare insurance company and individuals or groups purchasing the healthcare insurance that details the provisions of the healthcare insurance policy (also known as certificate of coverage, evidence of coverage, or summary plan description).

Charge Price assigned to a unit of medical or health service, such as a visit to a physician or a day in a hospital.

Charge capture The accounting for all reportable services and supplies rendered to a patient.

Charge code Hospital-specific internally assigned code used to identify an item or service within the charge description master. Alternative terms are *service code, charge description number, item code*, or *charge identifier*.

Charge description Hospital-specific explanatory phrase that is assigned to describe a procedure, service, or supply in the charge description master.

Charge description master (CDM) Data table used by healthcare facilities to manage required billing elements for all services provided to patients.

Charge status indicator Identifier used to indicate whether a charge description master line item charge is currently active or inactive.

Children's Health Insurance Program (CHIP) A state-federal partnership created by the Balanced Budget Act of 1997 that provides health insurance to children of families whose income level is too high to qualify for Medicaid but too low to purchase healthcare insurance.

Chronic condition special needs program (C-SNP) A form of Medicare Advantage plan for Medicare beneficiaries with severe disabling chronic conditions such as heart failure, diabetes mellitus, end-stage liver disease, and dementia.

Civilian Health and Medical Program of the Department of Veterans Affairs (CHAMPVA) A benefits program administered by the Department of Veterans Affairs for the spouse or widow(er) and children of a veteran who meets specified criteria.

Claim Request for payment, or itemized statement of healthcare services and their costs, provided by a hospital, physician's office, or other healthcare provider. Claims are submitted for reimbursement to the healthcare insurance plan by either the policyholder or the provider.

Claim denial The refusal of an insurance company or carrier to honor a request by an individual (or his or her provider) to pay for healthcare services obtained from a healthcare professional.

Classification system (1) A system for grouping similar diseases and procedures and organizing related information for easy retrieval. (2) A system for assigning numeric or alphanumeric code numbers to represent specific diseases and procedures.

Clean claim rate A measure of the coding unit's or organization's ability to comply with billing edits.

Clinical denial Type of denial issued when the insurance provider questions a clinical aspect of the admission, such as the length of stay of the admission, the level of service, if the encounter meets medical necessity parameters, the site of the service, or if clinical validation is not passed.

Clinical documentation integrity (CDI) Program that strives to initiate concurrent and retrospective reviews of health records to improve the quality of provider documentation.

Clinical validation denial Type of denial that indicates that there is insufficient clinical indicators or discussion points within the health record documentation to support the diagnosis assigned to the patient.

CMS hierarchical condition categories (CMS-HCC) model Risk adjustment model that uses patient demographic characteristics and medical conditions to predict the patient's healthcare costs. This model is used in Medicare Advantage and Medicare value-based purchasing programs.

CMS program transmittal Documents used by CMS to communicate policies and procedures for prospective payment systems' program manuals.

Coding compliance plan A component of a health information management compliance plan or a corporate compliance plan that focuses on the unique regulations and guidelines with which coding professionals must comply.

Coding management Management unit responsible for organizing the coding process so healthcare data can be transformed into meaningful information required in claims processing.

Coinsurance Cost sharing provision which is a preestablished percentage of eligible expenses to be paid by the beneficiary after the deductible has been met.

Community rating Method of determining healthcare premium rates by geographic area (community) rather than by age, health status, or company size. This method increases the size of the risk pool. Costs are increased to younger, healthier individuals who are, in effect, subsidizing older or less healthy individuals.

Comorbidity Pre-existing condition that, because of its presence with a specific diagnosis, causes an increase in length of stay by at least one day in approximately 75 percent of the cases (as in complication and comorbidity [CC]).

Compliance Managing a coding or billing department according to the laws, regulations, and guidelines governing it; performing job functions according to the laws, regulations, and guidelines set forth by Medicare and other third-party payers.

Complication (1) A medical condition that arises during an inpatient hospitalization (for example, a postoperative wound infection). (2) A condition that arises during the hospital stay that prolongs the length of stay at least one day in approximately 75 percent of the cases (as in complication and comorbidity [CC)]).

Complications and comorbidities (CCs) Diagnosis codes that when reported as a secondary diagnosis have the potential to impact the MS-DRG assignment by increasing the MS-DRG severity up one level. CC codes represent an increase in resource intensity for the admission.

Comprehensive Error Rate Testing (CERT) program Measures improper payments for the Medicare fee-for-services payment systems as mandated by the Improper Payments Elimination and Recovery Improvement Act of 2012.

Computer-assisted coding (CAC) The process of extracting and translating dictated and then transcribed free-text data (or dictated and then computer-generated discrete data) into diagnostic and procedural codes of varying classifications for billing and coding purposes.

Contractual allowance The difference between the actual charge and allowable charge.

Conversion factor (CF) National dollar multiplier that sets the allowance for the relative values; a constant.

Coordination of benefits (COB) Method of integrating benefits payments from multiple healthcare insurers to ensure that payments do not exceed 100 percent of the covered healthcare expenses.

Copayment Cost sharing measure in which the beneficiary pays a fixed dollar amount per service, supply, or procedure that is owed to the healthcare facility by the patient.

Cost report Report required from institutional providers on an annual basis for the Medicare program to make a proper determination of amounts payable to providers under its provisions in various prospective payment systems.

Cost sharing provisions Policy points that require the beneficiary to pay for a portion of their healthcare services; a cost-control mechanism.

Cost-of-living adjustment (COLA) Alteration that reflects a change in the consumer price index (CPI), which measures purchasing power between time periods. The CPI is based on a market basket of goods and services that a typical consumer buys.

Coverage gap Period of expanded cost sharing based on prescription drug utilization and cost experienced by beneficiaries enrolled in Medicare Part D.

Covered condition Health condition, illness, injury, disease, or symptom for which the healthcare insurance company will pay for treatment.

Covered service Specific service for which a healthcare insurance company will pay. *See* Benefit.

CPT Assistant Official monthly newsletter for Current Procedural Terminology (CPT) coding issues and guidance published by the American Medical Association (AMA).

Current Procedural Terminology (CPT) Coding system created and maintained by the American Medical Association that is used to report diagnostic and surgical services and procedures.

Days in accounts receivable The result of dividing the ending accounts receivable balance for a given period by the average revenue per day.

Deductible Annual amount of money that the policyholder must incur (and pay) before the health insurance plan will assume liability for the remaining charges or covered expenses.

Demand letter Letter issued by an improper payment review contractor that requests a specific amount to be repaid, provides a detailed rationale for the improper payment, and includes instructions for adjudication or appeal.

Denial rate A measure of how well a facility or practice complies with billing rules and regulations for all payers. Specific to coding management, it is a metric used to determine if the coding unit complies with coding requirements.

Department code Hospital-specific number that is assigned to each clinical or ancillary department that provides services to patients and has at least one charge item in the charge description master. Alternative terminology for this data element is *general ledger number*.

Dependent An insured's spouse, children and young adults until they reach age 26, and dependents with disabilities without an age limit. The definition of children includes natural children, legally adopted children, stepchildren, and children who are dependent during the waiting period before adoption. Children and young adults are eligible regardless of any, or a combination of any, of the following factors: financial dependency, residency with parent, student status, employment, and marital status; except for employer-based plans existing before March 23, 2010, which may state that young adults can qualify for dependent coverage only if they are not eligible for an employment-based health insurance plan. Some healthcare insurance policies also allow same-sex domestic partners to be listed as dependents.

Discharge status code Code reported on an inpatient claim to identify where the patient is being discharged or transferred to at the end of their stay.

Discharged, not final billed (DNFB) A measure of the health of the claims generation process. The measure can be displayed in days or in dollars.

Disease management Program focused on preventing exacerbations of chronic diseases and on promoting healthier lifestyles for patients and clients with chronic diseases.

Disproportionate share hospital (DSH) Healthcare organizations meeting governmental criteria for percentages of indigent patients. Hospital with an unequally (disproportionately) large share of low-income patients. Federal payments to these hospitals are increased to adjust for the financial burden.

Dual eligible special needs program (D-SNP) A form of Medicare Advantage plan for Medicare beneficiaries who qualify for both Medicare and Medicaid.

Eligibility Set of stipulations that qualify a person to apply for healthcare insurance; examples include percentage of the appointment or duration of employment.

Employer-based health insurance Coverage obtained by an individual or family as part of an employment benefit package.

Encoder Software program used to facilitate the assignment of diagnostic and procedure codes according to the rules of the coding system.

Enrollment Initial process in which new individuals apply and are accepted as beneficiaries of healthcare insurance plans.

Evaluation and management (E/M) codes HCPCS codes used to report levels of service for various healthcare settings.

Evidence-based clinical practice guideline Explicit statement that guides clinical decision making and has been systematically developed from scientific evidence and clinical expertise to answer clinical questions. Systematic use of guidelines is termed *evidence-based medicine*.

Exclusion Situation, instance, condition, injury, or treatment that the healthcare plan states will not be covered and for which the healthcare plan will pay no benefits.

Explanation of benefits (EOB) Report sent from a healthcare insurer to the policyholder that describes the healthcare service, its cost, applicable cost sharing, and the amount the healthcare insurer will cover.

False Claims Act Legislation passed during the Civil War that prohibits contractors from making a false claim to a governmental program; used to reinforce healthcare against fraud and abuse.

Family coverage Healthcare insurance coverage for dependents of the policyholder, such as spouses and children.

Federal Employees' Compensation Act of 1916 (FECA) A benefit program that ensures that civilian employees of the federal government are provided medical, death, and income benefits for work-related injuries and illnesses.

Federal Register The daily publication of the US Government Printing Office that reports all regulations (rules); legal notices of federal administrative agencies, of departments of the executive branch, and of the president; and federally mandated standards, including Healthcare Common Procedure Coding System (HCPCS) and *International Classification of Diseases, Tenth Revision, Clinical Modification* (ICD-10-CM) codes.

Fee schedule Third-party payer's predetermined list of maximum allowable fees for each healthcare service.

Final rule Regulation published by an agency, commented on by the public, and published in its official form in the *Federal Register*. Has the force of law on its effective date.

Formulary A list of prescription drugs that a health insurance plan will cover or allow to be reimbursed.

Fraud Healthcare provider requesting payment or reward when the requester knows it is against healthcare rules and regulations.

Gatekeeper Healthcare provider or entity responsible for determining the healthcare services a patient or client may access. The gatekeeper may be a primary care provider, a utilization review or case management agency, or a managed care organization.

Geographic practice cost index (GPCI) Index based on relative difference in the cost of a market basket of goods across geographic areas. A separate GPCI exists for each element of the relative value unit (RVU), which includes physician work, practice expenses, and malpractice. GPCIs are a means to adjust the RVUs, which are national averages, to reflect local costs of service.

Geometric mean length of stay (GMLOS) The *nth* root of a series of *n* length of stay observations.

Global payment method Method of payment in which the third-party payer makes one consolidated payment to cover the services of multiple providers who are treating a single episode-of-care.

Grouper Computer program using specific data elements to assign patients, clients, or residents to groups, categories, or classes.

Guaranteed issue Federal requirement that a healthcare insurer allow individuals to enroll in the health plan regardless of their health, age, sex, or other factors that might predict use of health services.

Guarantor Person who is responsible for paying the bill or guarantees payment for healthcare services. Patients who are adults are often their own guarantor. Parents guarantee payments for the healthcare costs of their children and are therefore the guarantor for minors.

Hard coding Use of the charge description master to code repetitive or noncomplex services.

Health Insurance Portability and Accountability Act of 1996 (HIPAA) Significant piece of legislation aimed at improving healthcare data transmission among providers and insurers; designated code sets to be used for electronic transmission of claims.

Health maintenance organization (HMO) Entity that combines the provision of healthcare insurance and the delivery of healthcare services. Characterized by (1) organized healthcare delivery system to a geographic area, (2) set of basic and supplemental health maintenance and treatment services, (3) voluntarily enrolled members, and (4) predetermined fixed, periodic prepayments for members' coverage. Prepayments are fixed, without regard to actual costs of healthcare services provided to members.

Health professional shortage areas (HPSAs) Areas that have a shortage of providers in medical care, dental care, or mental health, or some combination of these as designated by the US Health Resources and Service Administration.

Healthcare Common Procedure Coding System (HCPCS) Coding system created and maintained by the Centers for Medicare and Medicaid Services (CMS) that provides codes for procedures, services, and supplies not represented by a Current Procedural Terminology (CPT) code.

HCPCS code A code that is part of the **Healthcare Common Procedure Coding System**.

Hospital-issued notices of noncoverage (HINN) Patient financial responsibility form specific to the Medicare hospital inpatient settings that must be provided to Medicare beneficiaries prior to healthcare services delivery.

Hospital-acquired condition (HAC) Condition that developed during the hospital admission.

ICD-10-CM/PCS Coordination and Maintenance Committee Committee composed of representatives from the National Center for Health Statistics (NCHS) and the Centers for Medicare and Medicaid Services (CMS) that is responsible for maintaining the US clinical modification version of the *International Classification of Diseases, Tenth Revision, Clinical Modification (ICD-10-CM)* and *International Classification of Diseases, Tenth Revision, Procedure Coding System (ICD-10-PCS)* code sets.

Improper payment review Evaluation of claims to determine whether the items and services are covered, correctly coded, and medically necessary.

Incident to Services provided by nonphysician clinicians, such as a nurse or physician assistant, that are delivered to patients in a physician's office under the physician's direct supervision.

Indian Health Service (IHS) An agency within the Department of Health and Human Services (HHS) responsible for upholding the federal government's obligation to promote healthy American Indian and Alaskan Native people, communities, and cultures.

Indirect medical education (IME) Percentage increase in Medicare reimbursement to offset the costs of medical education that a teaching hospital incurs.

Individual health insurance Coverage that is purchased by an individual or family on their own as opposed to obtaining coverage through an employer.

Institutional special needs program (I-SNP) A form of Medicare Advantage plan for Medicare beneficiaries who live in an institution like a nursing home or who require nursing care at home.

Insurance System of reducing a person's exposure to risk of loss by having another party (insurer) assume the risk.

Integrated revenue cycle (IRC) The coordination of all revenue cycle activities, facility and physician, under a single leadership and team structure.

International Classification of Diseases, Tenth Revision, Clinical Modification (ICD-10-CM) Coding and classification system used to report diagnoses in all healthcare settings.

International Classification of Diseases, Tenth Revision, Procedure Coding System (ICD-10-PCS) Coding and classification system used to report inpatient procedures and services.

Key performance indicator (KPI) Quantifiable measure of performance over time for a specific objective.

Labor-related share Sum of facilities' relative proportion of wages and salaries, employee benefits, professional fees, postal services, other labor-intensive services, and the labor-related share of capital costs from the appropriate market basket. Labor-related share is typically 70 to 75 percent of healthcare facilities' costs. It is adjusted annually and published in the *Federal Register. See* Nonlabor share.

Limitation Qualification or other specification that reduces or restricts the extent of the healthcare benefit.

Line item Individual line of a charge description master that includes all the required data elements, such as charge code, description, revenue code, and charge.

Local coverage determination (LCD) Reimbursement and medical necessity policies established by Medicare administrative contractors (MACs). LCDs vary from contractor to contractor.

Major complication and comorbidity (MCC) Diagnosis codes that when reported as a secondary diagnosis have the potential to impact the MS-DRG assignment by increasing the MS-DRG up one or two levels. MCCs represent the highest level of resource intensity.

Major diagnostic category (MDC) First level in the hierarchical structure of the Medicare severity diagnosis-related groups (MS-DRG) classification system utilized by the federal inpatient prospective payment system (IPPS). The 25 MDCs are primarily based on body system involvement, such as MDC No. 06, Diseases and Disorders of the Digestive System. However, a few categories are based on disease etiology—for example, Human Immunodeficiency Virus Infections.

Malpractice (MP) element Element of the relative value unit (RVU); cost of the premiums for malpractice insurance and professional liability insurance.

Managed care Payment method in which the third-party payer has implemented some provisions to control the costs of healthcare while maintaining quality care. Systematic merger of clinical, financial, and administrative processes to manage access, cost, and quality of healthcare.

Maximum out of pocket Specific amount, in a certain time frame, such as one year, beyond which all covered healthcare services for that policyholder or dependent are paid at 100 percent by the healthcare insurance plan.

Measure (indicator) (1) The quantifiable data about a function or process. (2) An activity, event, occurrence, or outcome that is to be monitored and evaluated to determine whether it conforms to standards; commonly relates to the structure, process, or outcome of an important aspect of care; also called a *criterion*. (3) A measure used to determine an organization's performance over time. (4) Activity that affects an outcome (types include process measures and quality measures). (5) Compliance with treatment guidelines or standards of care.

Medicaid Part of the Social Security Act, a joint program between state and federal governments to provide healthcare benefits to low-income persons and families or those who meet other eligibility requirements.

Medically necessary Healthcare services and supplies that are proper and needed for the diagnosis or treatment of medical conditions; are provided for the diagnosis, direct care, and treatment of medical conditions; meet the standards of good medical practice in the local

area; and are not mainly for the convenience of the beneficiary or the doctor. Also called *medical necessity*.

Medically unlikely edit (MUE) Edit that identifies the maximum number of units of service that are allowable for an HCPCS code for a single beneficiary on a single date of service.

Medicare Federally funded healthcare benefits program for those persons 65 years old and older, as well as for those entitled to Social Security benefits.

Medicare administrative contractor (MAC) Contracting authority to administer Medicare Part A and Part B as required by section 911 of the Medicare Modernization Act of 2003. MACs process and manage Part A and Part B claims.

Medicare Advantage (Part C) Optional managed care plan for Medicare beneficiaries who are entitled to Part A, are enrolled in Part B, and live in an area with a plan. Types of plans available include health maintenance organization, point-of-service plan, preferred provider organization, and provider-sponsored organization. *See* Medicare Part C.

Medicare Claims Processing Manual Online publication that provides guidance for producing claims for all healthcare settings. Includes billing regulations, as well as service area-specific requirements.

Medicare Code Editor (MCE) Software that detects and reports errors identified on Medicare inpatient claims.

Medicare Integrity Program First comprehensive federal strategy to prevent and reduce provider fraud, waste, and abuse. This program includes the review of provider claims, cost reports, and payment determinations and ensures that ongoing compliance education is provided.

Medicare Part A The portion of Medicare that provides benefits for hospital inpatient services.

Medicare Part B An optional and supplemental portion of Medicare that provides benefits for physician services, medical services, and medical supplies not covered by Medicare Part A.

Medicare Part C A managed care option that includes services under Parts A, B, and D and additional services that are not typically covered by Medicare; Medicare Part C requires an additional premium. Also known as Medicare Advantage.

Medicare Part D Medicare drug benefit created by the Medicare Modernization Act of 2003 (MMA) that offers outpatient drug coverage to beneficiaries for an additional premium.

Medicare physician fee schedule (MPFS) The maximum amount of reimbursement that Medicare will allow for a service; consists of a list of payments for services defined by a service coding system (for example, the Healthcare Common Procedure Coding System [HCPCS]).

Medicare severity diagnosis-related group (MS-DRG) Medicare refinement to the diagnosis-related group (DRG) classification system, which allows for payment to be more closely aligned with resource intensity.

Medicare summary notice (MSN) Statement that describes services rendered, payment rendered, and benefits limits and denials for Medicare beneficiaries.

Modifier Two-digit alpha, alphanumeric, or numeric code that provides the means by which a physician or facility can indicate that a service provided to the patient has been altered by some special circumstance(s), but for which the basic code description itself has not changed.

Moral hazard When "policyholders as patients have an incentive to use more services than those on which their insurance premiums are based."

MS-DRG coding denial A denial where the payer believes there is a coding error that impact the MS-DRG assignment based on the *Official Guidelines for Coding and Reporting* or *Coding Clinic* guidance.

MS-DRG family A group of MS-DRGs that have the same base set of principal diagnoses with or without operating room procedures, which are divided into levels to represent severity of illness (SOI). There may be one, two, or three SOI levels in an MS-DRG family.

National Center for Health Statistics (NCHS) Organization that developed the clinical modification to the *International Classification of Diseases, Tenth Revision* (ICD-10); responsible for maintaining and updating the diagnosis portion of the *International Classification of Diseases, Tenth revision, Clinical Modification* (ICD-10-CM).

National correct coding initiative (NCCI) A set of coding regulations to promote correct coding in physician and hospital outpatient claims; specifically addresses unbundling and mutually exclusive procedures as well as proper reporting of units of service.

National coverage determination (NCD) National medical necessity and reimbursement regulations. Includes a description of the circumstances under which medical supplies, services, or procedures are covered nationwide by Medicare under title XVIII of the Social Security Act and other medical regulations and rulings.

National health service (Beveridge) model Method of health systems financing in which there is a single payer that owns the healthcare facilities, pays the healthcare providers, and is funded by a country's general revenues from taxes.

National unadjusted payment Product of the conversion factor multiplied by the relative weight, unadjusted for geographic differences.

New technology Advance in medical technology that substantially improves, relative to technologies previously available, the diagnosis or treatment of Medicare beneficiaries. Applicants for the status in new technology must submit a formal request, including a full description of the clinical applications of the technology and the results of any clinical evaluations demonstrating that the new technology represents a substantial clinical improvement, together with data to demonstrate that the technology meets the high-cost threshold.

Nonlabor share Facilities' operating costs not related to labor (typically 25 to 30 percent). *See* Labor-related share.

Nonparticipating physicians (nonPARs) Physicians who treat Medicare beneficiaries but do not have a legal agreement with the program to accept assignment of benefits for all Medicare services and who, therefore, may bill beneficiaries more than the Medicare reasonable charge on a service-by-service basis. Nonparticipating physicians receive 95 percent of the full Medicare physician fee schedule amount.

Office of Inspector General (OIG) A division of the Department of Health and Human Services (HHS) that investigates issues of noncompliance in the Medicare and Medicaid programs, such as fraud and abuse.

One-sided risk Type of risk used in accountable care organization (ACO) payment methodology where the ACO can share in any savings generated by the organization, but are not subject to any sharing of the cost if there is not savings or if the cost of care is higher while patients are attributed to the ACO.

Open enrollment period Period during which individuals may elect to enroll in, modify coverage under, or transfer between healthcare insurance plans, usually without evidence of insurability or waiting periods (Medicare uses the term *election*).

Other party liability (OPL) Method of determining responsibility for health expenses when nonhealth insurance sources are involved.

Outlier Cases in prospective payment systems with unusually long lengths of stay or exceptionally high costs; day outlier or cost outlier, respectively.

Outpatient Code Editor (OCE) Software program designed to process data for OPPS pricing, including executing packaging and bundling logic. Additionally, the OCE edits the claim based on coding and billing requirements.

Outpatient service-mix index (SMI) The sum of the weights of ambulatory payment classification groups for patients treated during a given period divided by the total volume of patients treated.

Packaging Occurs when reimbursement for minor ancillary services associated with a significant procedure is combined into a single payment for the procedure.

Partial hospitalization Program (PHP) Program of intensive psychotherapy that is provided in an outpatient day setting and is designed to keep patients with severe mental health conditions from being admitted to an inpatient unit.

Participating physician (PAR) Physician who signs an agreement with Medicare to accept assignment of benefits for all services provided to Medicare beneficiaries for the duration of the agreement.

Pass-through Exception to the Medicare outpatient prospective payment methodology for high-cost supplies. Eligible supplies are not packaged under OPPS and are often reimbursed at or near cost.

Patient financial responsibility agreement Form that outlines an agreement between the provider and the patient. The agreement typically states that the provider will submit a claim for the service to the patient's insurance company, but the patient is responsible to pay any cost sharing amounts as well as the cost of any procedures that may be denied by the insurance company.

Patient portal Component of the electronic health record that allows a patient to send and receive information with a provider.

Patient registration Process which includes the collection of data regarding the patient's provisional diagnosis and planned treatment, insurance coverage, as well as agreement to fulfill any financial obligations.

Patient-driven payment model (PDPM) Reimbursement model used under the skilled nursing facility payment system that assigns residents to payment categories based on individual patient characteristics.

Payer identifier Code that is used in the charge description master to differentiate among payers that have specific or special billing protocol in place.

Payment The amount paid to a healthcare provider for services provided to a patient.

Payment status indictor (SI) Code that identifies how a service, procedure, or item is paid or not paid under the OPPS, including whether the service, procedure, or item is packaged or payment is made separately.

Per diem payment Type of retrospective payment method in which the third-party payer reimburses the provider a fixed rate for each day a covered member is hospitalized.

Per member per month (PMPM) The amount of money paid to the provider each month per individual enrolled in the health insurance plan under a capitation reimbursement methodology.

Percent of billed charges Type of retrospective reimbursement methodology where the payer negotiates to reimburse the facility or provider a percentage of the charge amount for a service, supply, procedure, or admission.

Performance achievement Comparison of a facility's performance with all other facilities' performance.

Performance improvement Comparison of a facility's current performance with the facility's baseline performance.

Pharmacy benefit manager (PBM) A specialty benefit management organization that provides comprehensive pharmacy services; PBMs administer prescription drug benefits for healthcare insurance companies or for self-insured employers.

Physician work (WORK) element Element of the relative value unit (RVU) that should cover the physician's salary. This work is the time the physician spends providing a service and the intensity with which that time is spent. The four elements of intensity are (1) mental effort and judgment, (2) technical skill, (3) physical effort, and (4) psychological stress.

Point-of-service plan Managed care plan where members choose how to receive services at the time they need them. Members can choose at the point of service whether they want an HMO, a PPO, or a fee schedule plan.

Policy Binding contract issued by a healthcare insurance company to an individual or group in which the company promises to pay for healthcare to treat illness or injury.

Policyholder Individual or entity that purchases healthcare insurance coverage.

Post-acute-care transfer (PACT) Under IPPS, a transfer to a nonacute-care setting for designated MS-DRGs is treated as an IPPS-to-IPPS transfer when established criteria are met.

Practice expense (PE) element Element of the relative value unit (RVU) that covers the physician's overhead costs, such as employee wages, office rent, supplies, and equipment. There are two types: facility and nonfacility.

Preferred provider organization (PPO) Entity that contracts with employers and insurers, through a network of providers, to render healthcare services to a group of members. Members can choose to use the healthcare services of any physician, hospital, or other healthcare provider. Members who choose to use the services of network providers have lower out-of-pocket expenses than members who choose to use the services of out-of-network providers.

Premium Amount of money that a policyholder or beneficiary must periodically pay a healthcare insurance company in return for healthcare coverage.

Present on admission (POA) indicator Code used to indicate if the condition or disease was present before the admission or developed during the hospital admission. Required data element for designated diagnosis codes for claims submission.

Price transparency Readily available information on the price of healthcare services that, together with other information, helps define the value of those services and enables patients and other care purchasers to identify, compare, and choose providers that offer the desired level of value.

Primary care provider (PCP) Healthcare provider who provides, supervises, and coordinates the healthcare of a member. The PCP makes referrals to specialists and for advanced diagnostic testing. Family and general practitioners, internists, pediatricians, and obstetricians/gynecologists are primary care physicians. Other PCPs include nurse practitioners and physician assistants.

Primary insurer Entity responsible for the greatest proportion or majority of the healthcare expenses. *See* Secondary insurer.

Principal diagnosis Reason established after study to be chiefly responsible for occasioning the admission of the patient to the hospital for care.

Prior authorization Process of obtaining approval from a healthcare insurance company before receiving healthcare services. Also known as pre-certification and preauthorization.

Private health insurance model Method of health systems financing in which many competing private health insurance companies exist, collect premiums to create a pool of money, and pay for healthcare claims of their subscribers.

Procedure-to-procedure (PTP) edit Edit that identifies instances in which two procedure codes should not be reported together on the same date of service for a single beneficiary unless it is appropriate to append a modifier.

Program for Evaluating Payment Patterns Electronic Report (PEPPER) Hospital-specific report produced by CMS that provides statistics for discharges that are vulnerable to improper payments.

Programs of All-Inclusive Care for the Elderly (PACE) A joint Medicare-Medicaid venture that allows states to choose a managed care option for providing benefits to the frail elderly population.

Proposed rule Regulation published by a federal department or agency in the *Federal Register* for the public's review and comment prior to its adoption. Does not have the force of law.

Prospective reimbursement Type of reimbursement in which the third-party payer establishes the payment rates for healthcare services in advance for a specific time period.

Prudent layperson standard Standard for determining the need for emergency care based on what a prudent layperson (ordinary person) would believe or decide. A prudent layperson, possessing average knowledge about health and medicine, would expect that a condition could jeopardize the patient's life or seriously impair future functioning.

Qualifying life event (QLE) Changes in an individual's life that make him or her eligible for a special enrollment period. Examples include moving to a new state, certain changes in income, and changes in family size.

Quality Payment Program (QPP) Payment incentive program for physician and eligible clinicians that links physician payment to quality measures and cost-saving goals.

Quality reporting program Federal program in which the action of reporting data in the proper format within the given time frame is what allows facilities to receive full reimbursement.

Query Provider communication tool used concurrently or retrospectively to obtain documentation clarification.

Recovery audit contractor (RAC) Federal contractor that executes the provisions of the National Recovery Audit Program.

Recovery Audit Program Improper payment review program executed under the Medicare Integrity Program. This program began as a demonstration project but was made permanent due to its overwhelming success at recovering improper payments.

Referral Process in which a primary care provider or physician makes a request to a managed care plan on behalf of a patient to send that patient to receive medical care from a specialist or provider outside the managed care plan.

Reimbursement The amount paid to a healthcare provider for services provided to a patient.

Relative value unit (RVU) Unit of measure designed to permit comparison of the amount of resources required to perform various provider services by assigning weights to such factors as personnel time, level of skill, and sophistication of equipment required to render service. In the resource-based relative value scale (RBRVS), the RVU reflects national averages and is the sum of the physician work, practice expenses, and malpractice.

Relative weight (RW) Assigned weight that reflects the relative resource consumption associated with a payment classification or group. Higher payments are associated with higher relative weights.

Remittance advice (RA) Report sent by third-party payer that outlines claim rejections, denials, and payments to the facility; sent via electronic data interchange.

Resource intensity Measure of the amount of resources required to treat a patient. The resource intensity of a classification group is represented by the relative weight and is utilized to determine the final payment amount.

Resource-based relative value scale (RBRVS) Resource measurement system that assigns values to services performed by physicians and other health professionals based on the cost of furnishing services in different settings, the skill and training levels required to perform the services, and the time and risk involved.

Retrospective reimbursement Type of reimbursement in which the payer bases payment on the actual resources expended to deliver the service(s).

Revenue code Four-digit billing code that categorizes hospital charges based on type of service, supply, procedure, or location of service.

Revenue cycle The regular set of tasks and activities that produces reimbursement (revenue).

Revenue cycle management (RCM) The supervision of all administrative and clinical functions that contribute to the capture, management, and collection of patient service revenue.

Revenue integrity Performing revenue cycle duties to obtain operational efficiency, compliance adherence, and legitimate reimbursement.

Risk Likelihood of an individual to incur a healthcare expense or the probability of the cost of healthcare exceeding the amount paid to the health insurance company for coverage.

Risk adjustment Statistical process that considers the underlying health status and health spending of patients when examining their healthcare outcomes or healthcare costs.

Risk pool Group of individual entities, such as individuals, employers, or associations, who have a similar risk of loss and whose healthcare costs are combined for evaluating financial history and estimating future costs.

Scrubber Internal claim auditing system used to ensure that claims are complete and accurate before submission to third-party payers.

Secondary insurer Entity responsible for the remainder of the healthcare expenses after the primary insurer pays. *See* Primary insurer.

Severity of illness (SOI) The degree of illness and extent of physiological decompensation or organ system loss of function.

Single coverage Health insurance covering the policyholder or employee only.

Single path coding Process where one coding professional assigns the codes required for both facility and professional claims during the same coding session.

Single-payer health system One method of financing health systems' services. One entity acts as an administrator of a single insurance pool. "The entity collects all health fees (taxes or contributions) and pays all health costs for an entire population. The single entity can be an agency of the government or a government-run organization."

Skilled nursing facility (SNF) Facility that is certified by Medicare to provide 24-hour skilled inpatient nursing care and rehabilitation services in addition to other medical services for short-term care.

Skilled nursing facility value-based purchasing program (SNF VBP) Medicare value-based purchasing program that ties facility performance for established quality measures into the skilled nursing facility services prospective payment system.

Social insurance (Bismarck) model Method of health systems financing, based upon universal healthcare coverage, in which all workers and employers contribute, proportionate to their income, to a set of competing funds that collect and redistribute money for healthcare per government regulations.

Social Security Act Federal legislation established in 1935 to provide old-age benefits for workers, unemployment insurance, and aid to dependents and children with physical handicaps. It was amended by Public Law 89-97 on July 30, 1965, to create the Medicare program (Title XVIII).

Soft coding Process in which all diagnoses and procedures are identified, coded, and then abstracted into the HIM coding system by a coding professional.

Sole-community hospital Hospital that, by reason of factors such as isolated location, weather conditions, travel conditions, or absence of other hospitals (as determined by the Secretary of the Department of Health and Human Services [HHS]), is the sole source of patient hospital services reasonably available to individuals in a geographic area who are entitled to Medicare benefits.

Special enrollment period Period during which individuals may elect to enroll in, modify coverage under, or transfer between healthcare insurance plans, usually without evidence of insurability or waiting periods, because of specific work or life events, without regard to the healthcare insurance company's regular open enrollment period (Medicare uses the term *election*.)

Summary of Benefits and Coverage (SBC) Document that concisely details, in plain language, simple and consistent information about a health plan's benefits and its coverage of health services.

Supplemental insurance Additional healthcare insurance that fills in gaps (supplements) in comprehensive insurance or Medicare benefits; may be a cash benefit, per diem, or other form.

Third-party payer (1) Insurance company or health agency that pays the physician, clinic, or other healthcare provider (second party) for the care or services to the patient (first party). (2) An insurance company or healthcare benefits program that reimburses healthcare providers and patients for covered medical services.

Tier Level of healthcare benefit.

Total performance score (TPS) Measure of a facility's overall performance for the clinical domain measures and other requirements included in a value-based purchasing program.

Transfer An admission where the patient is moved to a different healthcare facility to complete their course of care.

TRICARE The healthcare program for active duty and retired members of one of the eight uniformed services administered by the Department of Defense; formerly known as Civilian Health and Medical Program of the Uniformed Services (CHAMPUS).

Two-sided risk Type of risk used in accountable care organization (ACO) payment methodology where the ACO must share in the loss if the cost of care for their attributed beneficiaries is greater than the benchmark as well as any savings if the cost of care is lower than the benchmark.

Unbundling The fraudulent process in which individual component codes are submitted for reimbursement rather than one comprehensive code.

Universal healthcare coverage Minimum level of healthcare insurance defined by the government, which may include coverage for preventive and primary care, hospitalization, mental health benefits, and prescription drugs.

Upcoding The fraudulent process of submitting codes for reimbursement that indicate more complex or higher-paying services than those that the patient actually received.

Utilization management Program that evaluates the healthcare facility's efficiency in providing necessary care to patients in the most effective manner.

Utilization review Process of determining whether a patient's medical care is necessary according to established guidelines and regulations. Cost containment measure that assesses the appropriateness of the setting for the healthcare service in the continuum of care and the level of service.

Value-based purchasing (VBP) Payment model that holds healthcare providers accountable for both the cost and quality of care they provide.

Variable day adjustment Adjustment in the skilled nursing facility services prospective payment system that adjusts the case-mix index value on specified days of the resident's stay for physical therapy, occupational therapy, and non-ancillary therapy components.

Veterans Health Administration (VA) Integrated healthcare delivery system dedicated to providing healthcare services to American veterans.

Vulnerability Claim type that poses a financial risk to the Medicare program because it is susceptible to improper payments.

Wage index Ratio that represents the relationship between the average wages in a healthcare setting's geographic area and the national average for that healthcare setting. Wage indexes are adjusted annually and published in the *Federal Register*.

Waiting period Period, generally not exceeding 90 days, between the availability of insurance and the ability to use the insurance for covered medical costs.

Withhold amount (1) Portion of primary care providers' prospective payments that managed care organizations deduct and hold to create an incentive for efficient or reduced use of healthcare services. (2) Portion of facility payments that are held back and then redistributed based on a facility's performance for the designated quality measures.

Workers' compensation Medical and income insurance coverage for employees who suffer from a work-related injury or illness.

World Health Organization (WHO) Organization that created and maintains the International Classification of Diseases (ICD) used throughout the world to collect morbidity and mortality information.

Appendix C

Answer Key for
Check Your Understanding Questions

Check Your Understanding 1.1

1. The US private health insurance model utilizes the Bismarck concept of workers and employers contributing to the cost of health insurance. Additionally, the entities that provide insurance are competitive. One component that is like the Beveridge model is that the federal government regulates and executes federal healthcare programs.

2. Health insurance was first utilized in 1929 for schoolteachers in Texas by Blue Cross Blue Shield. However, health insurance did not become widespread in the US until after World War II.

3. Insurance companies receive a premium in return for assuming the insureds' exposure to risk or loss.

4. c.

5. b.

Check Your Understanding 1.2

1. There are three components to revenue integrity. First, duties are completed in the most efficient way. Second is that all tasks are performed compliantly. Third is that only legitimate reimbursement is received for the services provided.

2. The payment systems are different for the revenue cycles. Additionally, a physician revenue cycle is smaller than a facility revenue cycle as there are fewer departments and ancillary services in the physician office setting.

3. Reduced cost to collect, performance consistency, and coordinated strategic goals.

4. Front-end processes, patient engagement; middle processes, resource tracking; back-end processes, claims production and revenue collection.

5. Patients have a narrow perspective of the revenue cycle as they are not aware of all the business practices required to request reimbursement. Examples are coding of medical records, auditing of claims, remittance advice receipt, and financial adjustments.

Check Your Understanding 2.1

1. Individual health insurance is obtained on one's own, not through employment. Employer-based health insurance is obtained as part of an employment benefit package.

2. Services or supplies that (1) are proper and needed for the diagnosis or treatment of the patient's medical conditions, (2) are provided for the diagnosis, direct care, and treatment of the patient's medical condition, (3) meet the standards of good medical practice in the local area, and (4) are not mainly for the convenience of the patient or the patient's doctor.

3. Loss of other healthcare coverage, marriage, divorce, birth, adoption.

4. a.

5. Outpatient surgery; diagnostic, interventional, and therapeutic outpatient procedures; physical, occupational, and speech therapies; behavioral health and substance use; inpatient care; home

health; private nurses; nursing home; and organ transplants.

Check Your Understanding 2.2

1. Benefits and services include any of the following: physician services, inpatient care, preventive care and wellness, prenatal care, emergency medical services, diagnostic and laboratory tests, and certain home health services.

2. Disease management focuses on preventing exacerbations of chronic diseases and promoting healthier lifestyles for patients with chronic diseases.

3. Financial incentives are used to prevent waste of financial resources through the prevision of excessive or unnecessarily expensive healthcare services.

4. Utilization review is a process that determines the medical necessity of a procedure and the appropriateness of the setting for the healthcare service in the continuum of care.

5. Community rating establishes healthcare premiums based on a geographic area rather than on beneficiary characteristics such as age or health status.

Check Your Understanding 3.1

1. a. Inpatient hospital services
   b. Physician services
   c. Medicare Advantage
   d Medicare drug benefit

2. The cost-sharing amount is $1,408, which is the inpatient deductible. Since Arnav has not exhausted his first 60 days of coverage, no daily copayment is required.

3. Examples include long-term care, dental care including dentures, eye exams including contacts and eyeglasses, fitness benefit, routine hearing care including hearing aids, transportation services, and meal benefits.

4. The Part D coverage gap is entered into when the beneficiary and their plan have spent $4,660 on prescription drugs. During the gap, the

beneficiary has to pay a higher coinsurance amount for prescription drugs. Once the beneficiary and plan have paid $7,400, the beneficiary leaves the coverage gap and enters into catastrophic coverage where 95 percent of prescription drug costs are covered.

5. Coverage differs among the states because Medicaid is a federal-state partnership rather than a federal-only program. Medicaid allows states to maintain a unique program adapted to state residents' needs and average incomes. Although state programs must meet coverage requirements for groups such as recipients of adoption assistance and foster care, other types of coverage, such as vision and dental services, are determined by the states' Medicaid agencies.

Check Your Understanding 3.2

1. a. TRICARE Young Adult
   b. TRICARE Select
   c. TRICARE Prime
   d. TRICARE for Life

2. PACE targets the frail, older adult population. The goal of the program is to enhance the quality of life for this population by allowing the frail, older adults to remain in their homes as long as safely possible.

3. Veterans are placed in priority plans based on established criteria. Examples of criteria include the level of their disability and awards or medals they have been awarded.

4. CHIP varies by delivery mechanism. CHIP can be part of Medicaid expansion or as a separate program. Each state has established income eligibility criteria. Each state can model their benefit package in different but regulated ways.

5. Over 9 million.

Check Your Understanding 4.1

1. a.

2. Even though the reimbursement amount for each service is established in advance, the type and number of services is unknown until after the services are delivered.

3. Case rate is provided to one provider for one admission or encounter. Bundled payment is for multiple services provided by multiple provides over a set period of time, which may include numerous encounters and admissions.

4.

Ancillary Services Lab tests	Supplies Injectable drugs Medical equipment Other supplies	Dialysis Services
One total reimbursement amount for services in all three categories		

5. Incentive to substitute less expensive diagnostic and therapeutic procedures; inappropriate elimination of laboratory radiological tests; delay or denial of procedures and treatments; inappropriate premature discharge in the inpatient setting.

Check Your Understanding 4.2

1. CMS-HCC model; RxHCC; HHS-HCC.

2. Diagnoses are used to establish the patient's health status. The patient's health status is assigned a risk score used in the risk adjustment algorithms.

3. Diagnoses are used to establish the patient's health status risk score. The health status risk score is combined with the demographic risk score to establish the patient's CMS-HCC risk score. CMS adjusts the Medicare Advantage PMPM rate based on the beneficiary's CMS-HCC risk score.

4. The one-sided model allows the organization to share in cost savings. The two-sided model allows the organization to share in cost savings, but the organization must also share in the losses if the costs are greater than the benchmark amount.

5. CMS uses a claims-based assignment process based on physician use and eligibility requirements.

Check Your Understanding 5.1

1. The quality reporting program requires healthcare facilities to report data for quality measures. Successful completion of this VBP program is based on participation, not on the quality of care. Payment rates are decreased for facilities that do not participate as required by the program.

2. Pre-MDC assignment; MDC determination; medical or surgical determination; refinement.

3. Examples include the following: Is an MCC present? Is a CC present? Did the patient have a certain disease or condition? Was the procedure performed for a neoplasm? What was the length of the coma? What is the patient's sex? What is the patient's discharge status code?

4. The labor portion represents the facilities' relative proportion of wages and salaries, employee benefits, professional fees, and other labor-intensive services.

5. MS-DRG relative weight times the facility's fully adjusted hospital-specific base rate.

Check Your Understanding 6.1

1. Physical therapy (PT), occupational therapy (OT), and speech-language pathology (SLP).

2. The variable day adjustment for PT and OT adjusts the CMI for days after day 21. Days 1 to 20 are not adjusted.

3. Acute Neurologic and Non-Neurologic.

4. Extensive services, clinical conditions, depression, number of restorative nursing services, and functional score.

5. Examples include drugs, laboratory tests, respiratory therapy, and medical supplies.

Check Your Understanding 7.1

1. Packaging occurs when reimbursement for minor ancillary services associated with a significant procedure is combined into a single payment for the procedure. Bundling occurs when payment for multiple significant procedures or multiple units of the same procedure related to an

outpatient encounter or to an episode-of-care is combined into a single unit of payment.

2. Packaging encourages hospitals to provide efficient care and manage resources with maximum flexibility; incentivizes hospitals to choose the most cost-efficient option when a variety of devices, drugs, items, and supplies could be utilized to meet the patient's needs; encourages hospitals to effectively negotiate with manufacturers and suppliers to reduce the purchase price for supplies and items; and influences hospitals to establish protocols to ensure the necessary services are provided, but scrutinize practitioner orders to maximize the efficient use of hospital resources.

3. 1 = K, 2 = J1, 3 = Q3, 4 = Q4.

4. The code with SI J1 is separately payable. The codes with T and S are packaged.

5. The code with SI T that has the highest relative weight is paid at 100 percent. All other codes with SI T are paid at 50 percent.

Check Your Understanding 8.1

1. RBRVS is a resource measurement system that assigns values to services performed by physicians and other health professionals based on the cost of providing services in different settings, the skill and training levels required to perform the services, and the time and risk involved.

2. Physician work (WORK).

3. Any three of the following: clinical payroll, administrative payroll, office expenses, medical material and supply expenses, medical equipment expenses, and all other expenses.

4. Geographic practice cost index.

5. 80 percent.

Check Your Understanding 9.1

1. Via patient portal or phone to provider office.

2. The healthcare provider.

3. Insurance information, copy of insurance card, and patient's medical history.

4. Payer portal, email, fax, telephone, or direct submission from the EHR.

5. When a service the patient is scheduled to receive may not be covered by Medicare.

Check Your Understanding 10.1

1. Reduce errors and improve patient safety; improve efficiency; improve reimbursements.

2. Barcoding allows the organization to track items, quality, and time of delivery in real time.

3. The CDM data can be used for utilization management and monitoring resource consumption levels.

4. Department code, hospital-specific; charge code, hospital-specific; charge description, hospital-specific; revenue code, national data element; HCPCS code, national data element; charge, hospital-specific; charge status indicator, hospital-specific; payer identifier, hospital-specific; modifier, national data element.

5. Charge codes must be unique to prevent the inadvertent submission of a wrong service or procedure on a claim.

Check Your Understanding 10.2

1. Health Insurance Portability and Accountability Act of 1996 (HIPAA).

2. Current Procedural Terminology (CPT).

3. The ICD-10-CM/PCS Coordination and Maintenance Committee comprised of the National Center for Health Statistics (NCHS) and CMS.

4. American Medical Association (AMA).

5. Healthcare Common Procedure Coding System (HCPCS) Level II.

Check Your Understanding 11.1

1. To ensure that claims are error-free prior to submission to the insurance company.

2. Accounts receivable are amounts owed to a facility by patients or insurance companies who received services but whose payments will be made at a later date.

3. Payment, suspend, reject, or deny.

4. Denial.

5. Medicare administrative contractor (MAC).

Check Your Understanding 12.1

1. The certified coding specialist: CCS is a coding professional who can classify medical data from patient records, and most often works in the hospital setting. They have expertise in ICD-10-CM, ICD-10-PCS, and CPT code sets. They have knowledge of medical terminology, disease processes, and pharmacology concepts.

2. Computer-assisted coding (CAC) is a coding tool used by organizations to improve coding efficiency and support code accuracy. CAC is the process of extracting and translating free-text data and EHR data into ICD-10-CM/PCS and HCPCS codes for billing and coding purposes.

3. CMI measures how effective coding management is in a healthcare organization.

4. Policies and procedures, education and training, and auditing and monitoring.

5. The CC/MCC capture rate is 57.1 percent. Calculation: (15/70)*100 = 21.4%; (25/70)*100 = 35.7%; 21.4% + 35.7% = 57.1%.

Check Your Understanding 13.1

1. Upcoding.

2. Proactively identify potential billing error patterns through data analysis and evaluation of other information, such as complaints; review CERT data, RAC vulnerabilities, and OIG reports; take action to prevent or provide education regarding identified errors; publish compliance guidance for the public and healthcare community.

3. CERT—measure improper payments; A/B MAC medical review—identify and prevent improper payments; DME MACs—identify and prevent improper payments; RAC—identify and correct improper payments; UPIC—develop investigations and take actions to prevent inappropriate payments; SMRC—lower improper payment rates and increase efficiencies of Medicare and Medicaid medical review; CRC recovery auditors—ensure Medicare reimburses appropriately as secondary payer; MEDIC—detect and prevent fraud, waste, and abuse; OIG—identify fraud and publish educational articles.

4. RACs are reimbursed on a contingency basis for issues identified rather than by a contractual rate.

5. Healthcare facilities can incorporate internal reviews based on active OIG Work Plan issues into their annual compliance plan. They can perform audits and proactively rectify issues.

Check Your Understanding 13.2

1. Internal audit is an audit that is initiated by the healthcare facility or provider practice. The internal audit can be conducted by a staff member or contracted out to a consulting firm. External audit is an audit that is initiated by a third-party payer and performed by employees of the insurance company.

2. Systematic random sampling.

3. Day-to-day operating instructions, policies, procedures based on statutes, regulations, guidelines, models, and directives.

4. NCDs are issued by CMS to identify which services are covered by Medicare for all beneficiaries nationwide. LCDs are issued by MACs to identify under which circumstances a service is covered by Medicare. LCDs apply only to the MAC jurisdiction that issued the LCD.

5. The NCCI includes two types of edits. Procedure-to-procedure edits identify two codes that should not be reported together on the same date of service for the same beneficiary. Medically unlikely edits identify the maximum number of units of service that are allowable for a HCPCS code for a single beneficiary on a single date of service. Both types of edits are issued for providers and facilities.

Appendix D
CMS 1500 Claim Form

HEALTH INSURANCE CLAIM FORM

APPROVED BY NATIONAL UNIFORM CLAIM COMMITTEE (NUCC) 02/12

☐☐ PICA   PICA ☐☐☐

1. ☐ MEDICARE (Medicare#) ☐ MEDICAID (Medicaid#) ☐ TRICARE (ID#/DoD#) ☐ CHAMPVA (Member ID#) ☐ GROUP HEALTH PLAN (ID#) ☐ FECA BLK LUNG (ID#) ☐ OTHER (ID#) | 1a. INSURED'S I.D. NUMBER (For Program in Item 1)

2. PATIENT'S NAME (Last Name, First Name, Middle Initial) | 3. PATIENT'S BIRTH DATE MM DD YY   SEX M☐ F☐ | 4. INSURED'S NAME (Last Name, First Name, Middle Initial)

5. PATIENT'S ADDRESS (No., Street) | 6. PATIENT RELATIONSHIP TO INSURED Self☐ Spouse☐ Child☐ Other☐ | 7. INSURED'S ADDRESS (No., Street)

CITY   STATE | 8. RESERVED FOR NUCC USE | CITY   STATE

ZIP CODE   TELEPHONE (Include Area Code) (   ) | | ZIP CODE   TELEPHONE (Include Area Code) (   )

9. OTHER INSURED'S NAME (Last Name, First Name, Middle Initial) | 10. IS PATIENT'S CONDITION RELATED TO: | 11. INSURED'S POLICY GROUP OR FECA NUMBER

a. OTHER INSURED'S POLICY OR GROUP NUMBER | a. EMPLOYMENT? (Current or Previous) ☐ YES ☐ NO | a. INSURED'S DATE OF BIRTH MM DD YY   SEX M☐ F☐

b. RESERVED FOR NUCC USE | b. AUTO ACCIDENT? ☐ YES ☐ NO   PLACE (State) | b. OTHER CLAIM ID (Designated by NUCC)

c. RESERVED FOR NUCC USE | c. OTHER ACCIDENT? ☐ YES ☐ NO | c. INSURANCE PLAN NAME OR PROGRAM NAME

d. INSURANCE PLAN NAME OR PROGRAM NAME | 10d. CLAIM CODES (Designated by NUCC) | d. IS THERE ANOTHER HEALTH BENEFIT PLAN? ☐ YES ☐ NO If yes, complete items 9, 9a, and 9d.

READ BACK OF FORM BEFORE COMPLETING & SIGNING THIS FORM.
12. PATIENT'S OR AUTHORIZED PERSON'S SIGNATURE I authorize the release of any medical or other information necessary to process this claim. I also request payment of government benefits either to myself or to the party who accepts assignment below.

SIGNED _____ DATE _____ | 13. INSURED'S OR AUTHORIZED PERSON'S SIGNATURE I authorize payment of medical benefits to the undersigned physician or supplier for services described below. SIGNED _____

14. DATE OF CURRENT ILLNESS, INJURY, or PREGNANCY (LMP) MM DD YY   QUAL. | 15. OTHER DATE QUAL. MM DD YY | 16. DATES PATIENT UNABLE TO WORK IN CURRENT OCCUPATION FROM MM DD YY   TO MM DD YY

17. NAME OF REFERRING PROVIDER OR OTHER SOURCE | 17a.   17b. NPI | 18. HOSPITALIZATION DATES RELATED TO CURRENT SERVICES FROM MM DD YY   TO MM DD YY

19. ADDITIONAL CLAIM INFORMATION (Designated by NUCC) | 20. OUTSIDE LAB? ☐ YES ☐ NO $ CHARGES

21. DIAGNOSIS OR NATURE OF ILLNESS OR INJURY Relate A-L to service line below (24E)   ICD Ind. | 22. RESUBMISSION CODE   ORIGINAL REF. NO.

A.   B.   C.   D.
E.   F.   G.   H.
I.   J.   K.   L.

| 23. PRIOR AUTHORIZATION NUMBER

24. A. DATE(S) OF SERVICE From MM DD YY To MM DD YY	B. PLACE OF SERVICE	C. EMG	D. PROCEDURES, SERVICES, OR SUPPLIES (Explain Unusual Circumstances) CPT/HCPCS MODIFIER	E. DIAGNOSIS POINTER	F. $ CHARGES	G. DAYS OR UNITS	H. EPSDT Family Plan	I. ID. QUAL.	J. RENDERING PROVIDER ID. #
1									NPI
2									NPI
3									NPI
4									NPI
5									NPI
6									NPI

25. FEDERAL TAX I.D. NUMBER SSN☐ EIN☐ | 26. PATIENT'S ACCOUNT NO. | 27. ACCEPT ASSIGNMENT? (For govt. claims, see back) ☐ YES ☐ NO | 28. TOTAL CHARGE $ | 29. AMOUNT PAID $ | 30. Rsvd. for NUCC Use

31. SIGNATURE OF PHYSICIAN OR SUPPLIER INCLUDING DEGREES OR CREDENTIALS (I certify that the statements on the reverse apply to this bill and are made a part thereof.) SIGNED _____ DATE _____ | 32. SERVICE FACILITY LOCATION INFORMATION   a. NPI   b. | 33. BILLING PROVIDER INFO & PH # (   )   a. NPI   b.

NUCC Instruction Manual available at: www.nucc.org   **PLEASE PRINT OR TYPE**   APPROVED OMB-0938-1197 FORM 1500 (02-12)

Clear Form

BECAUSE THIS FORM IS USED BY VARIOUS GOVERNMENT AND PRIVATE HEALTH PROGRAMS, SEE SEPARATE INSTRUCTIONS ISSUED BY APPLICABLE PROGRAMS.

NOTICE: Any person who knowingly files a statement of claim containing any misrepresentation or any false, incomplete or misleading information may be guilty of a criminal act punishable under law and may be subject to civil penalties.

REFERS TO GOVERNMENT PROGRAMS ONLY

MEDICARE AND CHAMPUS PAYMENTS: A patient's signature requests that payment be made and authorizes release of any information necessary to process the claim and certifies that the information provided in Blocks 1 through 12 is true, accurate and complete. In the case of a Medicare claim, the patient's signature authorizes any entity to release to Medicare medical and nonmedical information, including employment status, and whether the person has employer group health insurance, liability, no-fault, worker's compensation or other insurance which is responsible to pay for the services for which the Medicare claim is made. See 42 CFR 411.24(a). If item 9 is completed, the patient's signature authorizes release of the information to the health plan or agency shown. In Medicare assigned or CHAMPUS participation cases, the physician agrees to accept the charge determination of the Medicare carrier or CHAMPUS fiscal intermediary as the full charge, and the patient is responsible only for the deductible, coinsurance and noncovered services. Coinsurance and the deductible are based upon the charge determination of the Medicare carrier or CHAMPUS fiscal intermediary if this is less than the charge submitted. CHAMPUS is not a health insurance program but makes payment for health benefits provided through certain affiliations with the Uniformed Services. Information on the patient's sponsor should be provided in those items captioned in "Insured"; i.e., items 1a, 4, 6, 7, 9, and 11.

BLACK LUNG AND FECA CLAIMS

The provider agrees to accept the amount paid by the Government as payment in full. See Black Lung and FECA instructions regarding required procedure and diagnosis coding systems.

SIGNATURE OF PHYSICIAN OR SUPPLIER (MEDICARE, CHAMPUS, FECA AND BLACK LUNG)

I certify that the services shown on this form were medically indicated and necessary for the health of the patient and were personally furnished by me or were furnished incident to my professional service by my employee under my immediate personal supervision, except as otherwise expressly permitted by Medicare or CHAMPUS regulations.

For services to be considered as "incident" to a physician's professional service, 1) they must be rendered under the physician's immediate personal supervision by his/her employee, 2) they must be an integral, although incidental part of a covered physician's service, 3) they must be of kinds commonly furnished in physician's offices, and 4) the services of nonphysicians must be included on the physician's bills.

For CHAMPUS claims, I further certify that I (or any employee) who rendered services am not an active duty member of the Uniformed Services or a civilian employee of the United States Government or a contract employee of the United States Government, either civilian or military (refer to 5 USC 5536). For Black-Lung claims, I further certify that the services performed were for a Black Lung-related disorder.

No Part B Medicare benefits may be paid unless this form is received as required by existing law and regulations (42 CFR 424.32).

NOTICE: Any one who misrepresents or falsifies essential information to receive payment from Federal funds requested by this form may upon conviction be subject to fine and imprisonment under applicable Federal laws.

NOTICE TO PATIENT ABOUT THE COLLECTION AND USE OF MEDICARE, CHAMPUS, FECA, AND BLACK LUNG INFORMATION
(PRIVACY ACT STATEMENT)

We are authorized by CMS, CHAMPUS and OWCP to ask you for information needed in the administration of the Medicare, CHAMPUS, FECA, and Black Lung programs. Authority to collect information is in section 205(a), 1862, 1872 and 1874 of the Social Security Act as amended, 42 CFR 411.24(a) and 424.5(a) (6), and 44 USC 3101;41 CFR 101 et seq and 10 USC 1079 and 1086; 5 USC 8101 et seq; and 30 USC 901 et seq; 38 USC 613; E.O. 9397.

The information we obtain to complete claims under these programs is used to identify you and to determine your eligibility. It is also used to decide if the services and supplies you received are covered by these programs and to insure that proper payment is made.

The information may also be given to other providers of services, carriers, intermediaries, medical review boards, health plans, and other organizations or Federal agencies, for the effective administration of Federal provisions that require other third parties payers to pay primary to Federal program, and as otherwise necessary to administer these programs. For example, it may be necessary to disclose information about the benefits you have used to a hospital or doctor. Additional disclosures are made through routine uses for information contained in systems of records.

FOR MEDICARE CLAIMS: See the notice modifying system No. 09-70-0501, titled, 'Carrier Medicare Claims Record,' published in the Federal Register, Vol. 55 No. 177, page 37549, Wed. Sept. 12, 1990, or as updated and republished.

FOR OWCP CLAIMS: Department of Labor, Privacy Act of 1974, "Republication of Notice of Systems of Records," Federal Register Vol. 55 No. 40, Wed Feb. 28, 1990, See ESA-5, ESA-6, ESA-12, ESA-13, ESA-30, or as updated and republished.

FOR CHAMPUS CLAIMS: PRINCIPLE PURPOSE(S): To evaluate eligibility for medical care provided by civilian sources and to issue payment upon establishment of eligibility and determination that the services/supplies received are authorized by law.

ROUTINE USE(S): Information from claims and related documents may be given to the Dept. of Veterans Affairs, the Dept. of Health and Human Services and/or the Dept. of Transportation consistent with their statutory administrative responsibilities under CHAMPUS/CHAMPVA; to the Dept. of Justice for representation of the Secretary of Defense in civil actions; to the Internal Revenue Service, private collection agencies, and consumer reporting agencies in connection with recoupment claims; and to Congressional Offices in response to inquiries made at the request of the person to whom a record pertains. Appropriate disclosures may be made to other federal, state, local, foreign government agencies, private business entities, and individual providers of care, on matters relating to entitlement, claims adjudication, fraud, program abuse, utilization review, quality assurance, peer review, program integrity, third-party liability, coordination of benefits, and civil and criminal litigation related to the operation of CHAMPUS.

DISCLOSURES: Voluntary; however, failure to provide information will result in delay in payment or may result in denial of claim. With the one exception discussed below, there are no penalties under these programs for refusing to supply information. However, failure to furnish information regarding the medical services rendered or the amount charged would prevent payment of claims under these programs. Failure to furnish any other information, such as name or claim number, would delay payment of the claim. Failure to provide medical information under FECA could be deemed an obstruction.

It is mandatory that you tell us if you know that another party is responsible for paying for your treatment. Section 1128B of the Social Security Act and 31 USC 3801-3812 provide penalties for withholding this information.

You should be aware that P.L. 100-503, the "Computer Matching and Privacy Protection Act of 1988", permits the government to verify information by way of computer matches.

MEDICAID PAYMENTS (PROVIDER CERTIFICATION)

I hereby agree to keep such records as are necessary to disclose fully the extent of services provided to individuals under the State's Title XIX plan and to furnish information regarding any payments claimed for providing such services as the State Agency or Dept. of Health and Human Services may request.

I further agree to accept, as payment in full, the amount paid by the Medicaid program for those claims submitted for payment under that program, with the exception of authorized deductible, coinsurance, co-payment or similar cost-sharing charge.

SIGNATURE OF PHYSICIAN (OR SUPPLIER): I certify that the services listed above were medically indicated and necessary to the health of this patient and were personally furnished by me or my employee under my personal direction.

NOTICE: This is to certify that the foregoing information is true, accurate and complete. I understand that payment and satisfaction of this claim will be from Federal and State funds, and that any false claims, statements, or documents, or concealment of a material fact, may be prosecuted under applicable Federal or State laws.

According to the Paperwork Reduction Act of 1995, no persons are required to respond to a collection of information unless it displays a valid OMB control number. The valid OMB control number for this information collection is 0938-0999. The time required to complete this information collection is estimated to average 10 minutes per response, including the time to review instructions, search existing data resources, gather the data needed, and complete and review the information collection. If you have any comments concerning the accuracy of the time estimate(s) or suggestions for improving this form, please write to: CMS, Attn: PRA Reports Clearance Officer, 7500 Security Boulevard, Baltimore, Maryland 21244-1850. This address is for comments and/or suggestions only. DO NOT MAIL COMPLETED CLAIM FORMS TO THIS ADDRESS.

Appendix E
CMS 1450 (UB-04) Claim Form

1			2		3a PAT. CNTL #				4 TYPE OF BILL
					b. MED. REC. #				
					5 FED. TAX NO.	6 STATEMENT COVERS PERIOD FROM THROUGH		7	

8 PATIENT NAME	a		9 PATIENT ADDRESS	a				
b			b		c	d		e

| 10 BIRTHDATE | 11 SEX | 12 DATE | ADMISSION 13 HR | 14 TYPE | 15 SRC | 16 DHR | 17 STAT | 18 | 19 | 20 | CONDITION CODES 21 22 23 24 25 26 27 28 | 29 ACDT STATE | 30 |

31 OCCURRENCE CODE DATE	32 OCCURRENCE CODE DATE	33 OCCURRENCE CODE DATE	34 OCCURRENCE CODE DATE	35 CODE	OCCURRENCE SPAN FROM THROUGH	36 CODE	OCCURRENCE SPAN FROM THROUGH	37
a								a
b								b

38				39 CODE	VALUE CODES AMOUNT	40 CODE	VALUE CODES AMOUNT	41 CODE	VALUE CODES AMOUNT
			a						
			b						
			c						
			d						

42 REV. CD.	43 DESCRIPTION	44 HCPCS / RATE / HIPPS CODE	45 SERV. DATE	46 SERV. UNITS	47 TOTAL CHARGES	48 NON-COVERED CHARGES	49
1							1
2							2
3							3
4							4
5							5
6							6
7							7
8							8
9							9
10							10
11							11
12							12
13							13
14							14
15							15
16							16
17							17
18							18
19							19
20							20
21							21
22							22
23	PAGE ____ OF ____	CREATION DATE	TOTALS ➡				23

50 PAYER NAME		51 HEALTH PLAN ID	52 REL INFO	53 ASG. BEN.	54 PRIOR PAYMENTS	55 EST. AMOUNT DUE	56 NPI	
A							57	A
B							OTHER	B
C							PRV ID	C

58 INSURED'S NAME	59 P. REL	60 INSURED'S UNIQUE ID	61 GROUP NAME	62 INSURANCE GROUP NO.	
A					A
B					B
C					C

63 TREATMENT AUTHORIZATION CODES	64 DOCUMENT CONTROL NUMBER	65 EMPLOYER NAME	
A			A
B			B
C			C

66 DX	67	A	B	C	D	E	F	G	H	68
		I	J	K	L	M	N	O	P	Q	

69 ADMIT DX	70 PATIENT REASON DX a b c	71 PPS CODE	72 ECI a b c	73

74 PRINCIPAL PROCEDURE CODE DATE	a. OTHER PROCEDURE CODE DATE	b. OTHER PROCEDURE CODE DATE	75	76 ATTENDING NPI	QUAL
				LAST	FIRST
c. OTHER PROCEDURE CODE DATE	d. OTHER PROCEDURE CODE DATE	e. OTHER PROCEDURE CODE DATE		77 OPERATING NPI	QUAL
				LAST	FIRST
80 REMARKS	81CC a		78 OTHER NPI	QUAL
	b		LAST	FIRST
	c		79 OTHER NPI	QUAL
	d		LAST	FIRST

UB-04 CMS-1450   APPROVED OMB NO. 0938-0997   NUBC™ National Uniform Billing Committee LIC9213257   THE CERTIFICATIONS ON THE REVERSE APPLY TO THIS BILL AND ARE MADE A PART HEREOF.

UB-04 NOTICE: **THE SUBMITTER OF THIS FORM UNDERSTANDS THAT MISREPRESENTATION OR FALSIFICATION OF ESSENTIAL INFORMATION AS REQUESTED BY THIS FORM, MAY SERVE AS THE BASIS FOR CIVIL MONETARTY PENALTIES AND ASSESSMENTS AND MAY UPON CONVICTION INCLUDE FINES AND/OR IMPRISONMENT UNDER FEDERAL AND/OR STATE LAW(S).**

Submission of this claim constitutes certification that the billing information as shown on the face hereof is true, accurate and complete. That the submitter did not knowingly or recklessly disregard or misrepresent or conceal material facts. The following certifications or verifications apply where pertinent to this Bill:

1. If third party benefits are indicated, the appropriate assignments by the insured /beneficiary and signature of the patient or parent or a legal guardian covering authorization to release information are on file. Determinations as to the release of medical and financial information should be guided by the patient or the patient's legal representative.

2. If patient occupied a private room or required private nursing for medical necessity, any required certifications are on file.

3. Physician's certifications and re-certifications, if required by contract or Federal regulations, are on file.

4. For Religious Non-Medical facilities, verifications and if necessary re-certifications of the patient's need for services are on file.

5. Signature of patient or his representative on certifications, authorization to release information, and payment request, as required by Federal Law and Regulations (42 USC 1935f, 42 CFR 424.36, 10 USC 1071 through 1086, 32 CFR 199) and any other applicable contract regulations, is on file.

6. The provider of care submitter acknowledges that the bill is in conformance with the Civil Rights Act of 1964 as amended. Records adequately describing services will be maintained and necessary information will be furnished to such governmental agencies as required by applicable law.

7. For Medicare Purposes: If the patient has indicated that other health insurance or a state medical assistance agency will pay part of his/her medical expenses and he/she wants information about his/her claim released to them upon request, necessary authorization is on file. The patient's signature on the provider's request to bill Medicare medical and non-medical information, including employment status, and whether the person has employer group health insurance which is responsible to pay for the services for which this Medicare claim is made.

8. For Medicaid purposes: The submitter understands that because payment and satisfaction of this claim will be from Federal and State funds, any false statements, documents, or concealment of a material fact are subject to prosecution under applicable Federal or State Laws.

9. For TRICARE Purposes:

    (a) The information on the face of this claim is true, accurate and complete to the best of the submitter's knowledge and belief, and services were medically necessary and appropriate for the health of the patient;

    (b) The patient has represented that by a reported residential address outside a military medical treatment facility catchment area he or she does not live within the catchment area of a U.S. military medical treatment facility, or if the patient resides within a catchment area of such a facility, a copy of Non-Availability Statement (DD Form 1251) is on file, or the physician has certified to a medical emergency in any instance where a copy of a Non-Availability Statement is not on file;

    (c) The patient or the patient's parent or guardian has responded directly to the provider's request to identify all health insurance coverage, and that all such coverage is identified on the face of the claim except that coverage which is exclusively supplemental payments to TRICARE-determined benefits;

    (d) The amount billed to TRICARE has been billed after all such coverage have been billed and paid excluding Medicaid, and the amount billed to TRICARE is that remaining claimed against TRICARE benefits;

    (e) The beneficiary's cost share has not been waived by consent or failure to exercise generally accepted billing and collection efforts; and,

    (f) Any hospital-based physician under contract, the cost of whose services are allocated in the charges included in this bill, is not an employee or member of the Uniformed Services. For purposes of this certification, an employee of the Uniformed Services is an employee, appointed in civil service (refer to 5 USC 2105), including part-time or intermittent employees, but excluding contract surgeons or other personal service contracts. Similarly, member of the Uniformed Services does not apply to reserve members of the Uniformed Services not on active duty.

    (g) Based on 42 United States Code 1395cc(a)(1)(j) all providers participating in Medicare must also participate in TRICARE for inpatient hospital services provided pursuant to admissions to hospitals occurring on or after January 1, 1987; and

    (h) If TRICARE benefits are to be paid in a participating status, the submitter of this claim agrees to submit this claim to the appropriate TRICARE claims processor. The provider of care submitter also agrees to accept the TRICARE determined reasonable charge as the total charge for the medical services or supplies listed on the claim form. The provider of care will accept the TRICARE-determined reasonable charge even if it is less than the billed amount, and also agrees to accept the amount paid by TRICARE combined with the cost-share amount and deductible amount, if any, paid by or on behalf of the patient as full payment for the listed medical services or supplies. The provider of care submitter will not attempt to collect from the patient (or his or her parent or guardian) amounts over the TRICARE determined reasonable charge. TRICARE will make any benefits payable directly to the provider of care, if the provider of care is a participating provider.

Supporting Statement – Part A

Supporting Statement For Paperwork Reduction Act Submissions

Supporting Statement and Supporting Regulations Contained in 42 CFR 424.5 for the Uniform Institutional Providers Form -- CMS-1450 (UB-04)

Specific Instructions
A. Background

All hardcopy claims processed by Part A Medicare Administrative Contractors must be submitted on the UB-04 CMS-1450 after May 23, 2007. Data fields in the X12 837 data set are consistent with the UB-04 CMS-1450 data set.
We are requesting an OMB extension of the current approval for an additional three years.

B. Justification

1 . Need and Legal Basis

The basic authorities which allow providers of service to bill for services on behalf of the beneficiary are section 1812 (42 USC 1395d - http://www.gpo.gov/fdsys/granule/USCODE-2009-title42/USCODE-2009-title42-chap7-subchapXVIII-partA-sec1395d) (a) (1), (2), (3), (4) and 1833 (2) (B) of the Social Security Act). Also, section 1835 (42 USC 1395n) requires that payment for services furnished to an individual may be made to providers of services only when a written request for payment is filed in such form as the Secretary may prescribe by regulations. Section 42 CFR 424.5(a)(5) requires providers of services to submit a claim for payment prior to any Medicare reimbursement. Charges billed are coded by revenue codes. The bill specifies diagnoses according to the International Classification of Diseases, Ninth Edition (ICD-9-CM) code. Inpatient procedures are identified by ICD-9-CM codes, and outpatient procedures are described using the CMS Common Procedure Coding System (HCPCS). These are standard systems of identification for all major health insurance claims payers. Submission of information on the CMS-1450 permits Medicare intermediaries to receive consistent data for proper payment.

2. Information Users

The UB-04 is managed by the National Uniform Billing Committee (NUBC), sponsored by the American Hospital Association. Most payers are represented on this body, and the UB-04 is widely used in the industry.
Medicare receives 99.9 percent of the claims submitted by institutional providers electronically. Because of the number of small and rural providers who do not submit claims electronically, it is not possible to achieve total electronic submission at this time. Intermediaries use the information on the CMS-1450 to determine whether to make Medicare payment for the services provided, the payment amount, and whether or not to apply deductibles to the claim. The same method is also used by other payers.

CMS is also a secondary user of data. CMS uses the information to develop a data base which is used to update and revise established payment schedules and other payment rates for covered services. CMS also uses the information to conduct studies and reports.

3.   Use of Information Technology

Medicare receives 99.9 percent of the claims submitted by institutional providers electronically. CMS has simplified the claims submission process, effective July 1996, by accepting only national standard electronic claim formats except from small and rural providers. This means that CMS only accepts electronic claims in the American National Standards Institute (ANSI) Accredited Standards Committee (ASC) 837 HIPAA version format for institutional providers. Through the use of the uniform bill, we have been able to achieve a more uniform and a more automated bill processing system for fiscal intermediaries and providers. This form is consistent with the CMS electronic billing specifications, i.e., all coding data element specifications are identical. This has promoted and eased the conversion to electronic billing. Provider billing costs have decreased as a result of standardization of bill preparation, related training and other activities. The average cost to process a line 1 Part A claim in FY 2004 was $.92 per claim. In the electronic media claims process, the Medicare intermediary adjudicates the bill using its computer system after obtaining approval from CMS's Common Working File (CWF) system.

*To comply with the Government Paperwork Elimination Act (GPEA), you must also include the following information in this section:
- Is this collection currently available for completion electronically? **Yes. Medicare receives 99.9 percent of the claims submitted by institutional providers electronically.**
- Does this collection require a signature from the respondent(s)? **No.**
- If CMS had the capability of accepting electronic signature(s), could this collection be made available electronically? **N/A.**
- If this collection isn't currently electronic but will be made electronic in the future, please give a date (month & year) as to when this will be available electronically and explain why it can't be done sooner. **N/A.**
- If this collection cannot be made electronic or if it isn't cost beneficial to make it electronic, please explain. **N/A.**

4.   Duplication of Efforts

Most hospitals participate in both Medicare and many other insurance programs and, without use of the CMS-1450, would have to maintain distinct and duplicate billing systems to handle the billing form, the tape formats, and the diagnostic coding systems for the many programs. The purpose of the requirements in this package is to eliminate this duplication. There is no one form that can accommodate as much information as the CMS-1450 does; nor is there another that can handle a variety of services the way the uniform bill does.
The CMS-1450 is managed by the National Uniform Billing Committee, a standard's body sponsored by the American Hospital Association. Most major payers, such as the Blues network, the members of the Health Insurance Association of America, as well as the state hospital associations, are represented on this body.

5.   Small Businesses

Burden can be minimized by providing training materials and by obtaining assistance from the uniform bill coordinator designated by each CMS regional office.

6.   Less Frequent Collection

The use of the UB-04 will not result in less frequent collection under this extension than previously.

7.   Special Circumstances

There are no special circumstances.

8.   Federal Register/Outside Consultation

We published a notice with a 60-day comment period proposing the information collection on October XX, 2015.

9.   Payments/Gifts to Respondents

There are no payments and gifts to respondents.

10.   Confidentiality

Privacy Act requirements have already been addressed under a Notice Systems of Record entitled "Intermediary Medicare Claims Record" system number 09-70-0503, DHHS/CMS/OIS. Note that OIS has been renamed to the Office of Technology Solutions (OTS).

11.   Sensitive Questions

No questions of a sensitive nature are asked.

12.   Burden Estimates (Hours & Wages)

Currently 99.9 percent of all Medicare intermediary bill receipts are EMC. Application of this percentage to our calendar year 2014 volume of 204,138,881 bills results in the following estimate of burden:
Hardcopy bills at .1% = .1% x 204,138,881 bills = 204,139 bills
Hardcopy burden = 9 minutes per hardcopy bill x 204,139 = 30,621 hours
EMC bills at 99.9% = 99.9% x 204,138,881= 203,934,742 bills
EMC burden = 0.5 minutes per EMC bill x 203,934,742 bills = 1,699,456 hours
Total burden:
    30,621 Hardcopy burden hours

1,699,456 EMC burden hours

1,730,077 Total burden hours

Since the UB-04 will be completed by clerical staff or contractor billing staff, it is unclear of the total wages necessary to complete the form.

13. Capital Costs

There is no capital or operational costs associated with this collection.

14. Cost to Federal Government

The annual costs to the Federal government for the information collection activity include all aspects of the data collection function from the initial data entry to receipt/processing operations. The costs to the Federal Government for data collection can best be described as the total costs of processing the required billing information. Calculation of the precise costs for the data collection is not feasible for the purposes of the Paperwork Reduction Act without conducting a costly study. Therefore, aggregate costs have been developed taking into consideration programming, software, training, tapes, overhead costs, etc.

15. Changes to Burden

The number of hardcopy bills was greatly reduced and the number of electronic bill increased. We have adjusted the burden accordingly.

16. Publication/Tabulation Dates

The purpose of this data collection is payment to providers for Medicare services rendered. We do not employ statistical methods to collect this information, but rather all Medicare institutional providers generate this billing information subsequent to the delivery of services.

17. Expiration Date

Previous forms have been cleared without the expiration date present. Placing the expiration date of the form would require form changes. Since CMS is not responsible for the design and content of the UB-04 we would have to seek approval from the NUBC, which has responsibility for the UB-04, to make the change.

18. Certification Statement

There are no exceptions to the certification statement.

Appendix F
Medicare Summary Notice

Part A

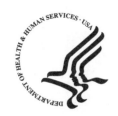

What is New on Your Redesigned "Medicare Summary Notice"?

You'll notice your "Medicare Summary Notice" (MSN) has a new look.
The new MSN will help to make Medicare information clearer, more accessible,
and easier to understand. Based on comments from people like you, we have
redesigned the MSN to help you keep track of your Medicare-covered services.

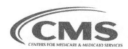

Your New MSN for Part A – Overview

Your Medicare Part A MSN shows all of the services billed to Medicare for inpatient care in hospitals, skilled nursing facility care, hospice care, and home health care services.

Each Page with Specific Information:

Page 1: Your dashboard, which is a summary of your notice,

Page 2: Helpful tips on how to review your notice,

Page 3: Your claims information,

Last page: Find out how to handle denied claims.

Bigger Print for Easy Reading

Page titles and subsection titles are now much larger. Using a larger print throughout makes the notice easier to read.

Helpful Tips for Reading the Notice

The redesigned MSN explains what you need to know with user-friendly language.

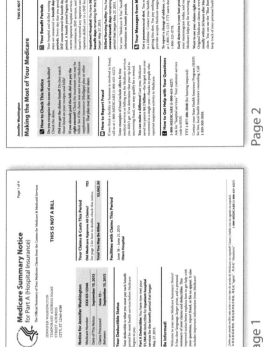

Page 1

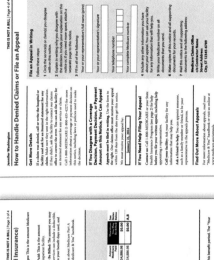

Page 2

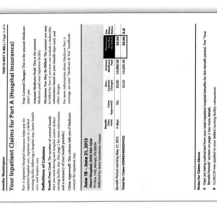

Page 3

Last Page

Page 1 – Your Dashboard

1 DHHS Logo
The redesigned MSN has the official Department of Health & Human Services (DHHS) logo.

2 Your Information
Check your name and the last 4 numbers of your Medicare number, as well as the date your MSN was printed and the dates of the claims listed.

3 Your Deductible Info
You pay a Part A deductible for services before Medicare pays. You can check your deductible information right on page 1 of your notice!

4 Title of your MSN
The title at the top of the page is larger and bold.

5 Total You May Be Billed
A new feature on page 1, this summary shows your approved and denied claims, as well as the total you may be billed.

6 Facilities You Went To
Check the list of dates for services you received during this claim period.

7 Help in Your Language
For help in a language other than English or Spanish, call 1-800-MEDICARE and say "Agent." Tell them the language you need for free translation services.

Page 1 of 4

1 **Medicare Summary Notice**
for Part A (Hospital Insurance)
The Official Summary of Your Medicare Claims from the Centers for Medicare & Medicaid Services

THIS IS NOT A BILL

JENNIFER WASHINGTON
TEMPORARY ADDRESS NAME
STREET ADDRESS
CITY, ST 12345-6789

2 Notice for Jennifer Washington

Medicare Number	XXX-XX-1234A
Date of This Notice	September 15, 2013
Claims Processed Between	June 15 – September 15, 2013

3 Your Deductible Status
Your deductible is what you must pay each benefit period for most health services before Medicare begins to pay.

Part A Deductible: You have now met your **$1,184.00 deductible for inpatient hospital** services for the benefit period that began May 27, 2013.

Be Informed!
Welcome to your new Medicare Summary Notice! It has clear language, larger print, and a personal summary of your claims and deductibles. This improved notice better explains how to get help with your questions, report fraud, or file an appeal. It also includes important information from Medicare!

5 Your Claims & Costs This Period

Did Medicare Approve All Claims?	YES
See page 2 for how to double-check this notice.	
Total You May Be Billed	**$2,062.50**

6 Facilities with Claims This Period

June 18 – June 21, 2013
Otero Hospital

7

¿Sabía que puede recibir este aviso y otro tipo de ayuda de Medicare en español? Llame y hable con un agente en español. **1-800-MEDICARE (1-800-633-4227)**
如果您希望获得帮助，请我电联用医疗保险, 请先说 "agent". 然后说" Mandarin".

Page 2 – Making the Most of Your Medicare

① Section Title
This helps you navigate and find where you are in the notice. The section titles are on the top of each page.

② How to Check
Medicare offers helpful tips on what to check when you review your notice.

③ How to Report
Help Medicare save money by reporting fraud!

④ How to Get Help
This section gives you phone numbers for where to get your Medicare questions answered.

⑤ Your Benefit Period
This section explains benefit periods.

⑥ General Messages
These messages get updated regularly, so make sure to check them!

Jennifer Washington   THIS IS NOT A BILL | Page 2 of 4

① Making the Most of Your Medicare

🔍 How to Check This Notice

Do you recognize the name of each facility? Check the dates.

Did you get the claims listed? Do they match those listed on your receipts and bills?

② If you already paid the bill, did you pay the right amount? Check the maximum you may be billed. See if the claim was sent to your Medicare supplement insurance (Medigap) plan or other insurer. That plan may pay your share.

📋 How to Report Fraud

If you think a facility or business is involved in fraud, call us at 1-800-MEDICARE (1-800-633-4227).

Some examples of fraud include offers for free medical services or billing you for Medicare services you didn't get. If we determine that your tip led to uncovering fraud, you may qualify for a reward.

③ You can make a difference! Last year, Medicare saved tax-payers **$4.2 billion**—the largest sum ever recovered in a single year—thanks to people who reported suspicious activity to Medicare.

📞 How to Get Help with Your Questions

④ 1-800-MEDICARE (1-800-633-4227) Ask for "hospital services." Your customer-service code is 05535.

TTY 1-877-486-2048 (for hearing impaired)

Contact your State Health Insurance Program (SHIP) for free, local health insurance counseling. Call 1-555-555-5555.

🏛 Your Benefit Periods ⑤

Your hospital and skilled nursing facility (SNF) stays are measured in **benefit days** and **benefit periods.** Every day that you spend in a hospital or SNF counts toward the benefit days in that benefit period. A benefit period begins the day you first receive inpatient hospital services or, in certain circumstances, SNF services, and ends when you haven't received any inpatient care in a hospital or inpatient skilled care in a SNF for 60 days in a row.

Inpatient Hospital: You have **56 out of 90 covered benefit days** remaining for the benefit period that began May 27, 2013.

Skilled Nursing Facility: You have **63 out of 100 covered benefit days** remaining for the benefit period that began May 27, 2013.

See your "Medicare & You" handbook for more information on benefit periods.

📨 Your Messages from Medicare ⑥

Get a pneumococcal shot. You may only need it once in a lifetime. Contact your health care provider about getting this shot. You pay nothing if your health care provider accepts Medicare assignment.

To report a change of address, call Social Security at 1-800-772-1213. TTY users should call 1-800-325-0778.

Early detection is your best protection. Schedule your mammogram today, and remember that Medicare helps pay for screening mammograms.

Want to see your claims right away? Access your Original Medicare claims at www.MyMedicare.gov, usually within 24 hours after Medicare processes the claim. You can use the "Blue Button" feature to help keep track of your personal health records.

Page 3 – Your Claims for Part A (Hospital Insurance)

1 Type of Claim

Claims can either be inpatient or outpatient.

2 Definitions

Don't know what some of the words on your MSN mean? Read the definitions to find out more.

3 Your Visit

This is the date you went to the hospital or facility. Keep your bills and compare them to your notice to be sure you got all the services listed.

4 Benefit Period

This shows when your current benefit period began.

6 Max You May Be Billed

This is the total amount the facility is able to bill you. It's highlighted and in bold for easy reading.

7 Notes

Refer to the bottom of the page for explanations of the items and supplies you got.

5 Approved Column

This column lets you know if your claim was approved or denied.

Jennifer Washington   THIS IS NOT A BILL | Page 3 of 4

1 Your Inpatient Claims for Part A (Hospital Insurance)

Part A Inpatient Hospital Insurance helps pay for inpatient hospital care, inpatient care in a skilled nursing facility following a hospital stay, home health care, and hospice care.

Non-Covered Charges: This is the amount Medicare didn't pay.

Amount Medicare Paid: This is the amount Medicare paid your inpatient facility.

2 Definitions of Columns

Benefit Days Used: The number of covered benefit days you used during each hospital and/or skilled nursing facility stay. (See page 2 for more information and a summary of your benefit periods.)

Claim Approved?: This column tells you if Medicare covered the inpatient stay.

Maximum You May Be Billed: The amount you may be billed for Part A services can include a deductible, coinsurance based on your benefit days used, and other charges.

For more information about Medicare Part A coverage, see your "Medicare & You" handbook.

3 June 18 – June 21, 2013
Otero Hospital, (555) 555-1234
PO Box 1142, Manati, PR 00674
Referred by Jesus Sarmiento Forasti

	Benefit Days Used	Claim Approved?	Non-Covered Charges	Amount Medicare Paid	Maximum You May Be Billed	See Notes Below
4 Benefit Period starting May 27, 2013	4 days	Yes	$0.00	$4,886.98	$0.00	
Total for Claim #20905400034102			$0.00	$4,886.98	**$0.00**	A,B

Notes for Claims Above
A Days are being subtracted from your total inpatient hospital benefits for this benefit period. The "Your Benefit Periods" section on page 2 has more details.
B $2,062.50 was applied to your skilled nursing facility coinsurance.

Last Page – How to Handle Denied Claims

1 Get More Details
Find out your options on what to do about denied claims.

2 If You Decide to Appeal
You have 120 days to appeal your claims.
The date listed in the box is when your appeal must be received by us.

3 If You Need Help
Helpful tips to guide you through filing an appeal.

4 Appeals Form
You must file an appeal in writing. Follow the step-by-step directions when filling out the form.

Jennifer Washington   THIS IS NOT A BILL | Page 4 of 4

How to Handle Denied Claims or File an Appeal

1 Get More Details

If a claim was denied, call or write the hospital or facility and ask for an itemized statement for any claim. Make sure they sent in the right information. If they didn't, ask the facility to contact our claims office to correct the error. You can ask the facility for an itemized statement for any service or claim.

Call 1-800-MEDICARE (1-800-633-4227) for more information about a coverage or payment decision on this notice, including laws or policies used to make the decision.

2 If You Disagree with a Coverage Decision, Payment Decision, or Payment Amount on this Notice, You Can Appeal

Appeals must be filed in writing. Use the form to the right. Our claims office must receive your appeal within 120 days from the date you get this notice.

We must receive your appeal by:

> January 21, 2014

3 If You Need Help Filing Your Appeal

Contact us: Call 1-800-MEDICARE or your State Health Insurance Program (see page 2) for help before you file your written appeal, including help appointing a representative.

Call your facility: Ask your facility for any information that may help you.

Ask a friend to help: You can appoint someone, such as a family member or friend, to be your representative in the appeals process.

Find Out More About Appeals

For more information about appeals, read your "Medicare & You" handbook or visit us online at www.medicare.gov/appeals.

File an Appeal in Writing   4

Follow these steps:

1 Circle the service(s) or claim(s) you disagree with on this notice.

2 Explain in writing why you disagree with the decision. Include your explanation on this notice or, if you need more space, attach a separate page to this notice.

3 Fill in all of the following:

Your or your representative's full name (print)

Your or your representative's signature

Your telephone number

Your complete Medicare number

4 Include any other information you have about your appeal. You can ask your facility for any information that will help you.

5 Write your Medicare number on all documents that you send.

6 Make copies of this notice and all supporting documents for your records.

7 Mail this notice and all supporting documents to the following address:

Medicare Claims Office
c/o Contractor Name
Street Address
City, ST 12345-6789

Index

Page references to online chapter 15 are indicated by 15. preceding the page number.